GLOBAL MIDWIFERY MENTORSHIP

The book begins by exploring the history of mentoring and its relationship to education and practice. Theories and models of mentorship, education and leadership within the context of midwifery will be discussed, along with the importance of critical thinking and reflection. The editors use the lens of global mentoring to focus on how mentoring in midwifery has developed and been implemented in 15 countries from North and Central America, Europe, Asia, Africa and Australasia. Each chapter explores regulation, professional accountability, education, leadership and career pathways in the country in question.

This international text draws on the perspectives of Australian mentors, mentees, healthcare organisations and academics to highlight the complexities of mentorship in real work midwifery practice, and includes a chapter discussing how to take cultural considerations into question. The final chapters draw on the previous discussion to make recommendations that will support midwifery to implement and sustain a successful and supportive mentorship program for the next generation of midwives.

In this book, authors often refer to midwives as women to reflect the gendered nature of subordination of midwifery. While most midwives globally are women providing care to women, not all midwives in Mexico or globally identify as women. We acknowledge and celebrate the diverse identities of midwives, as this is the best way to build an environment that guarantees enabling sexual and reproductive care for all people who need midwives. Further, the term First Nations which is used is a collective term that refers to Indigenous Australian and Aboriginal and Torres Strait Islander peoples of Australia. First Nations peoples will refer to themselves by any of these terms and may also identify through language groups. This term is used in acknowledgement that First Nations peoples have the right of self-determination to identify however they choose to do so.

This book is an invaluable read for midwifery students, educators and practitioners.

Dr Elaine Jefford, midwifery researcher, is an author and editor-in-chief for the *International Journal of Childbirth: Women's and Reproductive Health* and employed as a senior midwifery lecturer at the University of the Sunshine Coast, Queensland, and is Adjunct Associate Professor at Southern Cross University, Australia. Her research focus is within the field of midwifery decision-making and abdicating one's professional accountability. This research underpins midwifery education practice and policy, and leadership and mentorship, as the relationship of one or all on midwifery decision-making can impact risk, safety and quality of care provision. A programme of research has led to strong collaborations in national and international research, service development work and practitioner training initiatives. Other research interests include birth trauma, perinatal mental well-being, deteriorating women, childbirth for incarcerated women, self-compassion and women's health such as menopause. She led the validation of the Australian Birth Satisfaction Scale-Revised. This scale has been appraised by international opinion leaders and has been endorsed by the International Consortium of Health Outcome Measurement (ICHOM) as the measure of choice to assess 'birth satisfaction' worldwide within the ICHOM Standard Set for Pregnancy and Childbirth. She is now leading the Partner-Birth Satisfaction Scale-Revised (P-BSS-R) Australian validation team. She has also been involved in national and international midwifery curriculum development and was a member of the Midwifery Accreditation Committee, which is part of the Australian Nursing and Midwifery Accreditation Council. She is also Chair of the Trans-Tasman Midwifery Education Consortium.

Dr Lyn Ebert is a registered nurse and midwife, a women's health and midwifery education researcher and Associate Professor in Midwifery at the Southern Cross University (SCU). She is the Midwifery Work Integrated Learning Academic Coordinator (WILAC) for SCU. The WILAC role entails managing and administering the work integrated learning (WIL) or Midwifery Professional Experience (MPE) of a programme and ensures academic, clinical and strategic oversight and coordination of the WIL for the programme. She is committed to supporting the development of innovative health education strategies, curriculum teaching and learning methods that support student learning, childbearing women's safety and improved midwifery workforce culture.

GLOBAL MIDWIFERY MENTORSHIP

Building Capacity Through Connection

Edited by Elaine Jefford and Lyn Ebert

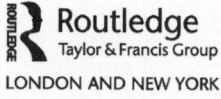

Routledge
Taylor & Francis Group

LONDON AND NEW YORK

First published 2026
by Routledge
4 Park Square, Milton Park, Abingdon, Oxon OX14 4RN

and by Routledge
605 Third Avenue, New York, NY 10158

Routledge is an imprint of the Taylor & Francis Group, an informa business

British Library Cataloguing-in-Publication Data
A catalogue record for this book is available from the British Library

ISBN: 978-1-032-87647-4 (hbk)
ISBN: 978-1-032-87635-1 (pbk)
ISBN: 978-1-003-53373-3 (ebk)

DOI: 10.4324/9781003533733

Typeset in Sabon
by KnowledgeWorks Global Ltd.

CONTENTS

PART III
**Guiding Hands Across Borders: Midwifery Mentorship
Around the World**

PART IV
Embedding Mentorship in Australian Midwifery —
Perspectives, Practice, and Impact

LIST OF CONTRIBUTORS

Rondi Anderson is a certified nurse–midwife who has dedicated her life to providing quality, evidence-based maternal and newborn health services to the poorest women. She has worked in both clinical service delivery and reproductive health programme management, serving marginalized communities in the US, Sierra Leone, Somalia, India, Syria, Rwanda and Bangladesh. She was an international midwifery specialist with UNFPA Bangladesh from 2015 to 2022 and served as an emergency coordinator for sexual and reproductive health programmes with UNFPA in Aleppo, Syria, throughout 2023. She holds a PhD from Lancaster University and has published more than 20 articles in peer-reviewed journals on the midwifery practice and evidence-based midwifery care. She is a leading voice on the development of international standard midwives and the provision of quality maternity care in low-resource health systems.

Fiona Arundell has been employed since 1994 at Western Sydney University and has held several positions including lecturer, Academic Programme Advisor, Deputy Director of Midwifery Professional Experience and Director of Academic Programme. She is enthusiastic about the future of midwifery education at a local and national level. Research interests include clinical decision-making; simulation; midwives as preceptors and mentors; and the experience of midwifery students on clinical placement. She has been a team member on several grants. Prior to working at Western, she held clinical roles as a clinical midwife and midwifery educator. She maintained clinical practice experience working as a midwife in a hospital in complex antenatal, postnatal and birth unit. She is currently enrolled in a PhD.

Cara Baddington is Senior Lecturer at the Otago Polytechnic School of Midwifery in Aotearoa New Zealand working with learners across undergraduate and postgraduate programmes. She has worked as a Lead Maternity Carer (LMC) midwife and a casual core midwife in primary and tertiary facilities in the Porirua and Wellington areas. She mentors new graduate midwives within the Midwifery First Year of Practice programme. She has varied research interests including sustainability of LMC midwifery practices, quality assurance processes and the experience of a large baby prediction in pregnancy.

Dr Sam Bassett is Head of Department, Midwifery and Lead Midwife for Education (LME) at King's College London. An experienced midwife and educationalist her ongoing centre of clinical practice is high-risk pregnancies completing her doctorate in 2016 focusing on maternal high dependency care. As LME, she is deemed an expert in midwifery education with the knowledge and skills to develop curricula and policy. As such, she represents midwifery education strategically both internally within the university and externally with all stakeholders, including the NMC. She has also taken an active role in developing midwifery clinical assessment documents and was part of the steering group that created the pan London Assessment Document (MPAD), now adapted to form the Midwifery Ongoing Record of Achievement (MORA) used by all midwifery students across England and Northern Ireland.

Hannah Borboleta is a feminist midwife and director of midwifery centre Morada Violeta in México City. As such, she provides sexual, reproductive and nonreproductive health care for women and people with vaginas and uteri – including pregnancy, birth and postpartum, STI testing, menopause, menstrual health and imbalances, vaginal health and imbalances as well as contraceptives and abortion care. She has been a mentor for several midwives and has extensively written and spoken about the midwifery model of care in México.

Dr Nicole Borg Cunen is a lecturer at University of Malta and Senior Midwife at Mater Dei Hospital, Malta.

Vivienne Brady is Assistant Professor in the School of Nursing and Midwifery, University of Dublin, Trinity College, and is Director of Midwifery and Head of Discipline. She was awarded a PhD from Trinity College and degrees of MSc in Midwifery and BSc in Midwifery from University College Dublin. Vivienne has expertise in undergraduate and postgraduate teaching, assessing and curriculum design and development, and is a practising midwife in the Coombe Hospital Dublin. She has over 20 years of research activity with expertise in action research and qualitative research methods. Her main research interests include women's experiences and appraisal of services, spirituality and childbirth, and postnatal supports for women.

Dr Annette Briley is a UK-trained nurse and midwife (SRN, RM) currently registered in Australia. She completed a MSc and PhD at King's College London (2005 and 2014). She has worked continuously in research since 1996, whilst maintaining and extending her clinical expertise. She has been involved in many clinical trials and other research methodologies that have informed guidelines and practice. In 2018, she became a Fellow of the Royal College of Midwives (FRCM) in recognition of her contribution to women's health. She is currently in a clinical academic position with Flinders University and Northern Adelaide Local Health Network as Professor of Women's Health and Midwifery Research.

Stacey Butcher (RN, RM, MMidwifery, GDip Healthcare Leadership) is a proud Dunghutti woman, a wife, a mother, a daughter and is currently a Clinical Midwifery Consultant for Growing Deadly families at Queensland health. Throughout her midwifery career, she has worked as a clinician, educator and academic in a variety of settings from region, rural and remote areas of Australia. She is keen to commence her PhD in the near future on the topic of First Nations midwifery workforce to explore what is working and want needs to be researched further. She is passionate in seeking better healthcare for all First Nations woman and their families no matter where they live and supporting the workforce to strengthen and grow.

Associate Professor Major General Saisamorn Chaleoykitti is focused on research in the areas of counselling psychology, mental health, psychiatric nursing and nursing administration.

Lisa Charmer is a registered nurse and midwife, a women's health, midwifery and education researcher, and a midwifery lecturer at Southern Cross University (SCU). She has worked in all areas of midwifery across rural, remote and metropolitan settings. She is committed to supporting the development of innovative health education strategies and curriculum teaching and learning methods that support student learning, transition to the workforce and improved midwifery workforce culture.

Deirdre Daly is an experienced midwife and midwife teacher/lecturer. She was awarded PhD and MA degrees from Trinity College Dublin; an MSc in Health Care Ethics and Law from the Royal College of Surgeons, Ireland; an MSc in Midwifery from Queen's University, Belfast; and a Postgraduate Diploma in Education (Midwifery) and BSc (Hons) in Professional Development in Nursing from the University of Ulster, Belfast. She is the Director of the Trinity Centre for Maternity Care Research (TCMCR) and a member of the national groups on severe maternal morbidity and maternal death in Ireland. She is the Principal Investigator on the Maternal health

And Maternal Morbidity in Ireland (MAMMI) study (https://www.tcd.ie/mammi/), a longitudinal study exploring the health of and health problems experienced by first-time mothers giving birth. She also leads several related studies on maternal health and has published widely on various aspects of maternal health.

Professor Linda Deravin is a proud Wiradjuri woman, a mother, a daughter, a sister, a nurse and an author and is currently the Head of School and Dean for the School of Nursing and Midwifery at the University of Southern Queensland. She completed her PhD studies at CSU, and her topic of interest was in Indigenous nursing and midwifery workforce issues. Throughout her nursing career, she has worked as a clinician, educator and both an executive nurse and health manager in a variety of settings. She continues to work with a variety of communities to pursue her research interests in Indigenous health, chronic care and health workforce issues.

Terri Downer has significantly shaped midwifery education, aligning it with best practices and future innovations in her role as Head of Discipline. Her leadership improves academic excellence and clinical growth, preparing students for the challenges of an evolving healthcare system. An advocate for integrating technology in education, she has led projects in the scholarship of teaching and learning, focusing on emerging digital technology. She introduced blended learning including ePortfolios, 3D visualization, QR codes, virtual reality and video assessments using simulation, thus enriching students' engagement and developing both practical and theoretical skills. These initiatives have not only improved midwifery education but also benefited other health programmes. As a mentor, she has guided students to become skilled, compassionate and culturally sensitive practitioners. Her leadership emphasizes collaboration, inclusivity and lifelong learning, creating a supportive environment where students and staff are empowered to excel and innovate.

Nicola Drayton is the Nurse Manager for Practice Development in the Nepean Blue Mountains Local Health District (NBMLHD) Nursing and Midwifery Directorate. She has a passion for working with clinicians using practice development to bring about meaningful insight and understanding about the way they care for patients, families and their team culture. This is achieved through a variety of practice development and appreciative inquiry approaches which includes the conduction of research. She has published articles in peer-reviewed journals and presented at conferences. She recently graduated from the Franklin Women Leadership programme and is now a member of their alumni group. She is also a member of the Person-centred Practice International Community of Practice.

Mieke Embo works and lives in Belgium. They studied Nursing, Midwifery, a Master's in Health Sciences and Management and defended their PhD at the University of Maastricht (NL) on competency-based workplace learning. They are Visiting Professor at the Antwerp University (Advanced Midwifery), and post-doctoral researcher at the University of Ghent (Educational Sciences) and the Artevelde University of Applied Sciences (Healthcare). They previously managed the midwifery department and facilitated different competency-based midwifery curricula reviews. They also coordinated educational innovation projects to introduce ePortfolios in healthcare programmes in Ghent, Rwanda, Uganda and Ethiopia (www.sbo-scaffold.com/en). Mieke is a member of the Board of the Flemish Association of Midwives and the Belgian Planning Committee for Midwives (Belgian Health Ministry) and a representative expert of the Network of Experts Superior Health Council in Belgium and a Subject Matter Expert at the WHO.

Dr. Louise Gallagher is a registered nurse, midwife, midwife teacher, and a lactation consultant. She was awarded MA and PhD degrees from Trinity College Dublin; an MSc in Public Health Nutrition from Atlantic Technological University, Sligo; an MSc in Midwifery Education from the University of Dublin (UCD); and a BSc (Hons) in Midwifery from Kings College London. She is an experienced midwifery educator and researcher. Her expertise spans the areas of curriculum development, teaching and assessment, and research into maternity care and more specifically infant nutrition and breastfeeding. Additional research interests include the evaluation of the knowledge and skills of health practitioners and voluntary supporters in supporting breastfeeding women.

Dr. Bootsakon S. Guyot is focused on research in prenatal health promotion and nutrition among pregnant women with anaemia to improve birth outcomes. Another area of interest is the management of labour pain. She has clinical teaching experience in hospital labour rooms and RN-preceptor training. She is developing a midwifery simulation centre to train midwifery skills at the Faculty of Nursing, Kasetsart University.

Daniel K. Guyot, a science teacher and naturalist from Illinois, US, resides in Thailand with his wife and daughter, where he is pursuing a degree in clinical psychology. His interests include resiliency training, mindfulness and biofeedback learning.

Georgie Haver is Registered Midwife at Lismore Base Hospital, NSW, Australia. With experience in antenatal, intrapartum, and postnatal care in a regional hospital setting, she is a strong advocate for continuing education and sustainable midwifery practice. Committed to evidence-based care and professional growth, she is passionate about strengthening midwife-to-midwife relationships and promoting mentorship as a key factor in enhancing practitioner well-being, fostering a positive workplace culture and ultimately improving outcomes for women and families.

Riza Kadilar is Alumni of Stanford University and holds a PhD in media economics. His professional career includes senior-level bank management for almost 30 years in the UK, the Netherlands, France and Turkey. He served as the president of EMCC Global between 2017 and 2024. He contributes to the democratization of learning and development with his online platform (RK Academy) and with his EMCC Quality Award recipient training programmes on coaching and mentoring. He is a visiting professor in various universities and has delivered numerous motivational speeches during the last 20 years to tens of thousands of participants in more than 30 countries. He is the author of seven published books, and columnist at Harvard Business Review Turkey. He invests in technology startups and provides business development and financial advisory services through his company K Ventures.

Yuri Kasamatsu is a registered nurse and professor of fundamental nursing at Otemae University, Japan.

Jessica Lees is a PhD candidate at Deakin University. Her research project explores how technology features in the teaching of touch based physical examination for health professional students. She is also an early career lecturer in physiotherapy at the University of Melbourne. In this role, she teaches subjects relating to equity in health, health promotion, strength and conditioning and career readiness. She is also involved in projects addressing student mental health, diversity and inclusion, and creating safer spaces for student learning of peer physical examination.

Kelley Lennon is a nurse and midwife with over 30 years' experience, having worked in a variety of midwifery models of care. Over the last 15 years, she has held various leadership roles with local, District and State perspectives. It has been in these roles that a passion for midwifery leadership and mentoring has been developed. She has bought her woman-centred approach into all aspects of her career and has enjoyed incorporating appreciative inquiry into her leadership roles.

Yaredh Marín Vázquez researches sexual and reproductive health, women, midwifery, sexual and reproductive rights, and violence in urban contexts. She is currently working on two editorial projects. The first is "Germinating and sustaining life in a pandemic," a book about the experience of care during the pandemic provided by mothers and midwives in Mexico (as author). The second material is "Midwifery practices in Mexico and the border. Analytical training material for and by midwives," a teaching material that describes sexual and reproductive health care from the midwifery model written by autonomous, empirical and professional midwives (Editorial Coordinator).

Akemi Mochizuki is a qualified midwife, registered nurse and public health nurse. For over 10 years, worked as a midwife in clinical settings in Japan. She also has experience of living in Bangkok, Thailand and Michigan, US, where she provided breastfeeding support to Japanese people living there as a midwife. She is currently an associate professor in the field of midwifery practice science at the Graduate School of Global Nursing at Otemae University, and she enjoys being able to contribute to the training of future midwives. She always has an energetic attitude towards midwife education, and she tries to create a relationship where midwifery students can improve their skills and demonstrate the results of their studies in the practice setting. In her private life, she loves playing golf, and she enjoys spending peaceful time with her family and cooking Thai food herself.

Marianne Nieuwenhuijze is Professor of Midwifery at Maastricht University and Head of the Research Centre of Midwifery Science at Zuyd University in the Netherlands. She is the founder and lead of the research programme on *Physiological Childbirth and Midwifery Care* working with an enthusiastic multidisciplinary team of researchers from midwifery, health science, medicine, psychology, social science and epidemiology. In their research, the team closely collaborates with women, their partners, midwives and other stakeholders in maternity care to produce high-quality evidence and to translate this evidence into practice to promote the health and well-being of women, infants and their families throughout the perinatal period. They conduct research with numerous international partners. Marianne's main research interests are physiological childbirth, health promotion, ethics and (shared) decision-making in maternity care. She also involved in the Bachelor and Master Sc of Midwifery in Maastricht and supervises PhD students.

Gail Norris is part of the School's Senior Leadership team and holds the position of Associate Dean, International. Her research interests include obesity, particularly during childbirth and midwifery education. She is Senior Teaching Fellow and has a keen interest in Interpretative Phenomenological Analysis (IPA) research methodology and facilitates an IPA research group within the School of Health and Social Care. She has a strong interest in respectful midwifery care and is currently leading projects in respectful midwifery care working with midwives in Vietnam.

Maeve O'Connell is a leader in Midwifery education and research-based in the UAE, specializing in evidence-based practice and student-centred learning. She co-led the development of the UAE's first fully accredited direct-entry Bachelor's in Midwifery. Her expertise spans curriculum design, perinatal care, labour support and complex cases. An experienced writer, public speaker and event organizer, she serves as Associate Editor for *Women and Birth Journal* and Guest Editor for a 2024 special issue on planetary health. With 15 peer-reviewed papers, five editorials, and five book chapters, her ongoing research focuses on perinatal mental health and fear of childbirth, midwifery education, breastfeeding and climate change.

Musarrat Rani is enthusiastic dynamic well experienced nurse midwife and serving more than 30 years as "Reproductive Maternal Newborn Child Adolescent Health and Nutrition (RMNCAH &N)" Professional. She is CEO of Irshad Amtul Reproductive Health and Midwifery Services (IARH&MS). She is having of extensive experience in health, nursing and midwifery institutional development, programmes development and management, community development programmes, advocacy and coordination in academia clinical and in community. She is master/lead trainer of health, gender and climate training including midwifery and nursing faculty development training, clinical trainings, GTA & GBV and RMNCH & N training. She is part of midwifery curriculum development with the Pakistan Nursing and Midwifery Council.

Dr. Georgette Spiteri is Senior Lecturer at the University of Malta and Senior Midwife at Gozo General Hospital, Malta.

Jennifer R. Stevens works as attending midwifery faculty at Boston Medical Center. She works globally with Jhpiego as MNH Principle Technical Advisor supporting projects globally and as consultant for the WHO in the SEA region. She recently lived in Bangladesh with UNFPA for three years, as midwifery education specialist. She is co-founder of Goodbirth Network, supporting the quality of midwifery centres in LMIC through data collection and accreditation. Finally, she teaches at Boston University, Boston and City University, London UK, and is currently chair of the Board of Review for the Accreditation Commission for Midwifery Education in the US.

Virginia Stulz spent a year at University of Canberra as the Discipline Lead of Midwifery and is now working at the University of Newcastle. She worked in a conjoint position between Nepean Blue Mountains Local Health District and Western Sydney University for six and a half years prior to this. She worked in NSW across four Local Health Districts on a major research project in an effort to improve student midwives' experiences. From 2018 to 2022, Virginia led a pilot randomised control trial across six hospitals in NSW on evaluating a peanut ball for women having an epidural during labour. She mentored and supported midwives in the local health district with their research projects. She collaborates with other university academics across Australia and New Zealand as a member of the Trans Tasman Midwifery Education Consortium (TTMEC) and worked as the Chair for the TTMEC from 2021 to 2022 and will be working as the Chair from 2023 to 2024. She is currently leading a national research project with this consortium that explores the characteristics of support within new graduate programmes within Australia and has led another national research project that focused on midwives' experiences during COVID-19. In collaboration with other researchers, she has published 35 peer-reviewed journal articles over the past five years in areas of complementary therapies, midwifery education, factors affecting birth practices, gender-based violence, and women's health. Virginia is currently supervising one PhD research student as a primary supervisor and co-supervising three PhD students.

Akane Sugimoto Storey is an autonomous midwife and Doctor of Global Health (DrGH) candidate at the University of Washington. Her work focuses on increasing access to safe and compassionate care during childbirth and the spectrum of life-course sexual and reproductive health needs. With extensive experience in mentoring midwives both in and beyond Mexico, she previously served as the clinical director of a midwifery centre in the state of Chiapas, where she supported the professional development of midwives. Her research and advocacy centre on integrating midwifery within health systems to improve cultural safety and clinical outcomes, particularly in resource-limited settings. Dedicated to advancing evidence-based, respectful maternity care, she works to strengthen midwifery-led initiatives globally and ensure that all birthing people and newborns receive the type of care they want, need and deserve.

Professor Linda Sweet is a midwife with broad experience in clinical environments, education, management and research. She is the inaugural Chair in Midwifery with Deakin University and the Western Health Partnership. She is a life member of the Australian College of Midwives, a Fellow of the Australian and New Zealand Association of Health Professional Educators and a Flinders University distinguished scholar. She has over 160 peer-reviewed publications and is the Deputy Editor of the international journal *Women and Birth*. She is passionate about the midwifery profession and improving maternity care.

Olivia Tierney is a clinician, leader and healthcare manager. She has experienced in strategic and operational leadership, policy, project management, mentoring, facilitation, research and education. She is dedicated to enhancing midwifery care, developing and expanding the workforce, and facilitating positive change, driven by her passion for innovation and research. She is enthusiastic about promoting collaboration and empowering individuals to realize their full potential.

Deepali Y. Upadhyaya is Associate Professor and Academic Director of the Bachelor of Midwifery programme at Mount Royal University in Calgary, Alberta, located on Treaty Seven Territory, Canada. She has worked in perinatal and child health and in the education of healthcare providers across various regions globally. In addition to her academic role, she practices as a Registered Midwife in a collaborative practice in a rural setting. Her areas of focus include midwifery education, evidence-informed decision-making, cultural humility and interprofessional collaboration.

Tamar van Haaren-Ten Haken is a senior lecturer at the Academy of Midwifery Studies Maastricht, the Netherlands – Zuyd University of Applied Science. She teaches in both the bachelor's and master's programme for midwives. She also works as a scientific programme leader, focusing on the art and science of midwifery at the Research Centre for Midwifery Science. With this programme, she aims to contribute to the strong, autonomous position of the midwife as a reflective professional within the interprofessional maternity care network. In 2018, she obtained her PhD from Maastricht University on the preferences, attitudes and beliefs of women regarding the preferred place of birth. She has expertise in both quantitative and qualitative research. Her focus within the education programme is on the integration of research, education and the professional field of midwifery.

Alison Weatherstone is a contemporary dual-qualified Midwife and Registered Nurse, Adjunct Associate Professor, holds a Master of Primary Maternity Care and is the Chief Midwife for the Australian College of Midwives. She plays a key role in leadership, policy, advocacy and media at a local, national and international level and is the co-chair of the International Confederation of Midwives Global Chief Midwives Community of Practice. With lived clinical midwifery experience across Australia and internationally, she is drawn to rural and remote midwifery and has a keen interest in midwives well-being, equitable access to culturally responsive midwifery and sexual reproductive healthcare for all, breech birth and global maternal health. She draws on extensive leadership experience working in the private and public healthcare sectors, not-for-profit member organizations, executive-level leadership and clinical research projects.

FOREWORD

It gives me great pleasure to introduce the first midwifery-specific textbook edited by and some chapters written by two leaders within midwifery academia with research areas such as midwifery decision-making and abdication, deteriorating woman and woman-centred care for all childbearing women regardless of the midwifery context in which their care is provided. This textbook is a global collaboration drawing on midwifery leadership across diverse areas of practice with an aim to demonstrate to midwives, and future midwives, how education and leadership are fundamental aspects of mentoring.

It provides insights into how effective mentorship can empower and guide the next generation of midwives. Working with midwives collaboratively across the world (13 countries and 42 authors) the chapters draw on national and international research and literature within the field of midwifery, incorporating creative midwifery-specific activities to engage readers in reflective practices and consolidate knowledge that can impact mentoring in the future.

The chapters provide valuable insights into the approaches being taken to support midwives within their practice, and just as importantly, the difference that workforce engagement and support make to the way that midwifery teams come together to support woman-centred care.

We know that when midwives feel empowered to make decisions about how they engage, work with women and work as part of a team, this translates into high-functioning teams and effective workplace cultures where everyone can thrive. We also know from our work in Australia and specifically within New South Wales (NSW) Health that midwives want to mentor and share their knowledge and skills, leaving a lasting legacy for those who come after them.

We need to provide the insights, approaches and shared experiences connecting midwives through a community of learning. This ensures the midwifery workforce more broadly is supported to develop the tools and confidence to engage in meaningful ways. Making connections with each other to truly understand the strengths, lived experiences, knowledge and opportunities that will enable them to learn and support one another in their practice, irrespective of where they are located around the world.

When we understand each other as individuals, our shared values and our combined strengths will support the development of workplace cultures where we are able to be our best selves, engage in reflective practice, think critically and creatively and most importantly provide evidenced-based care which meets the expectations of women and their families.

Jacqui Cross PSM
Chief Nursing and Midwifery Officer
NSW Health

INTRODUCTION

Elaine Jefford and Lyn Ebert

As academics, we teach mentorship within the context of midwifery and its relationship to midwifery leadership and education in our undergraduate and graduate programs. Yet, we have found no midwifery-specific textbooks related to mentorship to support our teaching or students/midwives in practice. There are texts in nursing or generic ones applied to all healthcare practitioners that are too old to be applicable in today's healthcare environment and/or tend to focus solely on the country of the authors and/or do not include leadership or education. As the need for such a book became more crystalised in our teaching, the concept of the book was conceived. Rather than developing a book that focuses solely on Australia (country of the editors/authors), we wanted to share with our global midwifery family and students the notion that education and leadership are fundamental aspects of mentorship. We wanted to demonstrate how effective mentorship can empower and guide the next generation of midwives to take over the midwifery baton. So, working collaboratively with some global partners (13 countries and 42 authors) and drawing on national and international research and literature within the field of midwifery, as well as creative midwifery-specific activities the book has transversed the journey from conception to birth.

In this book, authors often refer to midwives as women to reflect the gendered nature of subordination of midwifery. While most midwives globally are women providing care to women, not all midwives globally identify as women. We acknowledge and celebrate the diverse identities of midwives, as this is the best way to build an environment that guarantees enabling sexual and reproductive care for all people who need midwives. Furthermore, the term First Nations which is used is a collective term that refers to Indigenous Australians and Aboriginal and Torres Strait Islander peoples of Australia.

DOI: 10.4324/9781003533733-1

First Nations peoples will refer to themselves by any of these terms and may also identify through language groups. This term is used in acknowledgement that First Nations peoples have the right of self-determination to identify however they choose to do so.

The book is in five parts.

Part I Foundations of Mentorship: Historical and Theoretical Perspectives on Education and Leadership in Healthcare, explores the history of midwifery and mentoring. The first chapter, exploring the history of midwifery, shows us the skills and knowledge of the women supporting the birthing woman were passed from generation to generation, through what we know is mentorship, yet we might call, a form of apprenticeship, as well as through their stories. Critical review of 10 relevant theories for midwifery and health professions education, their potential applications, how they may support/ interact with one another is presented. The next chapter explores the vital role of leadership in midwifery, examining how effective leadership enhances maternity care, contributes to maternity service reform, and influences outcomes for mothers, newborns, and families.

Part II Contextualising Midwifery Mentorship – Attributes, Environments, and Strategic Support explore the context within which midwifery is situated and the contextual requirements in which midwifery mentorship might flourish. Some of the professional and personal attributes a mentor should role model are explored and how the environment, or workplace culture, in which the midwife works, teaches, and mentors impacts or influences these and the environment, or workplace culture, in which the midwife works, teaches, and mentors.

Part III Guiding Hands Across Borders: Midwifery Mentorship Around the World of the book offers insight into mentorship within 14 countries around the globe. Their legislation/regulation and professional accountability underpinning midwifery mentoring and the models used are discussed as is how midwives are educated to become a mentor and their ongoing professional development. The relationship of mentorship to midwifery education, relationship to midwifery leadership, and career pathways are interwoven. The chapters are from all income countries and diversity of midwifery. This diversity comes from midwifery being recognised formally as a profession for more than a century, yet in others, for example Mexico, we learn how midwifery training is scarce, and it occurs in spaces of conflict. The European Mentoring Coaching Committee offers a global perspective on mentoring and on its role in inclusive leadership development and their role within that. The need to consider critical thinking and reflection as they related to mentorship is also explored.

Part IV Embedding Mentorship in Australian Midwifery – Perspectives, Practice, and Impact, although this section of the book has an Australian focus, the content can be applied to any context worldwide. Midwifery mentorship with midwifery curricula is explored. Next cultural considerations concerning Australia's First Nations peoples and their relevance to mentorship in the midwifery profession is highlighted. An overview of the impact of colonisation and how these historical factors may shape mentoring relationships is presented. Additionally, practical suggestions for fostering successful mentorship within culturally safe spaces are provided. We then move into a chapter on how midwifery leaders can effectively foster, implement, and sustain mentorship programs that benefit both individual midwives and positively affect organisations. Two chapters present findings from recent studies exploring the experiences of those participating in a mentoring program. The first study presented explores midwifery students' experiences using an appreciative inquiry approach that enabled the research team to discover what matters and works well from the perspective of midwifery students, midwives, and midwifery managers. The findings were used to create enhanced experiences in the future. The second study explores mentees and mentor's expectations of, and experiences (pre- and post-mentoring program). Again, this knowledge can be used to support sustainable mentoring programs to enhance midwifery practice and professional development. The final chapter in this section looks at the context in which mentorship and supervision are applied.

Part V Shaping the Future of Midwifery Mentorship – Global Insights and Strategic Directions offers global recommendations for the future of mentorship.

As you progress through the chapters of this book, you will see how mentorship shapes and underpins midwifery practice and ultimately the quality and safety of care we provide to women, babies, and their family (however they define it) cannot be underestimated. You will also become aware of the complexity around the implementation and sustainability of mentorship in the healthcare context and the challenges to ensuring midwives have access to mentorship.

We hope this book provides you with a broad perspective on mentorship, along with the knowledge and skills to add into your midwifery professional development toolbox, wherever you are around the world. Remember, that you are not alone rather you are part of a global family of midwifery who have, and will continue to support and nurture each other and the next generation of midwives.

1

HISTORY OF MIDWIFERY EDUCATION AND MENTORSHIP

Elaine Jefford

Introduction

When researching for this chapter, it became apparent there are different definitions of the term 'Mentor' and when the term was first introduced. For example, in the journal of Mentoring & Tutoring: Partnership in Learning, authors claim mentoring was 'born' (published) in the late 18th century (Irby & Boswell, 2016). However, most writers agree with the date line below:

Between 800 - 600 BCE Homer's Poem, the Odyssey, tells us that an old man called Mentor was given the responsibility by Odysseus, King of Ithica, to act as a guardian, advisor, teacher, and friend to his son Telemachus, whilst he was away fighting the Trojan Wars. Telemachus was a baby when his father left, but as Telemachus grew into a young man, he wanted to find his father. Apparently, Mentor didn't always provide the needed guidance for Telemachus and so, the daughter of Zeus, Athena, the Goddess of Wisdom and War and the patroness of the Arts and Industry impersonated the old man Mentor and accompanied Telemachus on his quest to find his father. Father and son were reunited and defeated the would-be usurpers of Odysseus's throne and Telemachus' birthright.

(Butcher & Lang, 1890; Roberts, 1999)

While we do not wish to disparage males (midwives), it is interesting to note a woman, one of the most known mythological goddess Athena, steps into the role of mentor when an 'old man' fails in his mentorship role and responsibilities. In other words, it could be suggested Athena demonstrated her innate ability to nurture and support and applied these qualities to the role of

DOI: 10.4324/9781003533733-2

mentor and leader as early as 800–600 BC (Christos-Thomas & Alexander-Stamatios, 2019).

In all societies and cultures across the world, from ancient times until the present day, guiding, advising, and supporting the next generation of people (midwives) to survive and prosper in life has been an expected and accepted role of the older generations. Historically, the mentor's role and responsibility came with no instruction book rather evolving over time as one generation learnt from the one before. This process was essential to enable an individual (midwife) to grow and develop, yet in most societies, that guidance, advice, and support also meant the survival of that individual within their family; however, they defined it as well as their extended community. Historically, the role of the woman, within communities around the world, focused on family, caring for their children and all domestic household duties, which most of the time, excluded the financial aspect of a household. Women were respected for and entrusted with that role and were supported by a network of other women.

Thus, over the last 3000 years, the word mentor evolved to mean trusted advisor, friend, teacher and wise person, with the aim of supporting a less experienced person (midwife) to develop the skills and knowledge to progress in their chosen direction in life and specifically in their career or education (midwifery). This will become clearer as you read this book and specifically what different countries define mentor(ship) to mean in their specific context and how the term mentor is applied within midwifery. While the role of a mentor is to be a thoughtful and skilled partner, they must first understand what the mentee wants to achieve and then assist that person to draw out or develop the required skills to move in their desired direction. The history and evolution of the profession in which the mentor and the mentee work, influence the guidance, advice and support necessary. As does the psychosocial, professional or occupational context, and the cultural norms and expectations of the society in which they live and work. Understanding the history of the profession (midwifery) in which they work assists the mentor/mentee relationship and provides understanding and context. It can help the mentee find their way and direction in their profession and may provide, not only an explanation of why that profession is where it is, but also a way forward.

History of Midwifery

The history of midwifery is recognised as one of the oldest occupations/professions which can be traced back to the Paleolithic era, or Stone Age, approximately 2.5 million years ago to 40,000 BC (Australian College of Midwives, 2021; International Confederation of Midwives, 2022). Midwives are cited in the Old Testament (Bibles Net. Com – Online Christian

Library, 2008). Midwives were noted during the Greek, Roman and Saracenic eras (Murphy, 1864). World history shows us from the beginning of time women essentially supported each other to birth their babies at home with the help of women who had experience assisting others to birth. Further, these women or *'(lay) midwives'* were acknowledged, respected and paid for their services, albeit not always in money. One cannot, however, forget the witch's era (15, 16 and part of the 17 century). A terrible time for midwifery and midwives where demonologists wrote how midwives used newborn babies to conduct magic in the book published around 1473 titled *Formicarius* by Johannes Nider as noted by Harley (1990). The author further notes the book, *The Malleus Maleficarum's* published by Spregner and Kraemar in 1489, intense focus on children, impotence and infanticide can be seen as stemming either from a profound fear of women's (lay midwives) perceived power or from anxiety over the widespread medieval practices aimed at limiting family size (Forbes, 1962; Harley, 1990) or from the church and/or royal and government power at the time (Forbes, 1962).

Murphy (1864) notes in 1565 a book was published by Dr Ranaldi titled *The Birthe of Man-kind*: or the *Woman's book*. Interestingly, this book contained recipes for midwives to use, wearing of cosmetics in childbirth. It is suggested the author thought this text as an aid for midwives, which was rejected by midwives, feeling doctors were interfering with what was their business or women's business. Yet, the debate of when men insidiously moved into what was and arguably is still women's business, differs from country to country, and it is outside the scope of this chapter to provide the reader with each country's unique history of midwifery.

REFLECTIVE ACTIVITY 1

The unique history, culture, local traditions, challenges, and triumphs of each country shape the birthing environment, political context and midwifery ways of supporting women.

- Have you ever explored the story of midwifery in your own country? Take some time to explore how past generations cared for women, mothers and babies.

Understanding this history can offer insights and inspire a deeper appreciation for the journey midwifery and midwives have taken to be where they are today.

Informal Midwifery Education and Mentorship

England

History notes midwifery, in some form or another, in England for millenniums, and as requiring episcopal licensing as early as the 16th century, although an exact date is not clear (Fox & Brazier, 2020). A key role of a midwife at that time was administering baptism to fragile infants who were unlikely to survive until a priest's arrival and supporting birthing women. These midwives were usually married, had given birth themselves and learnt their skills and knowledge through what could be termed an apprenticeship model. Some midwives would establish their own practices by attending to women in labour when their mentors were unavailable, gradually gaining popularity among local women as news of their skill and competence spread. It is also suggested friends and neighbours came to observe 'the midwife' (Fox & Brazier, 2020). Yet, when talking about midwifery in England, one cannot forget to mention the 'The Midwives Book of the Whole Art of Midwifery Discovered' which was written by Jane Sharp in 1671 with thirty years' experience of midwifery practice. In this book, the author notes that midwifery was not learnt at university rather through 'long and diligent practice' and was 'communicated to others of our own sex' (Sharp, 1671). Nevertheless, like other countries England midwives succumbed to medicine, and the maternal and infant mortality was attributed to untrained midwives calling for scientifically trained doctors to replace them stating they alone could improve the wellbeing of mother and baby (Cahill, 2000).

Holland

Some midwives in Netherlands history served extensive communities and documented their work. For instance, the translated memoirs of Catharina Schrader, a 17th-century Dutch midwife, reveal her extensive professional practice, including detailed records maintained in her diary. Schrader established a midwifery practice that also encompassed surgical procedures. It is suggested her gynaecological and maternal expertise was acquired through studying midwifery literature and through mentorship from her husband, a barber-surgeon (Marland, 1984).

America

History shows America adapted their model of maternity healthcare along the same lines as England and other European countries. Yet, unlike some countries, American midwives were well respected, during the early colonisation period. Capitulo (1998) notes that some of these midwives were provided free accommodation and a salary. Things changed, however. Thomas (1933) in his book about American obstetrics talks about a midwife, Anne Hutchinson, who gained notoriety around the mid-1600s who was accused of being a witch after helping a woman birth an anencephalic baby. By the early 1700's midwives, or 'granny midwives' as they were known, needed to be credentialed to provide care (Capitulo, 1998). A 'granny midwife' from 1785 to 1812, named Martha Ballard, in the Hallowell district of Maine, United States, meticulously documented her work spanning several years. Historian Laurel Thatcher Ulrich (1990) highlighted Ballard's crucial role in her community, emphasising her comprehensive knowledge of birth, illness and death, which interconnected the lives of residents. Ballard's career also reflects the importance of mentorship, as knowledge and skills were often passed through hands-on learning and guidance within the community. Yet, as males began studying obstetrics in the 1800s the art of midwifery got subsumed into the science of medicine and the midwife began to lose popularity. This was compounded in 1843 as Mitford (1992) notes, the puerperal fever was rampant and doctors were saying as *'gentlemen and scholars' they could not 'be the cause of disease in their patients* (p. p34)', thus implying it was the 'granny midwives'.

Australia

Prior to the colonisation of Australia, First Nation people transversed the land living a simple, yet some might suggest a hard life due to the changing landscape and seasons, fishing, hunting and gathering just enough food and resources to live, thus permitting the land to regenerate season to season. First Nation women spoke about and conducted *'women's business'* with other women as discussing matters considered to be within the realm of women's affairs with men was often regarded as inappropriate or impolite. Childbirth was part of *'women's business'* (Bell, 1998). Traditionally, First Nation women birthed on the land of which they lived, and care was provided from within their mob (term used to denote a family group, clan group or wider community group or place). The skills and knowledge of the women supporting the birthing woman were passed from generation to generation, through what we might call, a form of apprenticeship, as well as through their stories. Post colonisation the lives and practices of the First Nation people were irrevocably changed as new governments emerged and policies developed (Dowd et al., 2010).

In 1788, the first ship left England bound for Australia to establish a penal colony. On board the 11 ships was John White a naval surgeon who went on to become the Surgeon-General in Australia, two assistant surgeons and one naval surgeon (Australian College of Midwives, 2021; Ford, 1972), it is not certain if their expertise included maternity care.

According to historical resources 187 women convicts and 33 sailors' wives made this journey. History does not record who helped the women who birthed 18 babies, including two stillbirths and one miscarriage, during the eight-month one-week journey, although supposition suggests it was other convict women and sailors wives (Australian College of Midwives, 2021). Burrows (2018) notes a convict called Ann Colpitts, entered on the travel log as a servant, acted as a 'midwife' to those convicted pregnant women and later when living in Australia. Again, it is assumed the knowledge and skills of women, such as Ann Colpitts, were passed on through stories and observation, a form of generational and intergenerational knowledge transfer that preserves the wisdom of birthing as most of these women could not read or write. Such mentorship helped other women take on the role of midwife, many unnamed in historical literature, during the early period of Australia's colonisation and the development of penal colonies and ex-pat communities (Australian College of Midwives, 2021).

Hannah Jane 'Grannie' Watts

Hannah Jane 'Grannie' Watts represented a class of women of her time. 'Hannah left Ireland to travel to Australia in 1854 and it is believed learnt her midwifery skills en route'. She was the daughter of a farmer but worked as a supervisor in a linen mill and survived the great famine. Then newly married, she set sail for Australia, birthing her first baby five weeks after arrival. Settling in the Melton area she farmed and worked as a midwife, walking the district attending births. She was twice widowed and had six children and 'progressed from helpful neighbour to grannie to registered midwife, and when she opened her home for care it became the first registered private hospital in the district'. Hannah kept a book of births she attended. 'She attended her last birth just a few months before her death in 1921, just short of her 90th birthday'. When her great-great granddaughter, Rebecca Hart researched her life and work, she learned of the extent and scope of her great-great-grandmother's practice. It is a source of pride in the Melton area to have ancestors who were 'Grannie born' and the community commemorates her 'in the Hannah Watts Park and the local electoral ward of Watts is named for her' (Hart, 2022).

While females and midwives largely were ignored in early medical literature, males and medicine took the lead in maternity care publications. Ford (1972) notes William Sherwin, the first native-born Australian medical author published an eight-page pamphlet in Sydney (1844) titled *On the Primum Mobile of the Blood to the Lungs at Birth; its Complete Vitalization or Animalization; and its Subsequent Circulation*. This publication is the earliest known medical publication by a native-born Australian. It explores the changes in foetal circulation at birth and reveals the first published evidence of males and medicine entering the field of maternity care in Australia.

As you can see, from the few examples presented here midwifery has navigated a difficult terrain to become the midwifery we know today, irrespective of geographical location around the world. Yet, the fundamental elements of midwifery have not changed. The first is to assist, support and prepare the environment for the baby's birth, while also safeguarding the woman's space to allow her to concentrate on *'women's business'* of bringing her baby into the world. The next is mentoring, where women through storytelling, observation, hands-on experience and sharing insights, gained through years of practice, pass down the critical knowledge and skills of midwifery. It is through the storytelling, brought to life through observing, that midwifery wisdom, has been passed intergenerationally.

Formal Midwifery Education and Mentorship

Midwifery began to reassert itself within the maternity care context through education. In Australia, the first midwifery training commenced in 1862 with the Diploma in Midwifery introduced in 1893. These midwives had to have completed a nursing qualification first (Barclay, 2008). The National College of Midwifery in Amsterdam was established in 1861, offering a two-year training program designed to enhance the quality of the profession and address the shortage of midwives. In England, the first Midwives *Act* came to pass in 1902, recognising midwifery as its own discipline yet like Australia one had to be a nurse. In 1931, American saw the introduction of the nurse–midwifery program in New York offered by the Maternity Center Association.

REFLECTIVE ACTIVITY 2

Explore when your country first starting formally teaching midwifery and if they had to be a qualified nurse first.

Midwives Supporting Midwives

Midwives have been meeting, to grow discipline-specific knowledge and skills to support each other and birthing women since the 1880s. These meetings were largely attended by midwives working in European countries and were the precursor to the International Confederation of Midwives (ICM), formed in 1954. The ICM's founding aim was to 'advance education in midwifery, and to spread knowledge of the art and science of midwifery, with the aim of improving the standard of care provided to mothers, babies and the family throughout countries of the world' (Wellcome Collection, n.d). Advancing the education and knowledge of midwifery practice involves passing on the skills to the next generation of midwives so that they may be with and support women to birth. If we refer to the definition of mentorship at the start of the chapter, passing on skills and knowledge is mentoring.

Irrespective, of when formal midwifery education came into being, or if one had to be a nurse first, a mentorship system would have existed, either formally or informally. Please go to Section II, *Mentorship, leadership and education: a global perspective* where country-specific chapters detail how midwifery mentorship is undertaken.

Other Resources

International Confederation of Midwives: The origins of Midwifery. https://uat.rcm.org.uk/news-views/news/2020/the-history-of-midwifery-how-far-weve-come/#:~:text=Midwifery%20and%20healthcare%20are%20constantly,next%20part%20of%20the%20journey

Royal College of Midwives: The History of Midwifery – how far we've come. https://uat.rcm.org.uk/news-views/news/2020/the-history-of-midwifery-how-far-weve-come

- Arnup, Katherine, Andree Levesque and Ruth Roach Pearson, eds. Delivering Motherhood: Maternal Ideologies and Practices in the 19th and 20th Centuries. London: Routledge, 1990.
- Cahill, Heather. "Male appropriation and medicalization of Childbirth: An Historical Analysis." Journal of Advanced Nursing. 33(3), 2000.
- Cook, William H. "Woman's Handbook of Health." 1871.
- Leavitt, Judith Walzer. Brought to Bed: Childbearing in America, 1750 – 1950. New York; Oxford UP, 1986.
- Davison, C. "Feminism, Midwifery and the Medicalization of Birth." BMJ. 28(12), 2020.
- Davison, C. Looking back and moving forward: A history and discussion of privately practicing midwives in Western Australia. PhD Thesis. Curtin University; 2019.

References

Australian College of Midwives. (2021). *Australian Midwifery History*. Australian College of Midwives. Retrieved 16 January from https://australianmidwiferyhistory.org.au/

Barclay, L. (2008). A feminist history of Australian midwifery from colonisation until the1980s. *Women & Birth*, 21(8), 3–8. https://doi.org/10.1016/j.wombi.2007.12.001

Bell, H. R. (1998). *Men's Business, Women's Business: The Spiritual Role of Gender in the World's Oldest Culture*. Inner Traditions.

Bibles Net. Com - Online Christian Library. (2008). *Easton's 1897 Bible Dictionary*. Bibles Net. Com - Online Christian Library. Retrieved 16 January from https://www.biblesnet.com/eastons_bible_dictionary/indexs.htm

Burrows, D. (2018). *Ann Colpitts: First Fleet Midwife*. NLA Publishing. https://australianmidwiferyhistory.org.au/first-fleet-1788-initial-contact/

Butcher, S. H., & Lang, A. (1890). *The Odyssey of Homer Done into English Prose*. Macmillian.

Cahill, H. (2000). Male appropriation and medicalization of childbirth: An historical analysis. *Journal of Advanced Nursing, 33*(3), 334–342. https://onlinelibrary.wiley.com/doi/pdf/10.1046/j.1365-2648.2001.01669.x

Capitulo, K. (1998). The rise, fall, and rise of nurse-midwifery in America. *The American Journal of Maternal/Child Nursing, 23*(6), 314–321. https://journals.lww.com/mcnjournal/fulltext/1998/11000/The_RISE,_FALL,_and_RISE_of_Nurse_Midwifery_in.8.aspx

Christos-Thomas, K., & Alexander-Stamatios, A. (2019). Goddess Athena as leader and mentor in Homeric epics. In Alexander-Stamatios, A., C. Cooper, & C. Gatrell (Eds.), *Women, Business and Leadership* (pp. 106–121). Edward Elgar Publishing Inc. https://china.elgaronline.com/edcollchap/edcoll/9781786432704/9781786432704.00013.xml

Dowd, T., Eckermann, A., Chong, E., Nixon, L., Gray, R., & Johnson, S. (2010). *Binan Goonj: Bridging Cultures in Aboriginal Health* (3rd ed.). Churchill Livingstone - Elsevier. https://books.google.com.au/books?hl=en&lr=&id=d-ZfzJNACu0C&oi=fnd&pg=PR9&ots=P8_tp3vwLM&sig=b6FjiTw5yawnsiH7ggvS8PovawM&redir_esc=y#v=onepage&q&f=false

Forbes, T. (1962). Midwifery and witchcraft. *Journal of the History of Medicine and Allied Sciences, XVII*(2), 264–283. https://doi.org/10.1093/jhmas/XVII.2.264

Ford, E. (1972). *Medical History*. Cambridge. https://www.cambridge.org/core/services/aop-cambridge-core/content/view/68EFCD0569DA93E930F72965E3FE061B/S0025727300017713a.pdf/div-class-title-some-early-australian-medical-publications-div.pdf

Fox, S., & Brazier, M. (2020). The regulation of midwives in England, c.1500–1902. *Medical Law International, 20*(4), 308–338. https://doi.org/10.1177/0968533220976174

Harley, D. (1990). Historians as demonologists: The myth of the midwife-witch. *The Society for the Social History of Medicine, 30*(1), 1–26.

Hart, R. (2022). A hundred year journey home: When family history becomes historic artifact. *Australian Midwifery News, 30*, 44–45. https://australianmidwiferyhistory.org.au/rebecca-hart-2/

International Confederation of Midwives. (2022). *Model of Care: The Origins of Midwifery*. International Confederation of Midwives. Retrieved 16 January from https://internationalmidwives.org/the-origins-of-midwifery/

Irby, B., & Boswell, J. (2016). Historical print context of the term, "Mentoring." *Mentoring & Tutoring: Partnership in Learning, 24*(1), 1–7. https://doi.org/http://dx.doi.org/10.1080/13611267.2016.1170556

Marland, H. (1984). Mother and child were save: The memoirs (1693-1740) of the Frisian midwife Catharina Schraders, (H. Marland, Trans.). In Marland, H., C. Kloosterman, & M. van Lieburg (Eds.), *The Art of Midwifery: Early Modern Midwives in Europe* (pp. 1–18). Rodopi. https://australianmidwiferyhistory.org.au/wp-content/uploads/2021/11/A-SUMMERS-THESIS-2021-11-15-at-6.18.03-pm.pdf

Mitford, J. (1992). *The American Way to Birth*. Penguin. https://www.amazon.com.au/American-Way-Birth-Jessica-Mitford/dp/0525935231

Murphy, E. W. (1864). Introductory lecture on the history of midwifery. *The British Medical Journal, 1*(1), 524–528. https://www.jstor.org/stable/pdf/25200790.pdf

Roberts, A. (1999). Duties fulfilled or misconstrued. *History of Education Journal, 5, 607–629.*

Sharp, J. (1671). *The Midwives Book, or, the Whole Art of Midwifery Discovered.* Oxford University Press.

Thomas, H. (1933). *Chapters in American Obstetrics.* Charles Thomas Publisher.

Ulrich, L. (1990). *A Midwife's Tale: The Life of Martha Ballard, Based on Her Diary, 1785 –1812.* Vintage Books Random House. https://archive.org/details/midwifestalelife00ulririch

Wellcome Collection. (n.d). *International Confederation of Midwives.* Retrieved 28th January from https://wellcomecollection.org/works/vexxs9ed

2

MIDWIFERY EDUCATION IN HEALTHCARE

Theories and Models

Linda Sweet and Jessica Lees

Introduction

As we explore various learning theories, it is important to recognise that midwifery practice, like other healthcare fields, is both a science and an art. Learning theories help us understand how to best bridge the gap between knowledge and practice, teach new skills, and nurture professional growth in midwifery to directly impact the well-being of mothers, infants, and families.

In the context of midwifery and other healthcare professions, the application of learning theories is essential for ensuring that students and professionals develop the knowledge, skills, and attitudes necessary to provide safe, effective, and compassionate care. Midwives must be able to continuously adapt to new information, technologies, and client needs. In this context, learning theories provide more than just a conceptual framework; they are the tools that shape the structure of education and professional development. By applying a range of learning theories, midwifery practitioners can create diverse, inclusive, and engaging learning experiences that not only enhance clinical expertise but also foster the development of compassionate and reflective practitioners.

The development of learning theories has been influenced by several academic disciplines that have shaped our understanding of how people learn, think, and develop over time. These disciplines have provided foundational knowledge that underpins the evolution of learning theories across various fields, including education, psychology, health professions, and sociology. The primary disciplines that have contributed to the development of learning theories include psychology, sociology, education, philosophy, and anthropology.

DOI: 10.4324/9781003533733-3

Behaviourism

Behaviourism is a learning theory that focuses on observable behaviours and the ways in which they are shaped by external stimuli and reinforcement. Key authors of behaviourism include Ivan Pavlov (1849–1936), Watson [1], and Skinner [2]. Behaviourism posits that learning occurs through interactions with the environment, where behaviours are learned through conditioning. In its simplest form, behaviourism suggests that new behaviours can be acquired through positive or negative reinforcement, repetition, and association. You may recall hearing of Pavlov's experiments in the 1890s with his dogs, where the dogs learned to associate food with the sound of a bell, triggering salivation.

Key Principles of Behaviourism Include

- *Conditioning:* Learning occurs through conditioning, which can be either classical (associating a neutral stimulus with a response) or operant (reinforcing behaviour with rewards or punishments).
- *Reinforcement:* Positive reinforcement (rewards) and negative reinforcement (removing unpleasant stimuli) strengthen desired behaviours, while punishment discourages undesired behaviours.
- *Stimulus–Response:* Behaviour is seen as a response to a specific stimulus. The connection between the stimulus and the response can be shaped through repeated exposure.
- *Observable Behaviour:* Behaviourism focuses on measurable, observable behaviour rather than internal thoughts or emotions.
- *Behaviour Modification:* The use of reinforcement or punishment to shape behaviour over time, making learning outcomes predictable and measurable.

Application in Health Professions Education

In health professions education, behaviourism is often used to teach practical skills where specific, measurable behaviours can be observed. For example, midwifery students learn technical procedures such as taking blood pressure or abdominal palpation through repetition and reinforcement. Positive reinforcement (e.g., praise or rewards for correct performance/assessment) encourages learners to repeat successful actions, while errors may be corrected through feedback and require further repetition. Simulations and drill-based training are commonly used, allowing learners to practise skills in a controlled environment with immediate feedback, reinforcing correct actions, and discouraging mistakes. Moreover, a midwife's ability to follow protocols or perform procedures may be assessed, and feedback may be provided to reinforce correct behaviours. If a midwife performs substandardly, behaviourism may underpin some directed guidance processes in mentoring and supervision.

Behaviourism in health profession education emphasises observable, measurable learning outcomes through conditioning, reinforcement, and repetition. Focusing on acquiring specific skills and behaviours, it offers a structured approach to teaching practical competencies and ensuring mastery in clinical settings. This theory is especially valuable in technical training, assessment, and developing professional behaviours in healthcare.

Further Reading

Baker-Rush, M. L., Pabst, A., Aitchison, R., Anzur, T., & Paschal, N. (2021). Fear in Interprofessional Simulation: The Role of Psychology and Behaviorism in Student Participation and Learning. *Journal of Interprofessional Education & Practice*, 24, 100432. https://doi.org/10.1016/j.xjep.2021.100432 [3].

Baker, L. R., Phelan, S., Woods, N. N., Boyd, V. A., Rowland, P., & Ng, S. L. (2021). Re-Envisioning Paradigms of Education: Towards Awareness, Alignment, and Pluralism. *Advances in Health Sciences Education*, 26(3), 1045–1058. https://doi.org/10.1007/s10459-021-10036-z [4].

Cognitivism

Cognitivism is a learning theory concentrating on the mental processes involved in learning and organising information. Key theorists of cognitivism include Piaget [5] and Bruner [6]. Unlike behaviourism, which focuses on observable behaviour, cognitivism is concerned with processes involved in learning, such as attention, memory, and problem-solving. The theory suggests that learners actively construct their understanding by processing information, connecting new and existing knowledge, and using mental strategies to store and retrieve information.

Key Principles of Cognitivism Include

- *Active Learning:* Learners are seen as active participants who process, organise, and interpret information rather than passive recipients of stimuli.
- *Schema Theory:* Knowledge is organised in mental frameworks or schemas. Learning involves linking new information to existing frameworks, helping individuals to integrate new knowledge into long-term memory.
- *Information Processing:* Cognitivism compares the mind to a computer, where information is received, processed, stored, and retrieved. Learning involves encoding new information and using strategies to make it retrievable when needed.

• *Metacognition:* Cognitivism emphasises the importance of thinking about one's thinking. Learners are encouraged to monitor and control their learning processes to enhance comprehension and retention.

Application in Health Professions Education

In health professions education, cognitivism is applied to enhance how students process and retain complex information. For example, midwives learn to integrate new knowledge with their prior understanding of anatomy, pharmacology, and clinical care through concept mapping and case-based or problem-based learning. By creating mental models and schemas, learners can organise information and make sense of clinical scenarios more effectively. This promotes active learning, encourages critical thinking, and helps learners develop problem-solving strategies by applying their knowledge to unfamiliar situations.

Cognitivist principles also inform simulation-based education in health professions. Through simulations, students are exposed to complex clinical scenarios, which require them to retrieve and apply their knowledge to solve problems, reinforcing their mental frameworks. Feedback and self-reflection are also integral to cognitivist strategies, allowing learners to refine their understanding and improve their clinical reasoning skills. Furthermore, metacognitive strategies are promoted to help students become more aware of their thinking processes and learning strategies, such as self-assessment, goal setting, and reflection on their clinical performance. These strategies foster deeper understanding and better retention of critical healthcare knowledge and are helpful in mentoring and peer support.

Further Reading

Finn, A., Fitzgibbon, C., Fonda, N., & Gosling, C. M. (2024). Self-Directed Learning and the Student Learning Experience in Undergraduate Clinical Science Programs: A Scoping Review. *Advances in Health Sciences Education.* https://doi.org/10.1007/s10459-024-10383-7 [7].

Servant-Miklos, V. F. C. (2019). Problem Solving Skills Versus Knowledge Acquisition: The Historical Dispute That Split Problem-Based Learning into Two Camps. *Advances in Health Sciences Education*, 24(3), 619–635. https://doi.org/10.1007/s10459-018-9835-0 [8].

Constructivism

Constructivism is a learning theory whereby learners actively construct their knowledge and understanding through experiences and reflecting on those experiences. Key theorists of constructivism include Piaget [5] and Vygotsky [9]. Unlike behaviourism and cognitivism, which emphasise passive reception or internal processing of information, constructivism emphasises the active role of learners in building their own mental models. According to this theory, learning is a process of adaptation, where individuals make sense of new information by connecting it with their prior experiences, creating new frameworks for understanding. This may be a self-directed process where learners engage with problems and reflect on their experiences to build understanding or collaborate with others.

Key Principles of Constructivism Include

- *Active Learning:* Learners actively construct their understanding with material, experiences, and social interactions.
- *Prior Knowledge:* Learners build on their knowledge, experiences, and cultural contexts. New information is integrated into existing cognitive structures or schemas.
- *Social Interaction:* Learning is often a social process. Interaction with peers, mentors, and instructors is crucial in helping learners refine and expand their understanding.
- *Problem-Solving and Inquiry:* Learners engage in inquiry and problem-solving, which leads to deeper understanding.
- *Contextual Learning:* Knowledge is best understood and retained when it is situated in real-life, meaningful contexts. Learning is often tied to authentic tasks or experiences.
- *Scaffolding:* Learners are supported through guided interactions with more knowledgeable others (teachers, peers, mentors, or experts), who help them reach higher levels of understanding through challenges that are just beyond the learners' current ability.

Application in Health Professions Education

In health professions education, constructivism encourages active engagement with complex clinical knowledge. For example, the use of problem-based or simulation-based learning enables midwives and health professions students to collaborate to solve authentic cases, fostering critical thinking and applying prior knowledge to new, context-rich problems in a safe environment. This approach emphasises the core constructivist principle of learning through experience.

Scaffolding, through mentorship and guidance from experienced professionals, helps learners build competence by gradually increasing the complexity of tasks. Mentors provide feedback and support, helping students improve over time. Additionally, constructivism promotes reflection and self-directed learning, encouraging learners to evaluate their experiences, identify knowledge gaps, and take ownership of their learning. This fosters lifelong learning habits and adaptability, essential qualities for healthcare professionals.

Further Reading

Arundell, F., Sheehan, A., & Peters, K. (2024). Strategies Used by Midwives to Enhance Knowledge and Skill Development in Midwifery Students: An Appreciative Inquiry Study. *BMC Nursing, 23*(1), 1–10. https://doi.org/10.1186/s12912-024-01784-5 [10].

Meen, A. (2021). From Theory to Practice. *British Journal of Midwifery, 29*(4), 186–188. https://doi.org/10.12968/bjom.2021.29.4.186 [11].

Social Learning Theory

Social learning theory, developed by Albert Bandura [12], posits that people learn not only through direct experience but also by observing others, making it a foundational theory for understanding how behaviour and knowledge are acquired in social contexts. Bandura introduced the concept that learning can occur through observation, imitation, and modelling, meaning that people learn by watching others and then mimicking their actions. Social learning theory relies on cognitive processes to mediate the observed into a response, and this consideration is called a mediational process.

Key Principles of Social Learning Theory Include

- *Observational Learning:* People observe others, particularly role models, and learn by watching the consequences of their actions. This can include direct imitation or adapting behaviours based on their observations.
- *Attention, Retention, Reproduction, and Motivation:* For learning to occur, individuals must pay attention to the model, remember the behaviour, be able to reproduce it, and have the motivation to do so. These processes underline that learning is both cognitive and behavioural.
- *Role of Reinforcement and Punishment:* Although Bandura argued that learning can occur without direct reinforcement, seeing someone else rewarded or punished for a behaviour influences whether an observer (learner) will replicate the behaviour or not.
- *Self-Efficacy:* A core aspect of Bandura's theory is self-efficacy—one's belief in their ability to succeed in specific situations. People are more likely to imitate behaviours if they feel capable of achieving the same success.

Application in Health Professions Education

Social learning theory has significant applications in fields of health professions education, supporting practices such as mentorship, role modelling, and peer learning. The theory emphasises the social context of learning, proposing that individuals are shaped not only by direct experience but also by the social and environmental cues around them. As a result, it highlights how learning and behaviour are profoundly influenced by the surrounding culture and interactions, bridging individual learning with the social environment.

Social learning theory has been widely applied in midwifery to enhance learning, behaviour change, and skill acquisition among healthcare professionals and women. It offers a framework for understanding how individuals in healthcare settings can learn by observing others, including mentors and peers.

In healthcare education, social learning theory underpins the concept of clinical placements and shadowing, where students learn by observing and modelling experienced professionals. This approach enables learners to develop practical skills by observing procedures, understanding patient (women's) interactions, and engaging in (women's) hands-on practice under supervision. Instructors serve as role models, demonstrating professional behaviours, clinical reasoning, and techniques that students imitate and refine. In continuing professional development for registered healthcare workers, social learning theory is a key theory to mentoring in the workplace.

Further Reading

McNeill, L., Gum, L., Graham, K., & Sweet, L. (2024). "Removing the Home Court Advantage": A Qualitative Evaluation of Lego® as an Interprofessional Simulation Icebreaker for Midwifery and Medical Students. *Nurse Education in Practice*, *80*, 104138. https://doi.org/10.1016/j.nepr.2024.104138 [13].

Folkvord, S. E., & Risa, C. F. (2023). Factors That Enhance Midwifery Students' Learning and Development of Self-Efficacy in Clinical Placement: A Systematic Qualitative Review. *Nurse Education in Practice*, *66*, 103510. https://doi.org/10.1016/j.nepr.2022.103510 [14].

Transformative Learning Theory

Transformative learning theory, developed by Jack Mezirow [15, 16], focuses on how individuals change their perspectives through critical reflection and dialogue. It emphasises not just acquiring knowledge but transforming one's worldview by questioning assumptions and beliefs. This process helps learners develop new ways of thinking and understanding the world.

Key Principles of Transformative Learning Theory Include

- *Critical Reflection:* Learners are encouraged to examine their assumptions and beliefs and challenge their existing views.
- *Disorienting Dilemma:* A challenging experience often prompts learners to question their current understanding, which, through this theory, may result in a life-changing event.

- *Dialogue and Interaction:* Transformation is often facilitated through conversation with others. Interacting with others helps learners to reconsider their perspectives and reexamine assumptions.
- *Perspective Transformation:* Individuals may transform their perspective after critical reflection and dialogue of a disorienting dilemma. This enables a shift in how learners view themselves or the world after reflection and dialogue.
- *Self-Awareness and Autonomy:* Through the transformative process, learners become more self-aware and take greater responsibility for their learning and actions. Ideally, with support, learners will gain autonomy in decisions based on critical reflection.
- *Cognitive and Emotional Growth:* Transformative learning leads to intellectual and emotional change.

Application in Health Professions Education

Transformative learning can have profound implications in the context of health professions education, particularly in fostering critical thinking, self-awareness, empathy, and the ability to adapt to complex, ever-changing healthcare environments. For example, through reflective practice, transformation learning can assist midwives in critically examining experiences that may contradict their preconceptions or beliefs, deepening their understanding, and developing cultural competence for woman-centred care. Applying the concepts of transformative learning can assist learners in managing the emotional aspects of healthcare, such as dealing with a loss or ethical challenge. The process of mentoring or peer support should have the goal of transformation, whereby significant support is required initially, and over time, the learner will adopt the strategies and gain autonomy in transforming their practice. Transformative learning theory enhances health professions education by promoting critical thinking, empathy, and adaptability, helping individuals to become thoughtful, compassionate, and resilient healthcare professionals.

Further Reading

Bass, J., Fenwick, J., & Sidebotham, M. (2017). Development of a Model of Holistic Reflection to Facilitate Transformative Learning in Student Midwives. *Women and Birth*, 30(3), 227–235 [17].

Wallace, H. J., & Harvey, T. M. (2024). 'Listen with an Open-Heart Always' – A Qualitative Study Exploring Transformational Learning Opportunities for Australian Midwifery Students Participating in a Virtual International Study Experience. *Nurse Education in Practice*, 81, 104174. https://doi.org/10.1016/j.nepr.2024.104174 [18].

Adult Learning Theory (Andragogy)

Adult learning theory (andragogy), primarily developed by Malcolm Knowles, [19, 20] is a framework that focuses on how adults learn differently from children. It emphasises that adults bring a wealth of life experience, knowledge, and self-direction to their learning process, which makes their learning needs distinct. The theory proposes that adult learners are motivated by practical, real-life applications and are often goal-oriented in their learning efforts. This theory is particularly relevant in health professions education, as it helps shape the design and delivery of training programmes for adult learners who may be pursuing new skills or knowledge while balancing professional and personal responsibilities.

Key Principles of Adult Learning Theory Include

- *Self-Directed Learning:* Adults are generally more self-directed in their learning. They prefer to take responsibility for their learning, setting their own goals, selecting learning methods, and assessing their progress.
- *Experience as a Learning Resource:* Adults bring a wealth of life and professional experience to the learning process, which can be valuable. They tend to connect new knowledge to their existing experiences, which helps them understand and retain information better.
- *Readiness to Learn:* Adults are generally motivated to learn when they perceive a need to solve a problem or fill a knowledge gap relevant to their personal or professional life.
- *Problem-Centred Learning:* Adults are more interested in problem-oriented learning rather than subject-oriented. They are motivated to solve specific, real-life problems rather than passively receiving content.
- *Internal Motivation:* While external rewards (like grades or certification) can be motivating, adults are often driven by internal factors such as career advancement, personal development, and the desire to make a meaningful contribution.
- *Respect for Adult Learners:* Adults expect to be treated as equals in the learning process. They appreciate being respected for their knowledge and experience, and they prefer to be involved in decision-making about their learning.
- *Immediate Application of Learning:* Adults prefer learning that can be immediately applied to real-life situations. They are less interested in theoretical knowledge unless it can be directly applied in practice.

Application in Health Professions Education

Adult learning theory provides a valuable framework for designing effective educational experiences for adult learners in health professions and is frequently used as one of the learning theories underpinning midwifery education programmes. By considering adult learners' need for self-direction, experience-based learning, and practical application, educators/peers can create learning environments that promote deeper understanding and competence. This approach ensures that healthcare professionals are well-prepared to meet the complex demands of professional practice while engaging in continuous personal and professional growth. For example, midwives and midwifery students may be encouraged to keep journals or participate in reflective debriefing with a mentor to improve their decision-making and care delivery [21].

Further Reading

Sweet, L., Bass, J., Sidebotham, M., Fenwick, J., & Graham, K. (2019). Developing Reflective Capacities in Midwifery Students: Enhancing Learning through Reflective Writing. *Women and Birth*, *32*(2), 119–126. https://doi.org/10.1016/j.wombi.2018.06.004 [21].

Sheehan, A., Dahlen, H. G., Elmir, R., Burns, E., Coulton, S., Sorensen, K., Duff, M., Arundell, F., Keedle, H., & Schmied, V. (2023). The Implementation and Evaluation of a Mentoring Program for Bachelor of Midwifery Students in the Clinical Practice Environment. *Nurse Education in Practice*, *70*, 103687. https://doi.org/10.1016/j.nepr.2023.103687 [22].

Gilkison, A., Giddings, L., & Smythe, L. (2016). Real Life Narratives Enhance Learning About the 'Art and Science' of Midwifery Practice. *Advances in Health Sciences Education*, *21*(1), 19–32. https://doi.org/10.1007/s10459-015-9607-z [23].

Competency-Based Learning

Competency-based learning focuses on learners acquiring specific competencies (measurable skills, knowledge, and attitudes) necessary to perform tasks and responsibilities effectively for professional practice. Unlike traditional education models that prioritise time spent in class or course completion, competency-based learning centres on learners demonstrating mastery of clearly defined competencies at their own pace. Two key writers in this area are Benjamin Bloom [24] and David Kolb [25]. In health professions education, including midwifery, competency-based learning ensures that students are fully prepared for clinical practice by focusing on the development of practical and professional skills, often through assessment-based progression.

Key Principles of Competency-Based Education Include

- *Mastery of Skills:* Learners must demonstrate mastery in specific competencies before moving forward. Mastery is often determined through assessments that evaluate the ability to apply skills in real-world situations.

- *Clear Competency Definition:* Competencies are clearly defined in terms of specific, measurable knowledge, skills, and attitudes required for practice in the healthcare field.
- *Self-Paced Learning:* Learners progress through the curriculum at their own pace, advancing once they demonstrate proficiency in a given competency. This allows for personalised learning pathways.
- *Assessment for Progression:* Learners' progression is determined by their ability to perform competencies rather than time spent in the programme. Continuous assessment, including both formative and summative evaluations, helps monitor progress.
- *Focused on Outcomes:* The goal of competency-based learning is to ensure that learners can perform the necessary tasks and functions in a healthcare setting effectively, enhancing clinical care and professional practice.
- *Continuous Feedback and Reflection:* Ongoing feedback and opportunities for reflection are integral to helping learners improve their performance and achieve competency.

Application in Health Professions Education

In health professions education, competency-based learning focuses on clear standards for essential clinical skills, such as patient/woman histories, physical exams, and clinical decision-making. Students' progress by demonstrating mastery of specific competencies rather than through time-based measures like credit hours. For example, midwifery students undertake clinical assessments, including Objective Structured Clinical Examinations (OSCEs), direct observation, and simulations, to evaluate real-world abilities, with feedback from academics, clinical educators, and/or mentor/peers helping learners improve. Validated assessment tools such as the Australian Midwifery Standards Assessment Tool (AMSAT) are ideal for these assessments [26]. Competency-based learning allows for personalised learning, enabling students to advance at their own pace and focus on areas needing further practice. It also supports interprofessional education, where students from different healthcare disciplines meet shared competencies in patient/women care, teamwork, and communication. Emphasising lifelong learning, competency-based learning ensures that healthcare professionals continually assess and develop their skills to adapt to evolving practices and patient/women's needs.

Competency-based learning theory in health professions education ensures that students acquire the practical and professional competencies needed to deliver effective care. By focusing on mastery, clear competency definitions, personalised progression, and continuous assessment, competency-based learning prepares students for real-world healthcare environments. It also fosters ongoing professional development, ensuring that healthcare workers are equipped to meet the demands of their evolving roles.

Further Reading

Sweet, L., Fleet, J., Bull, A., Downer, T., Fox, D., Bowman, R., Ebert, L., Graham, K., Bass, J., Muller, A., & Henderson, A. (2020). Development and Validation of the Australian Midwifery Standards Assessment Tool (AMSAT) to the Australian Midwife Standards for Practice 2018. *Women and Birth*, *33*(2), https://doi.org/10.1016/j.wombi.2019.08.004 [27].

Embo, M., Helsloot, K., Michels, N., & Valcke, M. (2017). A Delphi Study to Validate Competency-Based Criteria to Assess Undergraduate Midwifery Students' Competencies in the Maternity Ward. *Midwifery*, *53*, 1–8. https://doi.org/10.1016/j.midw.2017.07.005 [28].

Experiential Learning Theory

Experiential learning theory was developed by David Kolb [25]. Kolb emphasised that learning occurs through real-life direct experience and that education should focus on active participation. Experiential learning theory views learning as a continuous, dynamic process rather than a static outcome. It places the learner at the centre of this process, emphasising the active role that individuals play in constructing knowledge through personal experiences. The theory highlights the integration of cognition and emotion, recognising that learning involves the engagement of both thinking and feeling. Learners continuously develop new understanding and skills through active engagement with their environment and reflecting on those experiences. This holistic approach is theorised to foster deeper, more meaningful learning by connecting experiential insights with abstract concepts, connecting theory with practice.

Key Principles of Experiential Learning Theory Include

Kolb synthesised these ideas into a model highlighting the cyclical nature of learning through experience. Kolb [25] proposed a four-stage cycle of learning that consists of the following stages:

- *Concrete Experience:* This stage involves engaging in a direct experience where learners encounter a situation that challenges their existing knowledge.
- *Reflective Observation:* Here, learners step back from their experiences and reflect on them from different perspectives. It involves thinking about and analysing the experience and considering the outcome and processes.
- *Abstract Conceptualisation:* In this stage, learners conceptualise what they have experienced and reflect upon this, forming new ideas or modifying existing concepts and broadening knowledge.
- *Active Experimentation:* This stage focuses on applying new ideas or strategies in different situations and testing newly formed concepts, leading to new concrete experiences.

The cycle illustrates how individuals can learn effectively by repeatedly moving through these stages in a continuous loop (experience, reflect, conceptualise, experiment) refining their understanding with each cycle.

Application in Health Professions Education

In health professions education, experiential learning theory offers a means to bridge the gap between theory and practice. Students engage in hands-on clinical experiences, such as clinical placements, simulations, or role-play, which serve as a starting point for learning. Through reflective observation, learners critically analyse their experiences, considering what worked well and what could be improved. For example, in problem-based or case-based learning, midwifery students tackle authentic clinical cases, reflect on the problem and their problem-solving processes, refine their knowledge, and apply new strategies in subsequent scenarios. Experiential learning theory also supports interprofessional education by encouraging students from diverse healthcare disciplines to collaborate in real-world settings, fostering mutual learning and teamwork. Experiential learning theory supports the development of critical clinical skills, fosters lifelong learning, and prepares healthcare professionals to respond effectively to the dynamic nature of clinical care.

Further Reading

Yardley, S., Teunissen, P. W., & Dornan, T. (2012). Experiential Learning: Transforming Theory into Practice. *Medical Teacher*, *34*(2), 161–164. https://doi.org/10.3109/0142159X.2012.643264. [29]

Nicholls, D., Sweet, L., Hyett, J., & Müller, A. (2020). Push and Pull Factors Impacting the Pedagogical Approaches Used by Sonographers to Teach Scanning Skills. *Australasian Journal of Ultrasound in Medicine*, *23*(4), 220–226. https://doi.org/10.1002/ajum.12222 [30].

Rodríguez-Martín, S., Greig, Y., Shaw, E., McKellar, L., & Kuipers, Y. (2024). Strategies and Interventions Used to Provide Communication Education for Midwifery Students. A Scoping Review. *Nurse Education in Practice*, *78*, 103995. https://doi.org/10.1016/j.nepr.2024.103995 [31].

Situated Learning Theory

Situated learning theory, proposed by Jean Lave and Etienne Wenger [32], emphasises that learning occurs most effectively in a context that reflects how knowledge will be used in real social and physical environments. It suggests that learning is inherently social and occurs within a community of practice, where novices engage with experts and peers to acquire skills, knowledge, and values. In contrast to traditional views of learning as an individual and a decontextualised activity, situated learning emphasises the importance of context, interaction, and authentic tasks.

Key Principles of Situated Learning Theory Include

- *Community of Practice:* This is a core concept of situated learning theory. A community of practice is a group of individuals who share a common interest or profession and engage in shared activities. Learning occurs as individuals participate in the practices of these communities, gradually acquiring the skills, knowledge, and norms of the group.
- *Legitimate Peripheral Participation:* This concept refers to the process by which newcomers (novice learners) gradually become more involved in the activities of a community of practice. They start at the periphery, participating in less complex tasks, and as they gain more experience and knowledge, they take on more central roles within the community.
- *Authentic Activities:* Learning is most effective when it occurs in real-world contexts through authentic activities that mirror the kinds of challenges learners face in their professional lives. These activities are situated in the social context of the practice, ensuring they are relevant and meaningful.
- *Contextual Learning:* Situated learning emphasises the importance of context in the learning process. The learning environment, including the social and physical context, directly impacts how learners acquire knowledge and skills.
- *Social Interaction and Collaboration:* Knowledge is constructed through social interaction and collaboration within a community of practice. Learners interact with others, share experiences, and discuss challenges, all contributing to their learning process.
- *Co-Participation:* Learning is a shared process involving active participation between learners and more experienced practitioners. Through guided participation, learners gain insight into the community's practices, norms, and tacit knowledge.

Application in Health Professions Education

Situated learning theory provides a powerful framework for health professions education by emphasising the importance of context, social interaction, and authentic experiences in the learning process. Situated learning theory principles are applied in mentorship/preceptor and clinical apprenticeship models, where students learn through direct interactions with experienced practitioners in healthcare settings. This approach aligns with the idea of "cognitive apprenticeship," as learners observe, practice, and receive feedback on tasks performed in authentic contexts. For example, midwifery students shadow senior midwives, gradually moving from observation to more hands-on roles as they gain competence and confidence. This experiential learning approach helps novices internalise complex, tacit knowledge related to clinical care that would be challenging to learn in a classroom.

Interprofessional education aligns with situated learning by allowing students to develop collaborative skills and understand the roles of different healthcare team members in real or simulated environments. By engaging in team-based problem-solving and clinical care, students develop practical communication and collaboration skills that are crucial in healthcare settings. Interprofessional education has been widely used in simulations of complex patient/women cases requiring coordinated care across disciplines. This type of situated, collaborative learning enhances understanding of interprofessional dynamics and fosters effective teamwork.

Further Reading

Semple, L., & Currie, G. (2022). "It Opened up a Whole New World": An Innovative Interprofessional Learning Activity for Students Caring for Children and Families. *International Journal of Educational Research Open*, 3, 100106. https://doi.org/10.1016/j.ijedro.2021.100106 [33].

Renfrew, M. J., Bradshaw, G., Burnett, A., Byrom, A., Entwistle, F., King, K., Olayiwola, W., & Thomas, G. (2021). Sustaining Quality Education and Practice Learning in a Pandemic and Beyond: 'I Have Never Learnt as Much in My Life, as Quickly, Ever'. *Midwifery*, *94*, 102915. https://doi.org/10.1016/j.midw.2020.102915 [34].

Onda, E. L. (2012). Situated Cognition: Its Relationship to Simulation in Nursing Education. *Clinical Simulation in Nursing*, *8*(7), e273–e280. https://doi.org/10.1016/j.ecns.2010.11.004 [35].

Reflective Practice

Reflective practice, as a learning theory, emphasises the role of critical reflection in fostering deep, experiential learning. Developed notably by Donald Schön [36] in his work on "reflective practitioners," reflective practice suggests that individuals, especially in professional contexts, can improve their knowledge and skills through thoughtful reflection on their experiences. Schön categorised reflection into two main types. The theory also builds on earlier concepts, notably Kolb et al.'s Experiential Learning Cycle [37], which outlines a cyclic process of experience, reflection, conceptualisation, and experimentation. Reflective practice adds depth to this cycle by stressing the role of self-awareness, critical analysis, and evaluation. It is widely regarded as a key component in professional development, particularly in health professions, including midwifery, where adaptability and self-improvement are essential.

At its core, reflective practice as a learning theory highlights that learning is an ongoing, iterative process, with reflection acting as a bridge between theory and practice [38]. It promotes the idea that through systematic reflection, learners not only enhance their technical skills but also develop their critical thinking, emotional intelligence, and ethical decision-making abilities. The Bass Holistic Reflection Model [39] builds on the vast body of work about reflective practice, focusing solely on midwifery. The key difference of the Bass model [39] as compared to others, for example, the Gibbs model [38]. The Bass model is holistic, encompassing reflection as a continuum and incorporating critical reflection, reflexivity, critical thinking, and a whole-of-person approach.

Key Principles of Reflective Practice Include

- *Reflection-in-Action:* This involves thinking on one's feet or making adjustments in real-time while engaged in a task. Practitioners, for instance, adjust their approach during a clinical intervention or teaching session by assessing their immediate actions and outcomes. Reflection-in-action is often intuitive, relying on the practitioner's tacit knowledge.
- *Reflection-on-Action:* This occurs after the event, where individuals analyse their actions, outcomes, and the reasoning behind them. Reflection-on-action allows practitioners to identify what went well, what didn't, and what they might change in future scenarios.
- *Critical Thinking and Self-Awareness:* Reflective practice is closely linked to critical thinking, as it involves questioning assumptions, evaluating decisions, and recognising biases. It encourages practitioners to become more self-aware and understand how their thoughts, actions, and emotions influence their practice.
- *Experiential Learning:* Reflective practice ties closely to the theory of experiential learning, which emphasises learning through doing and reflecting on those experiences. Through reflection, professionals process and integrate new experiences into their knowledge base, which enhances their competence and understanding.

Application in Health Professions Education

Reflective practice is a critical component of health professions education, providing a structured approach for professionals and students to critically analyse their experiences, improve their skills, and enhance clinical care. By engaging in reflection-in-action and reflection-on-action, healthcare professionals can deepen their understanding of clinical practice, identify areas for growth, and develop the competencies required for effective, compassionate care. Integrating reflective practice into educational programmes, clinical supervision, mentorship, and self-directed learning enhances the lifelong development of healthcare professionals and promotes a culture of continuous improvement and excellence in professional practice.

Further Reading

Sweet, L., Bass, J., Sidebotham, M., Fenwick, J., & Graham, K. (2019). Developing Reflective Capacities in Midwifery Students: Enhancing Learning through Reflective Writing. *Women and Birth*, *32*(2), 119–126. https://doi.org/10.1016/j.wombi.2018.06.004 [21].

Bass, J., Fenwick, J., & Sidebotham, M. (2017). Development of a Model of Holistic Reflection to Facilitate Transformative Learning in Student Midwives. *Women and Birth*, *30*(3), 227–235. https://doi.org/10.1016/j.wombi.2017.02.010 [17].

Bass, J., Sidebotham, M., Sweet, L., & Creedy, D. K. (2022). Development of a Tool to Measure Holistic Reflection in Midwifery Students and Midwives. *Women and Birth*, *35*(5), e502–e511. https://doi.org/10.1016/j.wombi.2021.10.001 [39].

Carter, A. G., Creedy, D. K., & Sidebotham, M. (2018). Critical Thinking in Midwifery Practice: A Conceptual Model. *Nurse Education in Practice*, *33*, 114–120. https://doi.org/10.1016/j.nepr.2018.09.006 [40].

Conclusion

These theories and models guide the development of health professions education, ensuring that they are effective, relevant, and responsive to the needs of learners and the healthcare system. By integrating these frameworks, educators can enhance the learning experience and better prepare healthcare professionals for their roles. As described, many of the theories have similarities. However, there are also nuanced differences.

References

1. Watson JB. Psychology as the behaviourist views it. *Psychological Review* 1913; 20: 158–77.
2. Skinner BF. The operational analysis of psychological terms. *Psychological Review* 1945; 52(5): 270–77.
3. Baker-Rush ML, Pabst A, Aitchison R, Anzur T, Paschal N. Fear in interprofessional simulation: The role of psychology and behaviorism in student participation and learning. *Journal of Interprofessional Education & Practice* 2021; 24: 100432.
4. Baker LR, Phelan S, Woods NN, Boyd VA, Rowland P, Ng SL. Re-envisioning paradigms of education: Towards awareness, alignment, and pluralism. *Advances in Health Sciences Education* 2021; 26(3): 1045–58.
5. Piaget J. The role of action in the development of thinking. Knowledge and development. Springer US; 1977: pp. 17–42.

6. Bruner J. The process of education: Revised edition. Harvard University Press; 1960.

7. Finn A, Fitzgibbon C, Fonda N, Gosling CM. Self-directed learning and the student learning experience in undergraduate clinical science programs: A scoping review. *Advances in Health Sciences Education* 2024; 30(3); 973–1005.

8. Servant-Miklos VFC. Problem solving skills versus knowledge acquisition: The historical dispute that split problem-based learning into two camps. *Advances in Health Sciences Education* 2019; **24**(3): 619–35.

9. Pedapati K. Piagetian and Vygotskian concepts of cognitive development: A review. *Indian Journal of Mental Health* 2022; **9**(3): 227–39.

10. Arundell F, Sheehan A, Peters K. Strategies used by midwives to enhance knowledge and skill development in midwifery students: An appreciative inquiry study. *BMC Nursing* 2024; **23**(1): 1–10.

11. Meen A. From theory to practice. *British Journal of Midwifery* 2021; **29**(4): 186–88.

12. Bandura A. Social learning theory. Prentice-Hall; 1977.

13. McNeill L, Gum L, Graham K, Sweet L. "Removing the home court advantage": A qualitative evaluation of LEGO® as an interprofessional simulation icebreaker for midwifery and medical students. *Nurse Education in Practice* 2024; 80: 104138.

14. Folkvord SE, Risa CF. Factors that enhance midwifery students' learning and development of self-efficacy in clinical placement: A systematic qualitative review. *Nurse Education in Practice* 2023; **66**: 103510.

15. Mezirow J. Transformative learning: Theory to practice. *New Directions for Adult and Continuing Education* 1997; **74**: 1–8.

16. Mezirow J. Transformative learning as discourse. *Journal of Transformative Education* 2003; **1**(1): 58–63.

17. Bass J, Fenwick J, Sidebotham M. Development of a model of holistic reflection to facilitate transformative learning in student midwives. *Women and Birth* 2017; **30**(3): 227–35.

18. Wallace HJ, Harvey TM. 'Listen with an open-heart always' – A qualitative study exploring transformational learning opportunities for Australian midwifery students participating in a virtual international study experience. *Nurse Education in Practice* 2024; **81**: 104174.

19. Knowles MS, Holton EF, Swanson RA. The adult learner: The definitive classic in adult education and human resource development. Sixth edition. Elsevier Butterworth Heinemann; 2005.

20. Knowles MS. The modern practice of adult education: Andragogy versus pedagogy: Association Press; 1970.

21. Sweet L, Bass J, Sidebotham M, Fenwick J, Graham K. Developing reflective capacities in midwifery students: Enhancing learning through reflective writing. *Women and Birth* 2019; **32**(2): 119–26.

22. Sheehan A, Dahlen HG, Elmir R, et al. The implementation and evaluation of a mentoring program for Bachelor of Midwifery students in the clinical practice environment. *Nurse Education in Practice* 2023; **70**: 103687.

23. Gilkison A, Giddings L, Smythe L. Real life narratives enhance learning about the 'art and science' of midwifery practice. *Advances in Health Sciences Education* 2016; **21**(1): 19–32.

24. Bloom BS, Engelhart MD, Furst EJ, Hill WH, Krathowol DR. Taxonomy of educational objectives: The classification of educational goals. In Bloom BS (ed.), Handbook I: Cognitive domain. David McKay Company; 1956.

25. Kolb DA. Experiential learning: Experience as the source of learning and development. Prentice-Hall; 1984.

26. Sweet L, Henderson A, Fleet J, et al. Australian midwifery standards assessment tool: Revalidation to the midwife standards for practice 2018. *Women and Birth* 2019; **32**: S18.
27. Sweet L, Fleet J, Bull A, et al. Development and validation of the Australian Midwifery Standards Assessment Tool (AMSAT) to the Australian Midwife Standards for Practice 2018. *Women and Birth* 2020; **33**(2): 135–44.
28. Embo M, Helsloot K, Michels N, Valcke M. A Delphi study to validate competency-based criteria to assess undergraduate midwifery students' competencies in the maternity ward. *Midwifery* 2017; **53**: 1–8.
29. Yardley S, Teunissen PW, Dornan T. Experiential learning: Transforming theory into practice. *Medical Teacher* 2012; **34**(2): 161–64.
30. Nicholls D, Sweet L, Hyett J, Müller A. Push and pull factors impacting the pedagogical approaches used by sonographers to teach scanning skills. *Australasian Journal of Ultrasound in Medicine* 2020; **23**(4): 220–26.
31. Rodríguez-Martín S, Greig Y, Shaw E, McKellar L, Kuipers Y. Strategies and interventions used to provide communication education for midwifery students. A scoping review. *Nurse Education in Practice* 2024; **78**: 103995.
32. Lave J, Wenger E. Situated learning. Legitimate peripheral participation. University of Cambridge Press; 1991.
33. Semple L, Currie G. "It opened up a whole new world": An innovative interprofessional learning activity for students caring for children and families. *International Journal of Educational Research Open* 2022; **3**: 100106.
34. Renfrew MJ, Bradshaw G, Burnett A, et al. Sustaining quality education and practice learning in a pandemic and beyond: 'I have never learnt as much in my life, as quickly, ever'. *Midwifery* 2021; **94**: 102915.
35. Onda EL. Situated cognition: Its relationship to simulation in nursing education. *Clinical simulation in nursing* 2012; **8**(7): e273–e80.
36. Schön DA. Educating the reflective practitioner. Jessey-Bass; 1987.
37. Kolb DA, Fry R, Cooper AB. Toward an applied theory of experiential learning. MIT Alfred P Sloan School of Management; 1975.
38. Gibbs G. Learning by doing: A guide to teaching and learning methods. Great Britain Further Education Unit; 1988.
39. Bass J, Sidebotham M, Sweet L, Creedy DK. Development of a tool to measure holistic reflection in midwifery students and midwives. *Women and Birth* 2022; **35**(5): e502–e11.
40. Carter AG, Creedy DK, Sidebotham M. Critical thinking in midwifery practice: A conceptual model. *Nurse Education in Practice* 2018; **33**: 114–20.

3

MIDWIFERY LEADERSHIP IN HEALTHCARE

Theories and Models

Alison Weatherstone

Introduction

Midwifery needs leaders at all levels; however, midwifery leadership at an executive and national level is a significant lever for building capacity within the profession. Midwifery leadership, in recent times according to Adcock et al. (2022), must be visible, supported, effective and sustained. The International Confederation of Midwives (ICM), the global voice of midwives and midwives' associations for over a century, inspires similar messaging, which will be outlined in this chapter.

Australia introduced the first Bachelor of Midwifery three-year undergraduate degree in South Australia and Victoria in 2002. This was in line with international midwifery education (Kitschke, 2019), yet midwifery was not recognised in Australia as a separate profession from nursing until 2017 with the update of National Law (NMBA, 2017). The leadership that supports the midwifery profession has not evolved to recognise this significant legislative change and forms a key priority in many advocacy and workforce campaigns in recent times (ACM, 2023; CDNM, 2023; Homer et al., 2024). The State of the World's Midwifery Report confirms the limitation of leadership opportunities in countries where midwifery remains subsumed within nursing structures (Nove et al., 2021; UNFPA, 2021).

Midwifery leadership must be interpreted and effective within the context of the country and its healthcare system. Midwifery plays a key role in maternity services within healthcare, including maternity services, pregnancy, labour and birth care, sexual and reproductive healthcare and child, family and maternal health. To be effective, the midwifery profession requires

DOI: 10.4324/9781003533733-4

parity with other disciplines, with equivalent leadership, representation, delegation and decision-making ability to medical and nursing, with a clear distinction from both.

This chapter will outline ICM's principles and key elements of midwifery leadership, to enable readers to identify the midwifery leadership landscape in the Australian midwifery context, which can be applied to maternity care settings around the world. Furthermore, identify common leadership styles and theories in midwifery, list the characteristics of strong leadership, highlight some of the enablers and barriers to effective midwifery leadership, provide reflective practice on midwifery leadership in action and a call to action for the investment in midwifery leadership by demonstrating an argument for articulating a return on investment.

What Is Midwifery Leadership

Visible midwifery leadership is vital to the development and protection of the midwifery profession (ICM, 2022a).

According to the International Confederation of Midwives (ICM, 2022a), *'By ensuring that there are the right midwifery leadership systems, structures, roles and people in the right places, a country will ensure that its maternity services will go from strength to strength, improving the health of childbearing women and their families for generations to come'* (p1).

There are 10 elements to the ICM Midwifery Professional Framework (2025) (see Figure 3.1), and all elements are required to be in place to ensure an effective midwifery profession and service.

1 Midwifery Philosophy
2 Essential Competencies for Midwifery Practice
3 Education
4 Regulation
5 Association
6 Research
7 Continuity of midwife care model of practice
8 *Leadership*
9 Enabling Environment
10 Gender equality and justice, equity, diversity and inclusion (JEDI)

For midwifery leadership to be effective, it must be underpinned by the principles of effective leadership, that is, the skills to inspire, influence, advocate, collaborate, communicate, challenge the status quo, be accountable and demonstrate compassion (ICM, 2022a).

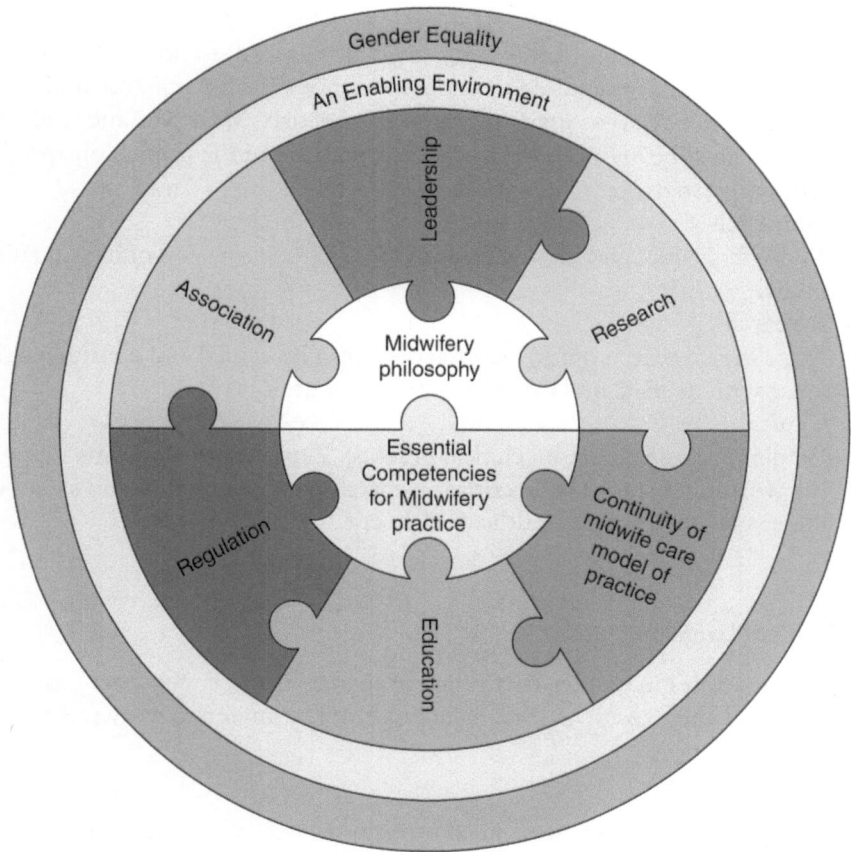

FIGURE 3.1 ICM Midwifery Professional Framework. Source: ICM (2025)

Leadership Pillars

There are six key areas to leadership within midwifery.

1 **Political strategic**
   All decision-making that has an actual or potential impact on maternity services and women's healthcare requires a midwifery leadership voice at the table. This includes local, regional, jurisdictional, national and whole of health system levels. Through policy, strategy, data, workforce planning, governance and service delivery, midwifery leadership is required across all levels. The Chief Midwife role represents political strategic leadership.

2 **Operational**
   Midwifery leadership roles are required to ensure strategic and professional issues are addressed, to liaise with key stakeholders and oversee high-quality service delivery.

3 **Regulatory**

Midwifery leadership roles within regulatory settings and within the national context are required to endure autonomy, safety, quality and midwives are working to their full scope of practice. Midwives and midwife leaders must be involved in setting the standards of the profession-specific sections of midwifery regulation.

4 **Education**

Midwifery educators play an essential role in the provision of high-quality midwifery care.

5 **Research**

Midwifery research (midwifery science) must be valued and considered on a par with medical and other healthcare research.

6 **Clinical**

Leaders are role models in clinical practice. Experienced clinicians support the workforce and provide critical leadership for the quality and safety of maternity services and healthcare delivery.

Midwifery Leadership Roles

Leadership roles may refer to a range of management, supervisory, clinical, non-clinical and executive titles, including and not limited to midwives working in:

- Ministry or Department of Health positions (e.g. Chief Midwife Officer, Chief Midwife, Midwife and/or Maternity Advisor, Director and Executive Director of Midwifery, Senior Midwifery Advisor)
- Leading rural, regional, remote and metropolitan maternity facilities (e.g. Midwife Director, midwives in charge of maternity units/wards)
- Leading professional midwives' associations (e.g. Chief Midwife, President, Chief Executive Officer)
- Leading midwifery regulatory authorities (e.g. Chair of Midwifery Council, Midwifery Regulatory Board roles)
- Leading midwifery education programs (e.g. Head of Midwifery School, Director of Midwifery, Head of Midwifery Program, Professor or Associate Professor of Midwifery).

State of the World's Midwifery Report

Global strategic directions for strengthening nursing and midwifery 2021–2025 (WHO, 2021b) identified four global strategic directions and policy priorities: education, jobs, leadership and service delivery. Furthermore, the

State of the World's Midwifery Report (2021) states that for midwives to achieve their potential, greater investment is needed in four key areas:

- Education and training
- Health workforce planning, management and regulation and the work environment
- *Leadership* and governance
  - Creating senior midwife positions
  - Strengthening institutional capacity for midwives to drive health policy advancements
- Service delivery

These investments should be considered at country, regional and global levels by governments, policymakers, regulatory authorities, education institutions, professional associations, international organisations, global partnerships, donor agencies, civil society organisations and researchers (UNFPA, 2021).

'Only half of reporting countries have midwife leaders within their national Ministry of Health. Limited opportunities for midwives to hold leadership positions and the scarcity of women who are role models in leadership positions hinder midwives' career advancement and their ability to work to their full potential' (p. viii, 49).

REFLECTIVE ACTIVITY 1:

How do you see the role of leadership in midwifery?

- What are your preconceptions about leadership in the context of midwifery?

Midwifery Philosophy and Leadership

As noted in Chapter 1, Midwifery practice can be traced back as far as 40,000 B.C. There is a long history of midwifery as a profession, and there are many papers, books, historical archives and unwritten words that hold the mystery, fascination, truth, trauma and evolution of birth, but what underpins almost all is the support of women by women based on mammalian behaviours, cultural practices, politics and most recently, the medicalisation of birth (ICM, 2022b). Midwifery is holistic, encompassing physical, social, emotional, spiritual and cultural aspects of birth. Today, we know this as woman-centred care or relational-based care or being 'with woman' (Bradfield et al., 2018). While this seeks to guide and inform contemporary midwifery practice, systems and institutional-based care can challenge a woman's true right to bodily autonomy, and research by Newnham (2019, 2023) throws a spotlight on the midwife-institution and midwife–woman relationship providing every healthcare provider an opportunity to critically reflect on their practice.

Chamberlain et al. (2016) presents a compelling paper on traditional midwifery or 'wise women' models of leadership which extends into Indigenous Aboriginal ways of Knowing, Being and Doing and non-Indigenous leadership theories and challenges the concept that there is no consensus about what midwifery leadership really is, identifying that leadership is more a process of influence rather than a person or position.

Traditional midwifery or 'wise women' models of leadership: Learning from Indigenous cultures: … Lead so the mother is helped, yet still free and in charge ….' Lao Tzu, 5th century BC (Chamberlain et al., 2016), identified four principles of midwifery leadership:

1 'Being a leader who empowers and frees others with "no one person wiser than the other".
2 Embodying wisdom and ethical practice which nurtures social, cultural and spiritual needs of women and mentors the next generation by "walking together".
3 Being competent and skilled as well as emotionally attuned ("feeling the job") to engender trust and calm which is crucial to birth, "depending on each other but looking to her to be in charge".
4 Paying attention and being responsive to emergent change and unfolding present reality rather than being prescriptive, "using her knowledge to adjust the situation" (pp. 346–363).

REFLECTIVE ACTIVITY 2:

What is your midwifery philosophy?

• Has your midwifery philosophy changed throughout your career?

Women in Leadership

Women are more likely to work part-time or have carer responsibilities and gender gaps in leadership. The State of the World's Midwifery Report (2021) and the World Health Organisation's (WHO) (2021a) Closing the Leadership Gap Policy Action Paper identify that more than 70% of the global healthcare workforce are women, increasing to 75% in Australia, yet women only hold 25% of senior or leadership roles (Monash Centre for

Health Research and Implementation, 2024). Women make up 98.8% of the midwifery workforce in Australia, according to the Nursing and Midwifery Board of Australia's 2023/2024 annual report (NMBA, 2024). This highlights a gender equity gap in leadership and systemic barriers to women's advancement, which enable policy actions to redress this gender imbalance impacting on health security and care delivery.

The WHO 2021 Policy Action Paper identified four action areas in 'A framework for change' to support women's leadership:

1 Build the foundation for equality.
2 Address social norms and stereotypes.
3 Address workplace systems and culture.
4 Enable women to achieve.

Furthermore, the chapter describes that beyond gender parity, improvements in global health will be addressed when leaders of all genders promote gender-transformative policies, defined as those that 'seek to transform gender relations to promote equality'. This type of leadership is grounded in the following principles (WHO, 2021a):

- A framework for gender equality, women's rights and human rights,
- Challenging privilege and power imbalances based on gender that undermine health,
- Intersectionality, addressing social and personal characteristics that intersect with gender – race, ethnicity, geography, etc., to create multiple disadvantages; and
- Being applicable to leaders of any gender, not exclusively women leaders.

The drivers for change for women in leadership include no shortage of women in the workforce (64.6% of the midwifery workforce in Australia in 2023/2024 were aged between 18 and 54 years, NMBA, 2024) and the ecological model in health. The ecological model (Figure 3.2) recognises environmental and policy contexts of individual behaviour, across multiple layers or factors of influence (e.g. attitudes, beliefs and personality).

Leadership Styles and Theories in Midwifery

The three most common leadership styles identified in midwifery research are situational leadership, transformational leadership and compassionate leadership; however, there exists an array of leadership styles that cross over or are evident in healthcare and caring professions including servant, transactional, authentic, behavioural, collaborative, trait, quiet, person-centred,

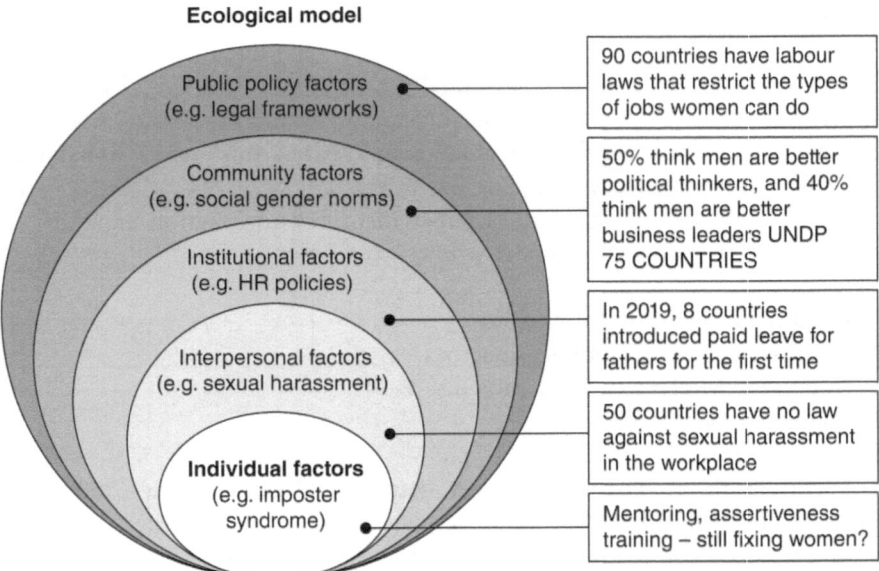

FIGURE 3.2 Ecological model. Source: WHO (2021a) Policy Action Paper

democratic, coaching, ethical and flat leadership styles (Jackston et al., 2021). You may wish to do some further research into these leadership styles as they all deserve a chapter of their own!

Situational Leadership

Situational leadership was developed by Paul Hersey & Kenneth Blanchard and applies a flexible approach which adapts according to the team's skills, knowledge, situation and maturity level. The four leadership styles are blended to meet diversity within the team and are described in the scoping review by Wang et al. (2024).

- Style 1 – Telling, directing or guiding.
- Style 2 – Selling, coaching, supporting or explaining.
- Style 3 – Participating, supporting, facilitating or collaborating.
- Style 4 – Delegating, empowering or monitoring.

Transformational Leadership

A traditional leadership theory, prevalent across health leadership and in particular, nursing as evidenced by the Florence Nightingale Foundation's leadership programs, applies continuous critical reflection to the way in which an individual sees themselves and the world in which they live. Transformational leadership challenges perspectives about self and differing perspectives of others and aims to elevate leaders through motivation. Transformational leaders communicate a vision, are inspirational and create a team who feel valued and invested in making a difference (Bond et al., 2023).

Compassionate Leadership

Compassionate leadership focusses on relationships through careful listening, empathising and supporting others to enable a feeling of value and respect and being nurtured to reach their full potential and provide high-quality work. Compassionate leadership engages and motivates team members who have demonstrated high levels of wellbeing, translating to high-quality care. Compassionate leaders are empathetic, inclusive and seek to understand challenges and adversity in colleagues. Compassionate leaders work towards shared solutions and outcomes to problems. The four behaviours of compassionate leadership are attending, understanding, empathising and helping (Atkins & Parker, 2012; Papadopoulos et al., 2021).

Servant Leadership

Servant leadership builds a sense of social identity in their followers in which team members assist and build the capacity of others in a holistic way. A systematic review of servant leadership spanning decades by Eva et al. (2019) suggests this modern-day approach to leadership considers challenges in the workplace while also considering team members needs of belonging. Servant leadership encompasses relational, ethical, emotional and spiritual dimensions, prioritising well-being and growth. Servant leaders focus on (followers) personal development while also prioritising performance and sustainability of the team or organisation.

REFLECTIVE ACTIVITY 3:

What leadership style do you align with or adopt in your role as a midwife?

• How does your personal value system guide your decision-making as a leader?

Curiosity in Leadership

Underpinning leadership styles and theories in midwifery, Medway and Rehayman (2024) and Pezaro et al. (2024) both identify that empathy and self-compassion are key attributes to leadership success. This when combined with curiosity enables midwives to provide holistic, contemporary evidence-based and individualised care to women and families. Weatherstone (2024) further suggests this creates pathways to excellence and innovation or going 'above and beyond' for the profession. As midwives, professional curiosity is embedded in the relational-based care we provide women and their families, with the application of critical evaluation to any information received while maintaining non-judgement and an open mind. As midwives in clinical practice, this comes quite naturally; however, when working in leadership and management roles, this curiosity can be diminished due to structural, system, workplace culture and staffing barriers.

Curiosity drives leaders to ask questions, seek new knowledge, challenge the status quo and remain open to different perspectives. Leaders who are curious are more likely to:

- Implement and embed evidence-based practice.
- Foster a learning culture.
- Promote innovation.
- Enhance communication and collaboration.

REFLECTIVE ACTIVITY 4:

- How can you promote innovation and change in midwifery through leadership?

Leadership Skills and Attributes

Medway and Rehayam (2024) call for strong and effective midwifery leadership, in all contexts of practice, across the career continuum and across Government, systems and organisations. This is required to drive meaningful change and maternity service reform, to ensure Australian maternity services are equitable, safe and focused on the needs of women. Yet this can be applied to maternity settings around the world.

While leadership skills can be learned, you must first be able to identify the key skills that make up effective leadership and then build capacity to support these skills. Leading by example and role modelling the qualities and characteristics we want to see in others and expect to receive in return contributes to positive workplace culture. A healthy workplace is the foundation for an environment in which a midwife will not only survive, but thrive, contributing to job satisfaction and sustainability and retention of the workforce.

Dr Lorri Sulpizio (2022) is an expert in gender and leadership and attributes the following seven key skills as a foundation for effective leadership:

- Flexibility,
- Sound decision-making,
- Effective feedback,
- Clear communication,
- Strategic thinking,
- Negotiation skills, and
- Accountability.

Each of the above skills require underlying capacity. For example, to make sound decisions, you require active listening, an openness to learn and critical reflection. Flexibility on the other hand requires tolerating a level of discomfort and uncertainty.

Characteristics of a Strong Midwife Leader

The principles of 'good' midwifery leadership were identified by Byrom and Downe (2010), indicating a move away from hierarchical models towards relational-based care. In a global study across 76 countries worldwide by Pezaro et al. (2024), clinical incident causation was attributed to poor leadership, and therefore, it was necessary to identify characteristics of strong leadership to improve patient safety, reduce morbidity and mortality and improve overall employee satisfaction. Similarly, in Australia, a study by Hewitt, Priddis and Dahlen (2019) identified the qualities required of Australian midwifery leaders to effectively manage a Midwifery Group Practice (MGP) continuity model of care, as even with the known benefits of this continuity model, it translates to less than 10% access by women. Both studies identify the need for midwifery leaders to have a vision and work towards a long-term goal.

The 10 characteristics of a strong midwifery leader identified in the Pezaro et al. (2024) study include:

1 Mediator,
2 Dedicated to the profession,
3 Evidence-based practitioner,
4 Effective decision maker,
5 Role model,
6 Advocate,
7 Visionary,
8 Resilient,
9 Empathetic, and
10 Compassionate.

The seven enablers identified were as follows:

1 Clear professional identity,
2 Increased societal value placed upon midwifery,
3 Ongoing research,
4 Professional development in leadership,
5 Interprofessional collaboration,
6 Succession planning, and
7 Self-efficacy.

The strong midwife leader must have the above skills to engage in:

• Effective conflict resolution,
• Demonstrate fairness and impartiality,
• Communicate respectfully and effectively,
• A genuine commitment and 'love' for the profession,
• A continuous learning and development approach,
• Apply research and evidence-based principles to practice,
• Think critically, and be calm and controlled under pressure,
• Inspire others to follow their leadership footsteps,
• Work collaboratively,
• Embody honesty, integrity and positivity,
• Celebrate and enable others success,
• Be adaptive to challenges, learn from mistakes and demonstrate self-care, and
• Foster psychological safety in the workplace.

REFLECTIVE ACTIVITY 5:

What leadership characteristics are important to you in a leader?

What leadership characteristics would you like to develop?

What personal qualities or skills do you bring to any leadership role in midwifery?

• How can these strengths benefit your practice and influence others?

Mentoring and Leadership

It is important to pass on professional knowledge, wisdom and learnings. Medway and Rehayman (2024) states that being generous with what we know is a powerful way to demonstrate leadership. Regardless of how long we have been in the profession, everyone brings something to the table. Everyone has life experience that is different from another, similarly every woman's birth journey and story will be different. Sharing knowledge, stories and expertise in meaningful ways can have many benefits individually, and on workplace culture collectively. Clinical supervision, mentoring and being mentored is an effective way to contribute to leadership.

REFLECTIVE ACTIVITY 6:

In what ways do I encourage and support others in the midwifery field?

- How can I enhance mentorship, collaboration or teamwork in my practice?

Building the Next Generation of Midwife Leaders – The Return on Investment of Midwifery Leadership

Midwives must be enabled to participate fully and effectively at every opportunity with equal opportunity for representation and leadership at all levels of decision-making, where decisions are made about sexual and reproductive health, midwifery, maternity, neonatal and child and family health. Through research, storytelling and showcasing exemplars, midwives can support the development of the next generation of leaders (Bradfield, 2023).

Armed with all this information about leadership, you may be thinking '*where to from here*'. There are many online and face-to-face leadership courses which follow a framework or leadership model or theory. Another way is to immerse yourself in opportunities to act at higher levels or undertake a supported project, participate in policy and procedure, quality improvement or guideline work and be active with your professional midwifery association.

REFLECTIVE ACTIVITY 7:

What is your vision for the future of midwifery, and how can leadership help you achieve it?

How does midwifery leadership contribute to improved outcomes for women, families and communities?

- How can I measure or evaluate the impact of leadership in my work?

Conclusion

In this chapter, we explored midwifery leadership from a local, national and international perspective, bringing together characteristics and leadership styles to be nurtured at all stages of a midwife's career. Midwifery is on the cusp of change, and it is as important as ever to invest in midwives' clear professional identity. There must be continued value placed on the midwifery profession, and we must not lose sight of the role of the midwife. You can be the change. Be curious. Midwifery leadership – for midwives, with women, for the future.

Acknowledgements

As a leader, I believe we should always acknowledge those who walked before us and those who will walk after us. Midwifery has always been in great hands, and we need to leave the profession better than we found it, for our children and our children's children. While there are always challenges, there is always boundless opportunity and shared success to be celebrated.

My clinical and midwifery leadership journey would not have been possible without acknowledging the following family members: My mum Brenda, my children Imogen, Brecon and Sage, and the following special colleagues, mentors and friends: Joan Wild, Nicki Bright, Kristy Wiegele, Kylie Ashton, Jocelyn Toohill, Nicky Leap, Sheena and Anna Byrom, Becky Reed, Jacqueline Dunkley-Bent, Paula Medway and Paula Evans. You have all in one way or another made me a better leader, midwife and person and for that I am grateful.

Further Reading

COAG Health Council. (2019). *Woman-centred care. Strategic directions for Australian maternity services.* Retrieved from https://www.health.gov.au/sites/default/files/documents/2019/11/woman-centred-care-strategic-directions-for-australian-maternity-services.pdf

International Confederation of Midwives. (2022). *Guide. Midwifery Leadership.* Retrieved from https://internationalmidwives.org/resources/guide-for-midwifery-leadership/

International Confederation of Midwives. (2022). *The Origins of Midwifery.* Retrieved from https://internationalmidwives.org/the-origins-of-midwifery/#:~:text=The%20practice%20of%20midwifery%20can,learned%20from%20observing%20other%20mammals

International Confederation of Midwives. (2025). *Professional Framework for Midwifery.* Retrieved from https://internationalmidwives.org/resources/professional-framework-for-midwifery/

Nursing and Midwifery Board. (2024). Midwifery futures: The Australian midwifery workforce project. *Final Report.* Retrieved from https://www.nursingmidwiferyboard.gov.au/News/Midwifery-Futures.aspx

World Health Organization (WHO). (2021). Closing the leadership gap: gender equity and leadership in the global health and care workforce. *Policy Action Paper,* June 2021. Licence: CC BY-NC-SA 3.0 IGO. Retrieved from https://iris.who.int/bitstream/handle/10665/341636/9789240025905-eng.pdf?sequence=1

References

Adcock, J. E., Sidebotham, M., & Gamble, J. (2022). What do midwifery leaders need in order to be effective in contributing to the reform of maternity services? *Women and Birth*, *35*(2), e142–e152. https://doi.org/10.1016/j.wombi.2021.04.008

Atkins, P. W. B., & Parker, S. K. (2012). Understanding individual compassion in organizations: The role of appraisals and psychological flexibility. *The Academy of Management Review*, *37*(4), 524–546. https://doi.org/10.5465/amr.2010.0490

Australian College of Midwives (ACM). (2023). *Position statement. Midwifery Leadership in Australia*. Retrieved from   https://www.midwives.org.au/common/Uploaded%20files/Position%20Statement%20-%20Midwifery%20leadership%20New%20June%206%202025.pdf

Bond, C., Stacey, G., Westwood, G., & Long, L. (2023). Evaluation of the impact of leadership development on nurses and midwives underpinned by transformational learning theory: A corpus-informed analysis. *Leadership in Health Services (2007)*, *37*(5), 1–12. https://doi.org/10.1108/LHS-09-2022-0092

Bradfield, Z. (2023). Advancing midwifery leadership through research. *Australian Midwifery News. Australian College Midwives*, *32*(1), 16–21.

Bradfield, Z., Duggan, R., Hauck, Y., & Kelly, M. (2018). Midwives being 'with woman': An integrative review. *Women and Birth: Journal of the Australian College of Midwives*, *31*(2), 143–152. https://doi.org/10.1016/j.wombi.2017.07.011

Byrom, S., & Downe, S. (2010). 'She sort of shines': Midwives' accounts of 'good' midwifery and 'good' leadership. *Midwifery*, *26*(1), 126–137. https://doi.org/10.1016/j.midw.2008.01.011

Chamberlain, C., Fergie, D., Sinclair, A., & Asmar, C. (2016). Traditional midwifery or 'wise women' models of leadership: Learning from indigenous cultures. *Lead so the Mother Is Helped, Yet Still Free and in charge…' Lao Tzu, 5th Century BC. Leadership*, *12*(3), 346–363. https://doi.org/10.1177/1742715015608426

Council of Deans of Nursing and Midwifery (ANZ) Midwifery Advisory Group. (2023). The Future of the midwifery workforce in Australia. *Position Paper*. Retrieved from   https://irp.cdn-website.com/1636a90e/files/uploaded/130723%20Midwifery%20workforce%20position%20paper%20AUS_v1.pdf

Eva, N., Robin, M., Sendjaya, S., van Dierendonck, D., & Liden, R. C. (2019). Servant leadership: A systematic review and call for future research. *The Leadership Quarterly*, *30*(1), 111–132. https://doi.org/10.1016/j.leaqua.2018.07.004

Folkvord, S., & Risa, C. (2023). Factors that enhance midwifery students' learning and development of self-efficacy in clinical placement: A systematic qualitative review. *Nurse Education in Practice*. *66*, 103510. https://doi.org/10.1016/j.nepr.2022.103510

Hewitt, L., Dahlen, H. G., Hartz, D. L., & Dadich, A. (2021). Leadership and management in midwifery-led continuity of care models: A thematic and lexical analysis of a scoping review. *Midwifery*, *98*, 102986. https://doi.org/10.1016/j.midw.2021.102986

Hewitt, L., Priddis, H., & Dahlen, H. (2019) What attributes do Australian midwifery leaders identify as essential to effectively manage a midwifery group practice? *Women Birth*. *32*(2), 168–177. https://doi.org/10.1016/j.wombi.2018.06.017

Homer CSE, Small K, Warton C, Bradfield Z, Baird K, Fenwick J, Gray JE, Robinson M. (2024). *Midwifery Futures – Building the future Australian midwifery workforce. A research project commissioned by the Nursing and Midwifery Board of Australia, Burnet Institute, Curtin University and the University of Technology Sydney*. Retrieved from https://www.nursingmidwiferyboard.gov.au/News/Midwifery-Futures.aspx

International Confederation of Midwives. (2022a). *Guide. Midwifery Leadership.* Retrieved from https://internationalmidwives.org/resources/guide-for-midwifery-leadership/

International Confederation of Midwives. (2022b). *The Origins of Midwifery.* Retrieved from https://internationalmidwives.org/the-origins-of-midwifery/#:~:text=The%20practice%20of%20midwifery%20can,learned%20from%20observing%20other%20mammals

International Confederation of Midwives. (2025). *Professional Framework for Midwifery.* Retrieved from https://internationalmidwives.org/resources/professional-framework-for-midwifery/

Jackson, C., McBride, T., Manley, K., Dewar, B., Young, B., Ryan, A., & Roberts, D. (2021). Strengthening nursing, midwifery and allied health professional leadership in the UK – A realist evaluation. *Leadership in Health Services. 34*(4), 392–453. https://doi.org/10.1108/LHS-11-2020-0097

Kitschke, J. (2019). The Australian bachelor of midwifery – How it all began. *Australian Midwifery News, 19*(1), 50–52. ISSN 1446-5612.

Medway, P., & Rehayam, A. (2024). Editorial: Midwifery leadership. *Women and Birth, 37*(1), 4–5. https://doi.org/10.1016/j.wombi.2023.09.001

Monash Centre for Health Research and Implementation. (2024). *Gender Equity and Equality Reporting for Leadership in Healthcare and Beyond: Towards a National Gender Equity and Equality in Leadership Data Framework.* MCHRI: Monash University. https://doi.org/10.26180/27926901

Newnham, E., & Buchanan, M. K. (2023). Being the change: How midwifery philosophy can redefine ethical practice to transform maternity care. *Women and Birth: Journal of the Australian College of Midwives, 36,* S36. https://doi.org/10.1016/j.wombi.2023.07.094

Newnham, E., & Kirkham, M. (2019). Beyond autonomy: Care ethics for midwifery and the humanization of birth. *Nursing Ethics, 26*(7–8), 2147–2157. https://doi.org/10.1177/0969733018819119

Nove, A., ten Hoope-Bender, P., & Boyce, M., et al. (2021). The state of the World's midwifery 2021 report: Findings to drive global policy and practice. *Human Resources for Health, 19,* 146. https://doi.org/10.1186/s12960-021-00694-w

Nursing and Midwifery Board of Australia. (October 2017). *National Scheme News.* Retrieved from https://www.nursingmidwiferyboard.gov.au/news/newsletters/october-2017.aspx#legislative

Nursing and Midwifery Board of Australia. (2024). Nursing and midwifery in 2023/24. *Annual Report.* Retrieved from https://www.nursingmidwiferyboard.gov.au/News/Annual-report.aspx

Papadopoulos, I., Lazzarino, R., Koulouglioti, C., Aagard, M., Akman, Ö, Alpers, L.-M., Apostolara, P., Araneda-Bernal, J., Biglete-Pangilinan, S., Eldar-Regev, O., González-Gil, M. T., Kouta, C., Krepinska, R., Lesińska-Sawicka, M., Liskova, M., Lopez-Diaz, A. L., Malliarou, M., Martín-García, Á, Muñoz-Solinas, M., & Zorba, A. (2021). The importance of being a compassionate leader: The views of nursing and midwifery managers from around the world. *Journal of Transcultural Nursing, 32*(6), 765–777. https://doi.org/10.1177/10436596211008214

Pezaro, S., Zarbiv, G., Jones, J., Feika, M. L., Fitzgerald, L., Lukhele, S., Mcmillanbohler, J., Baloyi, O. B., da Silva, K. M., Grant, C., Bayliss-Pratt, L., & Hardtman, P. (2024). Characteristics of strong midwifery leaders and enablers of strong midwifery leadership: An international appreciative inquiry. *Midwifery, 132*(2024), 103982. https://doi.org/10.1016/j.midw.2024.103982

Sulpizio, L. (2022). *Can Leadership Skills Be Learned*? Retrieved from https://www.lorrisulpizio.com/leadership-skills-learned/

United Nations Population Fund, International Confederation of Midwives, World Health Organization. *State of the World's Midwifery 2021*. New York: United Nations Population Fund; 2021.

Wang, X., Liu, Y., Peng, Z., Li, B., Liang, Q., Liao, S., & Liu, M. (2024). Situational leadership theory in nursing management: A scoping review. *BMC Nursing, 23*(1), 930–16. https://doi.org/10.1186/s12912-024-02582-9

Weatherstone, A. (2024). Cultivating curiosity in midwifery leadership. *The Practising Midwife: Australia, 03*(01), 8–12. https://doi.org/10.55975/LYYB2989

World Health Organization (WHO, 2021a). Closing the leadership gap: gender equity and leadership in the global health and care workforce. *Policy Action Paper*, June 2021. Licence: CC BY-NC-SA 3.0 IGO. Retrieved from https://iris.who.int/bitstream/handle/10665/341636/9789240025905-eng.pdf?sequence=1

World Health Organization (WHO, 2021b). *Global Strategic Directions for Nursing and Midwifery 2021–2025*. Geneva: World Health Organization; 2021. Licence: CC BY-NC-SA 3.0 IGO.

4

MIDWIFERY MENTORSHIP

The Context

Elaine Jefford, Jen Stevens, and Lyn Ebert

Introduction

As midwives, our practice is underpinned by our midwifery philosophical framework of woman-centredness. From here, we hold women's birthing space and embrace each woman's right to have choice over her body, and her childbearing journey. In other words, a midwife's fundamental role is to walk the childbearing journey alongside a woman advocating for her to have her optimal birthing experience. This, Parratt refers to as a 'genius birth' whereby the midwife supports the woman to enhance her innate power and her potential to centre herself to '... *experience the best possible, uniquely individual birth appropriate to that particular moment of her life...*' (Parratt, 2008, p. 53). This role is not dependent on the midwife being male or female, geographical location around the globe or as some would argue the model of care, rather it is embedded within the very essence of midwifery.

Midwifery as a Profession

Two definitions of what delineates a midwife and midwifery practice are offered, one being a non-midwifery-specific organisation and one being the key midwifery organisation for all midwives around the globe. The International Confederation of Midwives definition (2023a) does not include a midwives scope of practice or the philosophy of midwifery.

> A midwife is a registered health professional, and midwifery [an autonomous and independent from nursing] profession, grounded in woman-centred and evidence-based maternal health care – with midwives being an integral part of maternity care.
>
> *(Department of Health and Aged Care, 2024)*

DOI: 10.4324/9781003533733-5

A midwife is a person who has successfully completed a midwifery education programme based on the ICM Essential Competencies for Midwifery Practice and the framework of the ICM Global Standards for Midwifery Education, recognised in the country where it is located; who has acquired the requisite qualifications to be registered and/or legally licensed to practice midwifery and use the title 'midwife,' and who demonstrates competency in the practice of midwifery.

(International Confederation of Midwives, 2023a)

Guilliland and Pairman (2010) describe midwifery as a profession that facilitates 'the optimal experience of birth for pregnant women and their babies' (p. 38). Where the midwife, when working with-woman, is seen as a person who is responsible for optimising the individual woman's experience of childbirth and transition to parenthood. The midwifery profession, however, assumes a broader societal role in supporting women, their babies, and the family unit to improve community and population health. The midwife works with and for women, 'to strengthen women's confidence to care for themselves and their families' (Nursing and Midwifery Board of Australia, 2018, p. 4). Midwifery, while working at the individual woman's level and at the community level, works across professional boundaries related to maternal health, newborn health, and childbirth and reproductive health, and seeks to apply the professional body of midwifery knowledge in a collaborative and woman-focused manner. Midwives also work with and for students, mentees, and other staff, contributing to a 'culture that supports learning, teaching, knowledge transfer and critical reflection' (NMBA, 2018, p. 5). It is this (formal and informal) knowledge transfer that builds and strengthens the midwifery scope of practice and professional identity.

Professional identity, however, is not created within a culture free educational institution or health service. Teresa-Morales et al. (2022) argue that:

professions and professionals develop within a social context shaped by stereotypes that influence perceptions of the profession and affect its growth and development. [Midwifery, like] nursing has always been associated with components of gender, which relate to the origins of the profession and gender roles more broadly.

(p. 2)

While Teresa-Morales and colleagues (2022) research explored the nursing profession, midwifery is equally shaped by social perceptions and a society's, or the cultural, divide between men and women, and by the roles attributed to women working in the particular healthcare context. As such, this impacts midwives' perceptions of self and professional identity, before, during, and after commencing their career.

The midwifery profession, based in a gendered context, recognises the social circumstance of each woman is also different and meeting the individual woman's needs requires negotiation between the woman and midwife. This is also true for meeting the learning needs of less experienced midwives, mentees, students, and other staff. The foundation for quality services, and learning environments, lies in having an adequate competent midwifery workforce (World Health Organisation, 2013), and education is the key to a competent midwifery workforce. As noted by WHO (2013):

> Strong education institutions are needed to secure the numbers and quality of health workers as the performance of health care systems depends on the knowledge, skills and motivation of the people responsible for delivering services.
>
> *(p. 4)*

Equally, strong health institutions, and maternity services, with strong midwifery leadership are needed to build the level of quality midwives that can share their knowledge, skills, and professional motivation to those entering the profession. More information about the importance of midwifery leadership and mentorship is presented in Chapter 3.

The ICM (2023c) declares midwifery has its own unique body of knowledge which when taught provides the framework for midwives to provide professional, autonomous quality care for women and gender diverse people and their newborns. This is termed 'an enabling environment' and means that:

- Midwives can practise to their full scope,
- Are accountable for independent decisions within a health professional regulatory system that recognises and upholds their autonomy and accountability,
- Have access to continuing professional development, career pathways, and supportive professional mechanisms,
- Work within a functional health infrastructure with adequate human resources, diagnostic services, equipment, and supplies,
- Have access to timely and respectful consultation, collaboration, and referral, including transportation and communication systems,
- Are safe from physical and emotional harm, and
- Have fair and equitable compensation, including salary and working conditions (The International Confederation of Midwives, 2023, p. 6).

Only when an enabling environment is available for midwifery practice, can midwives work to their full scope of practice, act as role models, and teach midwifery ways of being 'with woman' to mentees, students, and less experienced maternity care staff. Viewing midwives as autonomous practitioners, with the ability to make independent decisions, within a health professional regulatory system is discussed in the next section.

Autonomy

The landscape of birth, place of birth, and model of care are shifting, so has its power base. The hospital environment remains medical dominant, with midwives having to defer to doctors and ask permission. Here, midwives advocate for physiological birth and women's choice, yet the final decision-maker tends to be a doctor. Within the shared space of a birth centre (however that is defined), doctors and midwives conduct the dance of collegiality and shared decision-making with the woman, prioritising minimal intervention. In the home environment, the power sits firmly with the woman. Here, the midwife waits to be invited in and respects the woman's space, and her choices. Irrespective of what environment a midwife works within, however, midwifery practice is governed by the legal, regulatory, and professional framework of the country. Fundamental within this framework is a midwife's accountability, which she cannot give away. The ICM defines professional accountability of the midwife as:

> ... midwives assume responsibility and accountability for their practice by applying up-to-date knowledge, skills and are responsible and accountable for clinical decision ... having a duty of care to the women and newborns they care for, and their own actions and professional advice. This accountability extends to those taken on the advice and orders of others ....
> *(International Confederation of Midwives, 2023b, p. 1)*

So how does professional accountability sit within a medically dominated environment where a midwife cannot or maybe limited in being autonomous and practice midwifery care as the guardian of birth as a natural physiological event?

This is without doubt a difficult terrain for a midwife to navigate, being woman-centred, and holding space for the woman while being asked to adhere to the social norms of medicalised birth or as Davis-Floyd (2017) termed it 'technocratic birth' and organisational policies. For a midwife to make decisions in such a contested space can lead to Midwifery Abdication (MA). This term was first introduced into the midwifery literature by Jefford (2012) and defined it as:

> ... a midwife surrenders one's voice and/or forsakes one's midwifery skills and/or knowledge, consciously or unconsciously, failing to fulfil and be accountable for one's own professional behaviour in accordance with professional frameworks as (primary) maternity care provider for the woman.
> *(p. 14)*

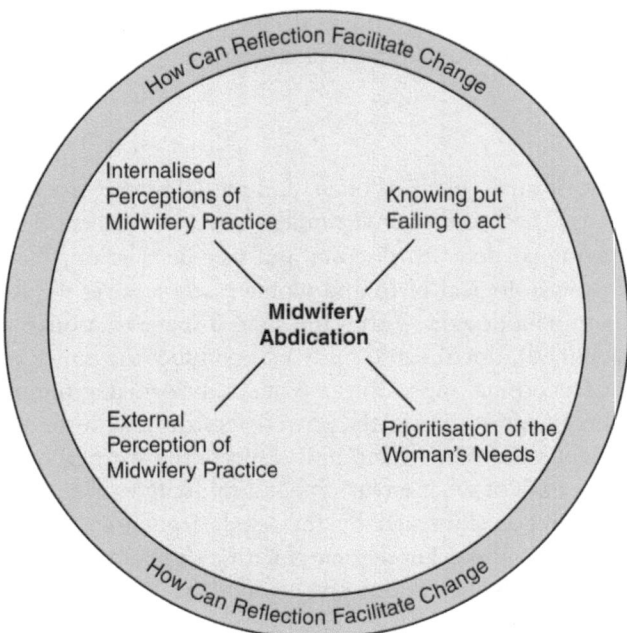

FIGURE 4.1 Constructs of Midwifery Abdication

Over time the concept of MA has been explored further locating evidence of it not only in Australia but internationally (Jefford & Jomeen, 2015). Evidence of MA was also noted within 41 cases of Australian midwifery practice cases that necessitated legal, coronial, and/or disciplinary procedures (Jefford et al., 2020). The constructs of MA are: *internalised perceptions of midwifery practice, knowing but failing to act, and prioritisation of the woman's needs, external perceptions of midwifery practice and how can reflection facilitate change?* (Figure 4.1).

An example of how MA might be evidenced in midwifery practice is:

In the antenatal period, Alisha (woman) imagined her perfect birth to be in the water, so she booked in early at her midwifery-led local birth centre (attached to a hospital). Alisha discusses her birthing wishes, at length, with her midwife (Jane). Jane, who had a water birth for her own child, expresses how wonderful this mode of birth is for mother and baby (*internalised perceptions of midwifery practice*) and agrees totally to support Alisha's choice.

Alisha's labour begins and she meets Jane at the birth centre. Labour progresses well, and Alisha is immersed in the bath. Spontaneously, Alisha's membranes rupture and there is meconium.

Jane knows Alisha really wants a water birth and research notes the benefits to mother and baby (*internalised perceptions of midwifery practice*). Jane decides to gate-keep the information from Alisha and her partner (Toni) hoping to 'rescue' the situation and ensure Alisha has her imagined birth (*prioritisation of the woman's needs*). Jane is aware of the organisational policies around meconium and its management, which should involve Alisha leaving the birthing pool. Yet, Jane decides to not ask Alisha to leave the water or inform her peers (*knowing, but failing to act*). Jane knows if her peers (or doctor) are aware they might not view Jane's actions favourably and doesn't meet the standard of expected midwifery care (*external perceptions of midwifery practice*). Or they might make Alisha leave the bath as per policy.

Jane, with no second midwife, facilitates the birth of baby Jacob in the birthing pool. Jacobs Apgar's are 4 and Jane calls for assistance. Jacob is transferred to NICU with meconium aspirate.

When reflecting on the case, Jane knows she went against polices yet believes she did the right thing because Alisha got her perfect birth (*how can reflection facilitate change?*)

A key question here must then be: if we consciously or unconsciously engage in MA or give away the power and control of being an autonomous midwife, how can we role model or mentor students, who are the next generation of midwives, or guard or protect the wellbeing of mother and/or baby?

REFLECTIVE ACTIVITY 1:

Reflecting on the example of Midwifery Abdication above, consider:

- How might mentorship have supported Jane to engage in clinical decision-making, while taking into account '*knowing, but failing to act*' and '*external perceptions of midwifery practice*'?

Becoming a Midwife and the Drive for Mentorship

We all remember the passion and excitement we had for midwifery when we first started as a student or graduated and became part of the local, national, and international midwifery family. We believed whole heartedly we would always be kind, gentle, compassionate, and involve the woman in every decision. We would create a safe space for women to experience empowering physiological (vaginal) births, and advocate for women, rejecting unwarranted medical interventions. We can achieve this some of the time and when we do it feeds our midwifery souls, yet sometimes we find women have complications which requires appropriate and necessary medical interventions some that fall outside our scope of practice, or babies that are not always cooperative, or women are offered 'social' medical interventions. In the United States, a conversation on quality of care is at the forefront to combat the rising maternal mortality. But it is challenged by the healthcare industry that is profit-driven and structural inequities (Kennedy-Moulton et al., 2023). This has the potential to result in less time to listen, and more interventions to control birth. Doing more makes us feel better, especially when we feel powerless, and in some countries, where interventions can be billed, it may provide motivation to intervene. But the poorer outcomes tell a different story, especially when listening to women's experiences of disrespect and abuse (Maung et al., 2021). Although an obvious issue in many low-income countries is the lack of dignity and respect in maternity care is omnipresent to different degrees (Stanton & Gogoi, 2022). It is at times like this we find ourselves in situations where we experience moral distress.

Moral Distress

First identified by Jameton (1984) and further expanded by Monteverde (2019). When exploring causes of moral distress in midwives within the literature, Rost et al. (2024) noted moral distress is when a midwife experiences a negative emotion or distress due to a situation that compromises moral agency or moral constraint. This can happen from external constraints such as culture, power asymmetries, hospital guidelines, a lack of resources, or our own conflicting moral standards such as women's autonomy vs foetal life. The authors did go on to note, midwifery is particularly at risk for moral distress not just from the bioethical complexity of maternal healthcare, but from socio-cultural, and structural factors such as gender inequities, power asymmetries, and the cultural norm of physician-based care that disregards midwifery values and women's agency (Rost et al., 2024).

Midwives commit to being with women, to partner with them, protect them, and help them in a patriarchal and hierarchal world of maternity care provision. The medical model was developed at the peak of patriarchy (Nisha, 2022). It plays an important role in healthcare when fast intervention is needed to save lives. Often, because patients are so sick and decisions are complicated, the medical model is weaker when attempting to partner with patients around health goals and decision-making (Hirsch, 2023). As such, the medical model, therefore, appears to be in opposition to the midwifery model of care provision where women are predominately well, are undertaking a normal physiological event and have agency over their decision-making. The World Health Organisation has created a quality of maternal health framework that puts equal value on the provision of care (Tunçalp et al., 2015). Midwifery works at a cultural and spiritual crossroads where women's desires, foetal life, and structural inequities push against each other every day, as noted above within the constructs of Midwifery Abdication (Jefford, 2012; Jefford & Jomeen, 2015; Jefford et al., 2020). Yet, looming in the back of every birth room is fear and the components of that fear may differ from country to country, model of care, and individually. For example, in high-income countries, fear may arise from the risk of litigation, while in both low- and high-income countries, fear maybe based around the risk of death. Irrespective of the type of fear, or who is feeling it, fear can be encapsulated by moral uncertainty (Dahlen & Caplice, 2014; Zondag et al., 2022). There is a link between moral distress and reduced clinical engagement (Rost et al., 2024). It could be hypothesised that if mentors create a safe space for students/mentees, mentoring may mitigate some of the impacts of moral distress.

Midwives are perfectly poised to demonstrate how the provision of care must centre around the woman and her values, optimising the experience of care for the woman. But this requires an enabling space for the midwife to listen and a system that values the midwifery model to make it possible. Midwives, therefore, need mentoring that considers the health system and what the midwife needs to honour her commitment to midwifery and the woman, especially in environments driven by the risk lens of medicine. This is the world midwives need to navigate intellectually, emotionally, and morally. The authors of this chapter, like many of the readers, have personal experiences which played an influencing role in developing our sense of midwifery self-worth, framing the type of midwife we chose to be. Two short narratives will be presented to highlight this journey, one through the American midwifery lens and one from the English lens.

American Lens

'Before becoming a midwife, I had two amazing births in the hospital and one powerful home birth, all with midwives. Those births woke up the feminist in me. I sought out stories of gentle births, midwives sitting and talking with women, helping them understand their bodies. I was excited about joining their ranks and cared deeply about women and being part of the mysteries of birth. Yet one scene from my midwifery education program haunts me to this day.

I was observing a woman in labour for hours. Someone made the decision she needed a vacuum extraction to assist 'delivery' of the baby. I don't remember anyone explaining things to her, discussing options, or offering support, I just remember her being wheeled into the theatre room, scared, in pain, yelling as a doctor with a large suction cup on a chain, attached it to the baby's head, and pulled. She screamed, he pulled, I froze. This felt all wrong. She seemed violated in a way that didn't fit with my understanding of healthcare, and certainly not with midwifery. No one explained what happened to me or helped me process my experience. None of my other rotations had a moment like this, a moment where we removed a person's rights, hurt them, and offered no support, no compassion, and no explanation.

Through my decades of experience since then, occasionally I'm reminded of that woman and her experience. Especially in moments where a gentle birth suddenly needs an intervention. A team swoops in and 'saves the day' and seems pleased with themselves when the baby has been delivered safely. But I still see the look on the woman's face, her confusion, her grief at losing a dream, her fear for her baby, or her panic as her body's memories surface and she is retraumatised from a moment in her past. And again, I stand frozen, powerless as a more powerful team makes decisions for her. I am left with so many questions. How do we fight a powerful system for what is considered 'soft' female skills? How can I protect the midwife in me, in awe of birth, wanting to provide gentleness, communication, compassion and support?'

REFLECTIVE ACTIVITY 2:

Reflecting on the Journey to midwifery from the American lens, consider:

1 Was professional dissonance apparent here?
2 How might mentorship have supported this student in her professional development and understanding of midwifery?
3 How might mentorship have reduced her moral distress?

English Lens

'As a student I had the privilege to work with two fantastic midwives who mentored me throughout my whole training. Both mentors embodied woman-centred care irrespective of acuity, type of birth or model of care. My midwifery focus became women-centred and working in partnership with women through their birthing journey. Some could argue this provided me with a limited view of what a midwife is, yet with my whole being some thirty years later I still defend the mentoring they provided me was the best I could have ever had.

Once I qualified as a midwife, I entered a birthing room as the second midwife. I observed the midwifery accoucheur, after the baby's head had birthed and before birth of the shoulders, push two fingers into the woman's vagina. The woman's hips briefly lifted off the bed and she said 'Ouch, what are you doing?' The midwife calmly said, 'Oh, I'm just feeling for the cord in case it's around your baby's neck.' This one midwifery action raised my awareness of how a midwife could medicalise birth: the normally self-determining woman became a patient, and the midwife alone was the decision-maker of care. Over time I observed other midwives doing the same. I believe such an invasive and often painful intervention violated women's right of choice, consent as well as social justice, and it led me to begin asking the following questions: Why did these midwives act as they did? What factors influenced and/or drove their practice? How did they reconcile the philosophy of woman-centred midwifery and 'checking for the cord' without the prior knowledge or permission of the woman? What also played on my mind was what these midwives were teaching students, and the importance a mentor, educator and leader can play in perpetuating such practice.

REFLECTIVE ACTIVITY 3:

Reflecting on the Journey to midwifery from the English lens, consider:

1 How did mentorship support this student in her professional development and understanding of midwifery?
2 How did mentorship shape her practice as a midwife?

As a senior midwife academic I have questioned, probed, challenged, and debated the incongruities of medicalised childbirth enacted by some midwives and medical staff and the truth of midwifery, its philosophy and feminism. I have taught midwives and continue to teach midwifery students the concept of women-centeredness and holism, which focuses on interconnections between mind, body, spirit, family, community, and environment. I pay attention to women's invisible energy flows, obstacles, and liberation. As midwives we connect with women, respecting and acknowledging their body's wisdom by providing them space to experience and value pregnancy and birth. I firmly believe midwifery should be emancipatory. To this end I have and will continue to challenge with conviction the concept of paternalism/maternalism and strive to create a safe environment for students to learn, make mistakes and grow. Yet in the clinical environment, if mentors are not creating a safe space for students/mentees, around the world, using the concepts of 'being available', 'feeling valued' and 'feeling safe' then how will they be able to take up the baton and move midwifery forward?

Requirements for Mentorship in the Midwifery Context

To ensure midwives are able to prove a safe environment to mentor students, midwives also need to *'feel safe'*, *'feel valued'*, and *'be available'* (Ebert, 2012).

Feeling Safe

Midwives face emotional and professional difficulties when their maternity service fails to provide appropriate resources, support, or time to continuously deliver individualised support for women, student midwife learning, mentoring of other staff, and their own professional development. The lack of support from maternity service management is seen as a failure to create a safe environment in which to cultivate the learning of self and others.

> Feeling safe within the maternity care encounter describes a state in which the woman and midwife can interact without fear of perceived or actual psychological (or physical) harm. The woman is guarded and guided by the midwife to experience maternity care encounters in a manner she chooses, free from controversy. The midwife offers the woman a sense of being protected against emotional or psychological harm during maternity care encounters.
>
> *(Ebert, 2012, p. 226)*

The midwife–mentor role models this behaviour, for two reasons: (1) So, mentees learn to create a safe space for the woman. (2) To create a safe space for students/mentees, so they understand they are guarded and guided by the midwife–mentor to learn to be a midwife. In other words, they are in a safe environment to learn, make mistakes, and grow.

Feeling Valued

Both the woman and midwife need to feel valued in their roles in the childbearing process. 'Feeling valued' within the midwifery context means – *being highly regarded; considered with respect or importance through the actions and reactions of the maternity care culture* (Ebert, 2012, p. 245). The woman, as the centre of decision-making processes, needs to feel she is heard, and her needs/wishes are important. The midwife, as the link between the woman and the health service provider, takes on the role of guide and guardian. For the midwife to feel valued within the maternity care environment, their professional identity, and ways of working with-woman need to be respected and valued. Midwives want to feel their professional knowledge and decision-making processes are valued by midwifery colleagues, management, and other healthcare professionals. Yet, communicate that managerial and medical control over midwifery models of care demonstrate not only a failure to value the needs of women but also demonstrated a failure to value midwifery as a profession. Professional survival, however, is often viewed as dependent on valuing and meeting the needs of the workplace culture, not the needs of the woman and or midwifery ways of working. This contrasts with the enabling environment as recommended by the ICM (2023) as facilitating quality and safe health care for childbearing women and a safe learning environment for students/mentees.

Equally, for the student midwife to feel valued, their need to learn and their future midwifery voice needs to be respectfully considered within the maternity care environment (Ebert, 2012). When student midwives/mentees feel unsupported in their clinical learning of midwifery, they may 'feel unsafe' to apply the midwifery understandings generated in their classroom to the maternity care environment. Students in Ebert's (2012) study recounted being ignored, dismissed, or intimidated into silence when they questioned observed practices. Their voices were not valued. Midwife–mentors therefore, who fail to question the status quo and practise in ways that maintain medical dominance and system-based work styles, enculture student midwives and/or their mentees to follow suit. This notion of enculturation into the profession or the need to belong has been understood in the nursing literature for more than 25 years. Levett-Jones and Lathlean (2008) explored the concept of belongingness in relation to student nurse learning. The authors concluded the behaviour of registered colleagues with whom students/mentees spent their workday with, formed the most influential determinant of student learning and their sense of professional belongingness. A student's need to belong took precedence over their need to be clinically competent. Cognitive impairment reduced critical thinking skills and a failure to question practice resulted when the student felt they did not belong and sensed a lack of respect and acceptance by their registered colleagues.

A few years later, in 2013, Australian researchers (McKenna et al., 2013) explored undergraduate midwifery students' sense of belongingness in their clinical practice using an adapted nursing questionnaire. Participants (66) were drawn from one university that provided both Bachelor of Midwifery degree and a double Bachelor of Nursing/Bachelor of Midwifery degree. Findings were similar to those found in nursing in that they felt comfortable and experienced a sense of belonging and feeling valued. Yet, they note much is not understood in the field of midwifery.

Being Available

The midwife needs to be available for the woman during maternity care encounters for the woman to feel she is safe to engage in decision-making and feel her needs are valued, taking precedence over autocratic institutionally dictated procedures. The concept of 'availability', or pledging oneself to another, was first introduced by the French philosopher Gabriel Marcel. Availability, within the midwifery context, assumes the carer, or midwife, is receptive and accepting of the woman and her family's experiences and needs (Lantz, 1994). The midwife actively participates with and for the woman so the woman's needs may be met. The midwife is non-judgemental and demonstrates empathy in standing alongside the woman, ready to support her in the way the woman requires. In doing so, the woman becomes aware that, in that moment, the midwife is focused on the woman and her needs. Being available within the mentor–mentee relationship equally requires the mentor to be non-judgemental, demonstrating empathy in standing alongside the mentee, ready to support them in the way they require. In doing so, the mentee becomes aware that, in that moment, the mentor is focused on them and their learning needs. The mentor is available for the mentee, which creates an enabling environment.

It is difficult, however, for the midwife–mentor to be available for the woman, or student/mentee, when support and resources for midwives are not available within their maternity service. Workplace needs often take precedence with pressure on midwives/mentors to complete tasks expected by organisational management. Task-centred midwifery work can result in midwives being available for things such as maternity ward routines, thus preventing midwives from being available for women or their mentees. When the maternity care workplace culture and management value decision-making processes based on evidence and the needs of the individual woman, the woman can feel safe to engage as an active partner in the decision-making process. In such a situation, the midwife can equally feel safe in their ability to guide and guard the woman, while role-modelling quality maternity care to their mentee. Midwifery leadership, woman-centred care, and ways of teaching and learning can be supported through the concepts 'being available', 'feeling valued', and 'feeling safe'. These concepts have the potential to facilitate meaningful woman–midwife interactions regardless of the midwifery context, to develop a sense of midwifery self-worth and support colleagues and mentees, enabling a midwifery mentorship model that is valued and sustainable.

Feminism, Midwifery, and Mentorship

Feminism has been described in waves: **First wave**, which focuses on gender equality with women suffragettes pioneering feminist activism; **Second wave**, focusing on women's work post war and gender roles and women's sexuality; **Third wave** linked with technological advances and a 'new consciousness' of the woman's role. It is at this juncture of feminism it met with strong antifeminism from both men and women. **Fourth wave** saw the re-emergence of past waves merging into one, bringing forth feminist values and voice (Malinowska, 2020). It could be suggested that we are entering/have entered a **Fifth wave** of feminism with the global movements such as 'Me Too' and the fight against sexual violence (Me Too, 2024). Liberation and equality for women, irrespective of race, religion, culture, social status, or location around the globe has been the call to arms for feminists. The historical sexist social construct of society and where women were placed within it, activated women to emancipation and became promoted within and synonymous with feminist theory (Lacan, 2002; Lerner, 1986). The patriarchal society came under scrutiny. Over time, for some women, their place within society changed and calls of equality and liberation were heard. Yet for many, there is still a long road to travel before all women can claim equality and liberation. The field of midwifery is one such area.

When looking through the lens of midwifery, one must see midwifery is the same lens as feminism which champions women's empowerment, equality (Oakley, 1974, 1998; Oakley et al., 1996), and their reproductive rights (Cook & Plata, 1994; Kaczor, 2022), rebelling against obstetric violence or termed by the United Nations, gendered violence (Keedle et al., 2024).

Midwifery is first noted as a role, in which women support women as early as 40,000 B.C., where women cared for women experiencing childbirth. Midwifery's more recent past, however, has involved patriarchal dominance. With doctors moving into the childbirth field of health, came the erosion of women caring for women in the community. Compounding this was the claim that the rising mortality rate (in Australia) was caused by those women who provided birthing support (Purcell, 1998). Birth was managed by doctors. To become a midwife, the only route was to become a nurse then undertake additional training to become a midwife. In some countries, this route remains. Midwives, however, began the push to reclaim their place with women in childbirth. The ability to become a midwife independent of nursing education (direct entry) was introduced in the 1960s (UK) and 1998 (Australia). Feminism was able to be taught within midwifery education (Davison et al., 2018; Jefford & Nolan, 2022), and it could be found within language used within key midwifery textbooks such as Myles Textbook for Midwives (Harkenss & Cheyne, 2019).

Feminist Foundations of Midwifery Mentorship

Mentorship is a critical component in the development of any profession, particularly for midwifery which is deeply rooted in relationship and the feminist ethos of care, dignity, and compassion for women (Barnes, 1999). It is vital to fostering a supportive environment for midwives to grow both personally and professionally. Jefford and Nolan (2022) argue feminism is embedded within midwifery education with '*concepts such as reciprocity, partnership, equality, emancipation and empowerment, of both women's belief in childbearing physiology, and childbirth as a powerful rite of passage (acknowledging there is a place for medical intervention, however it should not control or influence)*' (p. p105589). Feminist principles are naturally symbiotic with midwifery practice where mentee-focused mentorship can ensure students' knowledge of feminism transcends the theory–practice nexus to demonstrate the feminist principles that promote informed choice, partnership, and equality in childbirth practices. Embracing midwifery's feminist underpinnings are essential to combat the internalised oppression women share in patriarchal and hierarchal models. Mentorship can provide midwives with the tools and confidence to advocate for women and themselves. Yet, most of all it provides moments for reflection and validation of our experiences and values. Through guidance and support, mentors help students of midwifery and midwives navigate the challenges of working in the healthcare environment and ensure the feminist values of women's dignity and self-determination remain central to their practice (Hawke, 2021). This not only empowers midwives but also promotes emancipatory care for women, challenging the medicalised and technocratic approach that often dominates maternity care (Hawke, 2021).

Feminist-based mentorship echoes the midwifery model of care. Ideally, it will:

- Embrace midwifery and feminist foundations with mentor–mentee relationships that include reciprocity, partnership, and mutual respect when mentoring. This allows us to model the midwifery model of care between mentor and mentee (Jefford & Nolan, 2022).
- Create a space of safety for the new midwife. This allows her to reflect and explore her own personal approach, philosophy, and expression of midwifery.
- Allow the mentorship to develop as an intimate dance between two people. Like midwife and women, mentor and mentee must learn to trust each other, listen to each other, and identify each other's values.

What Mentorship Provides

In different countries and different contexts, mentoring will vary in how it is expressed and who is doing the mentoring, but the foundation remains the same for example, trust needs to be built to create a circle of safety that invites listening and reflecting. This variation makes midwifery strong and responsive to the needs to the woman and the system. Mentoring takes many forms, yet the goal of mentoring in midwifery is to support the students of midwifery and midwives find her/his midwifery path. Yet, it is important to note that as mentors guide students of midwifery and midwives, they too refine their perspectives, reflect on their practices, and stay updated with evolving feminist ideologies in midwifery. This mutual exchange not only strengthens the individuals involved but also reinforces a collective commitment to woman-centred care across generations of midwives. This model of partnership mirrors the midwife–woman relationship, fostering professional growth rooted in respect, equality, and shared responsibility.

How we struggle to do this – create a structure for mentoring to be done well, and be flexible to meet individual and contextual needs. Hopefully, this book can provide health services, education providers and midwives a resource to implement a sustainable model of midwifery mentorship.

References

Barnes, M. (1999). Research in midwifery – The relevance of a feminist theoretical framework. *Women & Birth, 12*(2), 6–10. https://doi.org/10.1016/S1031-170X(99)80013-0

Cook, R., & Plata, M. (1994). Women's reproductive rights. *International Journal of Gynaecology & Obstetrics, 46*, 215–220.

Dahlen, H., & Caplice, S. (2014). What do midwives fear? *Women & Birth, 27*(4), 266–270. https://doi.org/10.1016/j.wombi.2014.06.008

Davis-Floyd, R. (2017). *Ways of Knowing about Birth: Mothers, Midwives, Medicine, and Birth Activism.* Waveland Press Inc.

Davison, C., Geraghty, S., & Dobbs, K. (2018). The F word: Midwifery students' understanding of feminism. *British Journal of Midwifery, 26*(11), 731–737. https://doi.org/10.12968/bjom.2018.26.11.731

Department of Health and Aged Care. (2024). *Nurses and Midwives.* Australian Government, Department of Health and Aged Care. Retrieved 31 December from https://www.health.gov.au/topics/nurses-and-midwives

Ebert, L. (2012). *Woman-centred Care and the Socially Disadvantaged Woman: An Interpretative Phenomenological Analysis.* University of Newcastle. University of Newcastle Research Repository NOVA. http://hdl.handle.net/1959.13/936189

Guilliland, K., & Pairman, S. (2010). *The Midwifery Partnership: A Model for Practice* (2nd ed.). The New Zealand College of Midwives.

Harkenss, M., & Cheyne, H. (2019). Myles textbooks for midwives 1953 and 2014, a feminist critical discourse analysis. *Midwifery, 76*, 1–7. https://doi.org/10.1016/j.midw.2019.05.003

Hawke, M. (2021). Subversive acts and everyday midwifery: Feminism in content and context. *Women & Birth, 34*(1), e92–e96. https://doi.org/10.1016/j.wombi.2020.05.013

Hirsch, A. (2023). Relational autonomy and paternalism – Why the physician-patient relationship matters. *Zeitschrift für Ethik und Moralphilosophie, 6*, 239–260. https://doi.org/10.1007/s42048-023-00148-z

International Confederation of Midwives. *Advocacy, Enabling Environment, Regulation.* International Confederation of Midwives. Retrieved 31 December from https://internationalmidwives.org/resources/midwifery-an-autonomous-profession/

International Confederation of Midwives. (2023a). *International Definition of the Midwife.* 1. Retrieved 27 June 2024, from

International Confederation of Midwives. (2023b). *Professional Accountability of the Midwife.* (Vol. Position statement PS20008_014V2014, p. 2). Geneva: International Confederation of Midwives.

International Confederation of Midwives. (2023c). *Qualifications and ompetencies of Midwife Educators/Teachers, Position Statement*. International Confederation of Midwives. Retrieved 31 December from https://internationalmidwives.org/resources/qualifications-and-competencies-of-midwifery-educators/

Jameton, A. (1984). *Nursing Practice: The Ethical Issues*. Prentice-Hall.

Jefford, E. (2012). *Optimal Midwifery Decision-Making during 2nd Stage Labour: The Integration of Clinical Reasoning into Practice* [Research, Southern Cross University]. New South Wales. https://researchportal.scu.edu.au/esploro/outputs/doctoral/Optimal-midwifery-decision-making-during-2nd-stage/991012821111602368

Jefford, E., & Jomeen, J. (2015). "Midwifery abdication": A finding from an interpretive study [research]. *International Journal of Childbirth*, 5(3), 116–125. https://doi.org/10.1891/2156-5287.5.3.116

Jefford, E., & Nolan, S. (2022). Two parts of an indivisible whole - midwifery education and feminism: An exploratory study of 1st year students' immersion into midwifery. *Nurse Education Today*, 119, 105589. https://doi.org/10.1016/j.nedt.2022.105589

Jefford, E., Nolan, S., & Jomeen, J. (2020). Is the concept of midwifery abdication evident in Australian case law? A systematic review of legal literature, Court/Tribunal decisions, and coronial findings. *International Journal of Childbirth*, 10(4), 217–223. http://doi.org/10.1891/IJCBIRTH-D-20-00038

Kaczor, C. (2022). *The Ethics of Abortion* (3rd ed.). Routledge. https://doi.org/10.4324/9781003305217

Keedle, H., Keedle, W., & Dahlen, H. (2024). Dehumanized, violated, and powerless: An Australian survey of Women's experiences of obstetric violence in the past 5 years. *Violence Against Women*, 30(9), 2320–2344. https://doi.org/10.1177/10778012221140138

Kennedy-Moulton, K., Miller, S., Persson, P., Rossin-Slater, M., Wheery, L., & Aldana, A. (2023). *Maternal and Infant Health Inequity: New Evidence from Linked Administrative Data*. National Bureau of Economic Research. Retrieved 9 January from https://www.nber.org/papers/w30693

Lacan, J. (2002). *Écrits: A Selection 1948–1960* (B. Fink, Trans.). Norton.

Lantz, J. (1994). Marcel's 'availability' in existential psychotherapy with couples and families. *Contemporary Family Therapy: An International Journal*, 16(6), 489–501.

Lerner, G. (1986). *The Creation of Patriarchy*. Oxford University Press.

Levett-Jones, T., & Lathlean, J. (2008). Belongingness: A prerequisite for nursing students' clinical learning. *Nurse Education in Practice*, 8(2), 103–111. http://www.sciencedirect.com/science/article/pii/S1471595307000364

Malinowska, A. (2020). Waves of feminism. *The International Encyclopedia of Gender, Media, and Communication*, 1–7. https://doi.org/10.1002/9781119429128.iegmc096

Maung, T., Mon, N., Mehrtash, H., Bonsaffoh, K. A., Vogel, J. P., Aderoba, A. K., & Irinyenikan, T. (2021). Women's experiences of mistreatment during childbirth and their satisfaction with care: Findings from a multicountry community-based study in four countries. *BMJ Global Health*, 5(2), 1–11. https://doi.org/10.1136/bmjgh-2020-003688

McKenna, L., Gilmour, C., Biro, A., McIntyre, M., Bailey, C., Jones, J., Miles, M., Hall, H., & McLelland, G. (2013). Undergraduate midwifery students' sense of belongingness in clinical practice. *Nurse Education Today*, 33(8), 880–883. https://doi.org/10.1016/j.nedt.2012.09.009

Me Too. (2024). *Me Too*. Me Too. Retrieved 9 July from https://metoomvmt.org/get-to-know-us/history-inception/

Monteverde, S. (2019). Complexity, complicity and moral distress in nursing. *Ethik in Der Medizin*, 31(4), 345–360. https://doi.org/10.1007/s00481-019-00548-z

Nisha, Z. (2022). The medicalisation of the female body and motherhood: Some biological and existential reflections. *Asian Bioethics Review*, *14*, 25–40. https://doi.org/10.1007/s41649-021-00185-z

Nursing and Midwifery Board of Australia. (2018). *Midwife Standards for Practice*. Canberra: Nursing and Midwifery Board of Australia.

Oakley, A. (1974). *The Sociology of Housework*. Martin Robertson.

Oakley, A. (1998). Gender, methodology and people's way of knowing: Some problems with feminism and the paradigm debate in social science. *Sociology*, *32*(4), 707–731.

Oakley, A., Hickey, D., & Rajan, L. (1996). Social support in pregnancy: Does it have long-term effects? *Journal of Reproductive and Infant Psychology*, *14*, 7–22.

Parratt, J. (2008). Territories of the self and spiritual practices during childbirth. In K. Fahy, M. Foureur, & C. Hastie (Eds.), *Birth Territory and Midwifery Guardianship: Theory for Practice, Education and Research* (pp. 39–54). Butterworth Heinemann-Elsevier.

Purcell, N. (1998). Traditional midwifery and its influence on contemporary maternity care: A brief historical review of events in New South Wales. *Birth Issues*, *7*(2), 58–65. http://scu.rl.talis.com/items/F05D004C-oD70-7F10-247E-82BE512C5826.html?referrer=%2FDC6902BD12D1-6A94-806D-5EEB-F471CF57.html%23item-F05D004C=0D70-7F10-247E-82BE512C5826

Rost, M., Montagnoli, C., & Eichinger, J. (2024). Causes of moral distress among midwives: A scoping review. *Nursing Ethics*. https://doi.org/10.1177/09697330241281498

Stanton, M. E., & Gogoi, A. (2022). Dignity and respect in maternity care. *BMJ Global Health*, *5*(5), 1–4. https://doi.org/10.1136/bmjgh-2022-009023

Teresa-Morales, C., Rodríguez-Pérez, M., Araujo-Hernández, M., & Feria-Ramírez, C. (2022). Current stereotypes associated with nursing and nursing professionals: An integrative review. *International Journal of Environmental Research and Public Health*, *19*(13), 7640. https://doi.org/10.3390/ijerph19137640

The International Confederation of Midwives. (2023). *Midwifery: An Autonomous Profession*, accessed 11 June 2025. https://internationalmidwives.org/resources/midwifery-an-autonomous-profession/

Tunçalp, O., Were, W. M., MacLennan, C., Oladapo, T., Gulmezoglu, A. M., Bahl, R., Daelmans, B., Mathai, M., Say, L., Kristensen, F., Temmerman, M., & Bustreo, F. (2015). Quality of care for pregnant women and newborns – The WHO vision. *1*(8), 1045–1049. https://doi.org/10.1111/1471-0528.13451

World Health Organisation. (2013). *Midwifery Educator Core Competencies*. World Health Organisation. Retrieved 31 December from https://www.who.int/publications/i/item/midwifery-educator-core-competencies

Zondag, L. D. C., Maas, V. Y. F., Beuckens, A., & Nieuwenhuijze, M. J. (2022). Experiences, beliefs, and values influencing midwives' attitudes toward the use of childbirth interventions. *Journal of Midwifery & Women's Health*, *67*(5), 618–625. https://doi.org/10.1111/jmwh.13392

5

MIDWIFERY MENTORSHIP

Professional and Personal Attributes

Elaine Jefford

Introduction

At the outset of this chapter, it is important to acknowledge different countries use different terms, some interchangeably, when discussing mentorship. As you progress through this book, those terms will be clarified in the context of specific countries. The role of a mentor, in its generic form, which is the term used in this chapter is defined firstly as:

> dynamic, reciprocal, personal relationship in which a more experienced person (mentor) acts as a guide, role model, teacher, and sponsor of a less experienced person (mentee) ... and provides knowledge, advice, counsel, support, and opportunity in the mentee's pursuit of full membership in a particular profession.
>
> *(Johndon & Riley, 2018, p. XVIII)*

And when applied to nursing and midwifery within the Australian context, the term mentor is defined as:

> a relationship in which the mentor facilitates the personal and professional growth and development of another nurse or midwife (the mentee).
>
> *(Nursing and Midwifery Board of Australia, 2021)*

Although supervision of students or mentoring of new graduate or junior nurses/midwives is excluded from the scope of Nursing and Midwifery Board of Australia (NMBA) supervision guidelines for nursing and

DOI: 10.4324/9781003533733-6

midwifery (2021), we believe they are applicable. Mentors, within the clinical environment, facilitate students to convert theory to practise acquiring requisite professional skills, develop their professional identity, a sense of belonging and integration into the midwifery profession (Ebert et al., 2019; Mclukie & Kuipers, 2024). All key components to ensuring midwifery students use the lens of evidence to provide safe, quality competent woman-centred care, which supports the ability to work autonomously within their full scope of practice as a midwife.

Benner's (1984) claims, one can move from a beginner practitioner upon accumulating the pre-requisite knowledge and skill competencies and experience through to an advanced beginner, competent, proficient, and finally to expert practitioner. Ultimately, the same could be applied to being a mentor if one is using the objective lens of learning. A Japanese study published in 2016 argues that three overarching concepts are required to be a competent mentor (Hishinuma et al., 2016). The concepts identified include professional competencies, educator competencies, and personal characteristics. Participants in Hishinuma and colleagues' study were recruited through a cluster sample over a two-month period in one country and included 464 student midwives and midwives who had qualified as a registered midwife within the last year. The questionnaire return rate was 67.5%. Although some may argue that an eight-year-old study undertaken in one country is not relevant today, the resulting concepts appear singularly or in combination explicitly or opaquely within recent international mentoring literature (Bogren et al., 2022; Bradford et al., 2022; Neiterman et al., 2023; Nespoli et al., 2024; Nieuwenhuijze et al., 2020; Stephenson et al., 2023). What appears to be absent from Hishinuma et al.'s (2016) work is the influence of Environment, or workplace culture. The three concepts of professional, educational, and personal as well as environment will be discussed within this chapter. Please note although the concepts are presented as separate, they are in fact symbiotic parts of an indivisible whole.

REFLECTIVE ACTIVITY 1 YOUR PROFESSIONAL AND PERSONAL ATTRIBUTES

Reflect on what attributes you have, and then how do you role model them when working with student midwives using the three below headings:

1 Professional.
2 Personal.
3 Educator.

Professional

Irrespective of geographical location around the globe or one's social status or religious beliefs, women are entitled to safe high quality midwifery care by someone who has legitimate authority to call themselves a Midwife (Jefford et al., 2019). In other words to use the title Midwife, one should have completed an educational program based on the International Confederation of Midwives (ICM) Essential Competencies for Midwifery Practice (2019) and the program, as a minimum, meets the Global Standards for Midwifery Education (2021a). Furthermore, the midwife must demonstrate competency in the scope of practice as defined in the ICM International Definition of Midwife (2023), as well as any regulatory standards that are country specific. A midwifery mentor should exhibit high proficiency or expertise in both midwifery knowledge and skills (Bogren et al., 2022; Rooke, 2014; Sheehan et al., 2022) be current and demonstrate practice which is evidence-based (Australia, 2018; International Confederation of Midwives, 2019; Nursing and Midwifery Council, 2024).

Effective clinical decision-making demonstrates professional status and capability, both intra and interprofessionally. Good decision-making skills is an expectation of a midwife and therefore a midwifery mentor. Effective, collaborative decision-making ensures the safety of the public. Poor decision-making, however, can have devasting consequences for women, babies, the midwife, the midwifery profession, and the health provider (Ebert et al., 2022; Jefford et al., 2020). Clinical decision-making predominately utilises hypothetico-deductive theory. Jefford (2012), using etic and emic data developed a midwifery specific decision-making tool incorporating intuition and framed it within the midwifery philosophy. It is called Enhancing Decision-Making and Assessment in Midwifery (EDAM) which was psychometrically validated in 2016 (Jefford et al., 2016). Intuition is a valuable contributing factor within this model (see Table 5.1).

This model draws on medical clinical reasoning as it facilitates the midwife to engage in empirical, precise decision-making using a transparent, logical framework that offers provision for peer consensus and can be easily taught. Although intuition is an important part of decision-making, due to its opaqueness consensus of decision-making is not always possible and thus may or may not hinder how one is perceived professionally.

Critical thinking and reflective practice underpin decision-making. In 2022, Cater et al. sought to define a midwifery specific definition of critical thinking via international consensus. The results offered 14 'Habits of Mind' and 12 Skills that are the core of critical thinking in midwifery practice:

Skills:
- analysis, constructive application and contextualisation of best available evidence, problem solving, discriminating, predicting, evaluation of care, collect and interpret clinical cues, collaboration/negotiation, reflexivity, facilitates shared decision-making, communication, and transforming knowledge.

TABLE 5.1 EDAM

Clinical reasoning	
Clinical reasoning process	*Integration and intervention*
1 Cue acquisition† – appears to be comprehensive	6 Evaluates treatment options relevant to the diagnosis – if relevant
2 Cue clustering†† – appears to be comprehensive	7 Prescribes and/or implements planned care
3 Cue Interpretation††† – Generating multiple hypotheses – if relevant	8 Evaluates outcomes
4 Focused cue acquisition – if needed and relevant to hypothesis	9 Uses intuition to aid decision-making
5 Ruling in and Ruling out hypotheses – if relevant	

Midwifery Practice	
Woman's relationship with midwife	*General midwifery practice*
1 Stays in the room with the woman in labour	4 Honest and complete information sharing with woman/partner
2 Shares a common, known goal with the woman	5 Accountability for own professional behaviour in accordance with professional frameworks
3 Trusts the woman and her body	6 Skills in negotiating with medical staff or senior midwifery staff
	7 Assumes appropriate responsibility for woman/baby's well-being in labour
	8 Shows reflexive practice
	9 When the woman and midwife disagree about care takes appropriate action (documentation and consultation)
	10 The woman is the final decision-maker

Habits of mind:

• intellectual curiosity, reflective, holistic view, intellectual integrity, flexibility, questioning challenging, participatory, open mindedness, listening with understanding and empathy, cultural humility, woman centred, being brave, confidence, and creativity (Carter & Creedy, 2022).

In essence, critical thinking offers the ability to engage in higher-order thinking where inquisitiveness and questioning, alongside the skills and habits of mind noted above, are used to carefully define, analyse, and interpret an issue. In other words, a mentor needs to be able to demonstrate critical thinking using reason, and evidence to make sound clinical decisions. Yet, this needs to be done through the lens of the midwifery philosophy of partnership, being woman-centred and birth as a normal physiological process (Australian College of Midwives, 2024; Nespoli et al., 2024; Nieuwenhuijze et al., 2020). Critical thinking demands reflection in and on practice.

Educationalists have long recognised the importance of reflection. As noted in 1933, reflection provides the opportunity to continually evolve, challenge self-beliefs, values, and judgements that may, consciously or unconsciously, influence one's critically thinking and ultimately decision-making (Dewey, 1933). Midwifery drew on nursing's reflective models until 2017. In 2017, Bass et al. (2017) developed a six-phase model of midwifery holistic reflection as an educational tool to facilitate student midwives transformative learning. Critical thinking and decision-making are by default part of the Bass et al. model (Bass et al., 2017) as one needs to utilise critical thinking when reflecting and make a decision on how this awareness integrates and transforms oneself. Midwives in Australia are required to undertake 'ongoing processes of reflection to ensure professional judgements acknowledge how personal culture impacts on practice' (Nursing and Midwifery Board of Australia, 2018, p. 3). Student midwives in Australia must also demonstrate their capability in evaluating, monitoring, and reflecting on practice as part of their continuing professional development in the work integrated learning (WIL) environment (Australian College of Midwives, 2018). Consequently, student midwives are familiar with reflection and seek it in their mentors behaviour as well as, together, having time to reflect on their practice (Ball et al., 2022). Student midwives want their mentors to role model specific knowledge, skills, and behaviours and to share their professional wisdom (Bogren et al., 2022; Bradford et al., 2022). It is through creating an educational environment and undertaking such, mentor facilitated, activities student midwives explore and form their professional identity (Neiterman et al., 2023).

It is not surprising therefore reflection is evidenced in the UK Standards of Proficiency for the Midwife (Nursing and Midwifery Council, 2024) Standard 5.9 which denotes midwives *must contribute to team reflection activities to promote improvements in practice and service*, whilst Standard 6.88 notes midwives must '*reflect on own thoughts and feelings ...*' (p. 59). In Australia, critical reflection is noted in Standard 3.4 of the NMBA Midwife Standards for Practice (2018).

Educator

The next concept is that a mentor is an educator. Student midwives are the future workforce, so it is imperative midwives take on the role of educator within the clinical environment. The ICM (2021b) note the role of a clinical preceptor/teacher who is:

> ... an experienced midwife engaged in the practice of midwifery who is competent and willing to teach students in the clinical setting. A preceptor/clinical teacher works closely with the student midwife to provide

guidance, training, support, assessment, evaluation, and constructive feedback, and serves as a role model for the student midwife... Noting: Some programmes/schools use the term "clinical mentor." For the purposes of these standards, the clinical mentor should meet this definition ....

(p. 2)

Yet, in the ICM Essential Competencies for Midwifery excel toolkit (2024), there is no reference to the requirement of a midwife to take on the role of clinical preceptor/teacher/mentor. This exclusion is mirrored in some country's regulatory documents. Whilst the UK Standard 6.85 (Nursing and Midwifery Council, 2024) the words 'teaching and student' are noted and in Australia Midwife Standards for Practice: Standard 3.4 a midwife must *'contribute to a culture that supports learning, teaching, knowledge transfer ...'* (Nursing and Midwifery Board of Australia, 2018). However, such inclusions do not necessarily make a midwife a good educator (mentor) with the ability to teach and/or share one's knowledge and wisdom. Nevertheless, demonstrating appropriate educational strategies to promote learning including teaching and assessment skills are what student midwives wish to see mentors exhibit (Bogren et al., 2022; Neiterman et al., 2023). Further students want an educational learning environment whereby mentors provide protected time, effective formal and informal learning opportunities and hands on experiences where they can be effectively supervised and motivated to move from having embryonic clinical skills through to full integration of knowledge and skills (Ball et al., 2022; Nespoli et al., 2024). By mentors creating such a learning environment, it may help reduce the anxiety of clinical assessments, increase confidence and competence, promote the midwifery philosophy, and encourage students to become the guardians of normal physiological birth in the future.

Personal

One could suggest being professional and being educator are learnt skills, whilst the personal attributes a mentor requires are more innate. The word *'mid-wife'* means being with woman and as midwives we care for women, their babies, and the family however they define it. Consequently, words like compassion, empathy, emotional intelligence, approachability, nurturing, and kindness could be applied when considering a midwife's personal attributes. In 2020 displaying good interpersonal skills, conduct based on dignity and respect, trust empathy, emotional support, and continuous informational support were found to be important characterises of compassionate midwifery care in study undertaken on Facebook (Krause et al., 2020). Patience, flexibility and creativity, tolerance, and acceptance were noted in a Latvian study in 2024 exploring what their professional identity as a midwife meant (Ansule et al., 2024). What this list of personal attributes demonstrates is, irrespective of where a midwife practises midwifery they will possess some if not all of these personal attributes.

It is logical; therefore, the above personal attributes should or could transfer into the role of midwife mentor. This is important when considering how students perceive mentors as role models, someone to aspire to be (Nieuwenhuijze et al., 2020), someone to learn from, someone to help develop their confidence and competence (Nespoli et al., 2024), and professional identify (Sheehan et al., 2022).

Environment

Midwifery education has two elements, theory, and clinical practice or work integrated learning (WIL). Both are equally important, and both are critical in facilitating a positive learning environment for the student. It is vital for mentors to create a supportive WIL environment that positively impacts on a student's learning as the WIL environment has multiple influencing factors that can change daily or even hourly. It could be suggested a contributing element may be the dynamics between health professionals. It is widely acknowledged within history, midwifery and childbirth became medicalised and technocratic (Davis-Floyd, 2001; Willis, 1983). Over time midwifery became a profession is its own right, yet the dominance of obstetrics on a midwife's autonomy can impact one's feelings of confidence and competence and thus consciously or unconsciously control how one practices midwifery (Zolkefli et al., 2020). Further contributing to this is that the medicalisation of childbirth remains the dominant paradigm. The medical lens of risk and intervention is juxtaposed to the midwifery lens of birth being a normal physiological event (Davis-Floyd & Sargent, 2023). Navigating this tension may be difficult for a midwife as well as challenging for a student midwife to observe. Furthermore, teaching a student to be a midwife in this environment can hinder the students' understanding of their scope of practice as a midwife. Consequently, the model of care and the midwives' ability to work to their full scope of practice plays an important part in student's learning with midwifery led care having demonstrated benefits for the woman, the midwife, and the student (Evans et al., 2020; Sandall et al., 2015).

A fundamental role of a mentor, therefore, is to work collaboratively with medical colleagues to reduce any hierarchical or power differences (McKellar & Graham, 2017; Nespoli et al., 2024). By role modelling authoritative knowledge grounded within the philosophy of midwifery and understanding of physiological birth will positively impact student midwives learning experience, self-efficacy and how they wish to practice once qualified (Folkvord & Risa, 2023; Norris & Murphy, 2020). The environment, or workplace culture, in which the midwife works, teaches, and mentors, is impacted by and influences the personal attributes of the midwife. The next chapter explores the midwifery environment and the barriers and facilitators to mentoring.

REFLECTIVE ACTIVITY 2 MIDWIFERY WORKPLACE ENVIRONMENT

Reflect on the midwifery setting in which you currently work, and answer the following questions:

1 Is your midwifery workplace predominantly technocratic or woman-centred?
2 Does the workplace culture impact on your role as a mentor – if so, how and why?
3 Is there anything you do to 'protect' a student from the perceived workplace culture – if so, what and why?

Conclusion

In this chapter, we have explored some of the professional and personal attributes a mentor should role model. Through this role modelling, mentors become someone who shares their wisdom and demonstrates the philosophy of midwifery through the woman-centred care they provide. This is paramount as students begin to develop their professional identify. These mentors become someone midwifery students wish to aspire to, be someone to learn from, someone to help develop their confidence and competence. We have also explored the impact an environment, or workplace culture, in which the midwife works, teaches, and mentors within can consciously or unconsciously influence care.

References

Ansule, I., Flemming, V., & Millere, I. (2024). To be a midwife in Latvia – Midwives talking - pilot study. *Heliyon, 10,* e32504. https://doi.org/10.1016/j.heliyon.2024.e32504

Australia, N. M. B. (2018). *Midwife Standards for Practice.* Nursing and Midwifery Board of Australia.

Australian College of Midwives. (2018). *Australian Midwifery Standards Assessment Tool.* Australian College of Midwives. Retrieved 8 July 2024 from https://midwives.org.au/Web/Web/Professional-Development/AMSAT/Australian_Midwifery_Standards_Assessment_Tool.aspx

Australian College of Midwives. (2024). *Australian College of Midwives: Philosophy Statement for Midwifery.* Australian College of Midwives. Retrieved 1 July from www.midwives.org.au

Ball, K., Peacock, A., & Winters-Chang, P. (2022). A literature review to determine midwifery students' perceived essential qualities of preceptors to increase confidence and competence in the clinical environment. *Women and Birth, 35,* e211–e220. https://doi.org/10.1016/j.wombi.2021.06.010

Bass, J., Fenwick, J., & Sidebotham, M. (2017). Development of a model of holistic reflection to facilitate transformative learning in student midwives. *Women & Birth*, *30*, 227–235. https://doi.org/10.1016/j.wombi.2017.02.010

Benner, P. (1984). *From Novice to Expert, Excellence and Power in Clinical Nursing.* Addison-Wesley Publishing Company.

Bogren, M., Alesö, A., Teklemariam, M., Sjöblom, H., Hammarbäck, L., & Erlandsson, K. (2022). Facilitators of and barriers to providing high-quality midwifery education in South-East Asia—An integrative review. *Women & Birth*, *35*(3), e199–e210. https://doi.org/10.1016/j.wombi.2021.06.006

Bradford, H., Hines, H. F., Labko, Y., Peasley, A., Valentin-Welch, M., & Breedlove, G. (2022). Midwives mentoring midwives: A review of the evidence and Best practice recommendations. *Journal of Midwifery & Women's Health*, *67*(1), 21–30. https://doi.org/10.1111/jmwh.13285

Carter, A. M. S., & Creedy, D. K. (2022). International consensus definition of critical thinking in midwifery practice: A Delphi study. *Women and Birth*, *35*, e590–e597.

Davis-Floyd, R. (2001). The technocratic, humanistic, and holistic paradigms of childbirth. *International Journal of Gynecology & Obstetrics*, *75*(1), S5–S23. https://doi.org/10.1016/S0020-7292(01)00510-0

Davis-Floyd, R., & Sargent, C. (2023). *Childbirth and Authoritative Knowledge: Cross-Cultural Perspectives.* California Press.

Dewey, J. (1933). *How We Think: A Restatement of the Relation of Reflective Thinking to the Educative Process.* Health and Company.

Ebert, L., Levett-Jones, T., & Jones, D. C. (2019). Nursing and midwifery Students' sense of connectedness within their learning communities. *Journal of Nurse Education*, *58*(1), 47–52. https://doi.org/10.3928/01484834-20190103-08

Ebert, L., Massey, D., Flenady, T., Nolan, S., Dwyer, T., Reid-Searl, K., Ferguson, B., & Jefford, E. (2022). Midwives' recognition and response to maternal deterioration: A national cross-sectional study. *Birth*. https://doi.org/10.1111/birt.12665

Evans, J., Taylor, J., Browne, J., Ferguson, S. K., Atchan, M., Maher, P., Homer, C., & Davis, D. (2020). The future in their hands: Graduating student midwives' plans, job satisfaction and the desire to work in midwifery continuity of care. *Women & Birth*, *33*, E59–66. https://doi.org/10.1016/j.wombi.2018.11.011

Folkvord, S., & Risa, C. (2023). Factors that enhance midwifery students' learning and development of self-efficacy in clinical placement: A systematic qualitative review. *Nurse Education in Practice*, *66*, 103510. https://doi.org/10.1016/j.nepr.2022.103510

Hishinuma, Y., Horiuchi, S., & Yanai, H. (2016). Factors defining the mentoring competencies of clinical midwives: An exploratory quantitative research study in Japan. *Nurse Education Today*, *36*, 330–336. https://doi.org/10.1016/j.nedt.2015.08.024

International Confederation of Midwives. (2019). *Essential Competencies for Midwifery Practice.* International Confederation of Midwives. Retrieved 27 June from https://internationalmidwives.org/resources/essential-competencies-for-midwifery-practice/

International Confederation of Midwives. (2021a). *Global Standards for Midwifery Education* (pp. 1–11) Published by International Confederation of Midwives Netherlands, Accessed 11 June 2026. https://internationalmidwives.org/wp-content/uploads/global-standards-for-midwifery-education_2021_en.pdf

International Confederation of Midwives. (2021b). *Global Standards for Midwifery Education* (pp. 1–31). International Confederation of Midwives.

International Confederation of Midwives. (2023). *International Definition of the Midwife.* 1. Retrieved 27 June 2024, from https://internationalmidwives.org/resources/international-definition-of-the-midwife/

International Confederation of Midwives. (2024). *Essential Competencies – Self-Assessment Tool: Education, Essential Competencies.* International Confederation of Midwives. https://internationalmidwives.org/wp-content/uploads/ICM-V.1.0-Essential-Competencies-Assessment-guide-2024-EN-29112024-1.pdf

Jefford, E. (2012). *Optimal Midwifery Decision-Making during 2nd Stage Labour: The Integration of Clinical Reasoning into Practice* [Research, Southern Cross University].

Jefford, E., Alonso, C., & Stevens, J. R. (2019). Call us midwives: Critical comparison of what is a midwife and what is midwifery. *International Journal of Childbirth*, *9*(1), 39–50. https://doi.org/10.1891/2156-5287.9.1.39

Jefford, E., Jomeen, J., & Martin, C. (2016). Determining the psychometric properties of the enhancing decision-making assessment in midwifery (EDAM) measure in a cross cultural context [Research]. *BMC Pregnancy And Childbirth*, *19*, 95–106. https://doi.org/10.1186/s12884-016-0882-3

Jefford, E., Nolan, S., & Jomeen, J. (2020). Is the concept of midwifery abdication evident in Australian case law? A systematic review of legal literature, Court/Tribunal decisions, and coronial findings. *International Journal of Childbirth*, *10*(4), 217–223. https://doi.org/10.1891/IJCBIRTH-D-20-00038

Johndon, W., & Riley, C. (2018). *The Elements of Mentoring.* St. Martin's Press.

Krause, S., Minnie, C., & Knobloch Coetzee, S. (2020). The characteristics of compassionate care during childbirth according to midwives: A qualitative descriptive inquiry. *BMC Pregnancy & Childbirth*, *20*(1), 10. https://doi.org/10.1186/s12884-020-03001-y

McKellar, L., & Graham, K. (2017). A review of the literature to inform a best-practice clinical supervision model for midwifery students in Australia. *Nurse Education in Practice*, *24*, 92–98. https://doi.org/10.1016/j.nepr.2016.05.002

Mclukie, C., & Kuipers, Y. (2024). Discursive constructions of student midwives' professional identities: A discourse analysis. *Nurse Education in Practice*, *74*, 103847. https://doi.org/10.1016/j.nepr.2023.103847

Neiterman, E., Beggs, B., HakemZadeh, F., Zeytinoglu, I., Geraci, J., Plenderleith, J., & Lobb, D. (2023). Can peers improve student retention? Exploring the roles peers play in midwifery education programmes in Canada. *Women & Birth*, *36*(4), e453–e459. https://doi.org/10.1016/j.wombi.2023.02.004

Nespoli, A., Sacco, G. G. A., Bouhachem, F. Z., Motta, F., Paredi, S., Antolini, L., Panzeri, M., Pellegrini, E., & Fumagalli, S. (2024). Assessment of the psychometric properties of the Italian version of the midwifery student evaluation of practice (MIDSTEP-IT): A validity and reliability study. *Midwifery*, *133*, N.PAG-N.PAG. https://doi.org/10.1016/j.midw.2024.103991

Nieuwenhuijze, M., Thiompson, S., Gudmundsdottir, E., & Gottfreosdottir, H. (2020). Midwifery students' perspectives on how role models contribute to becoming a midwife: A qualitative study. *Women and Birth*, *33*, 433–439. https://doi.org/10.1016/j.wombi.2019.08.009

Norris, S., & Murphy, F. (2020). A community of practice in a midwifery led unit. How the culture and environment shape the learning experience of student midwives. *Midwifery*, *86*, 102685. https://doi.org/10.1016/j.midw.2020.102685

Nursing and Midwifery Board of Australia. (2018). *Midwife Standards for Practice.* Canberra: Nursing and Midwifery Board of Australia.

Nursing and Midwifery Board of Australia, A. (2021). *Supervision Guidelines for Nursing and Midwifery* (pp. 1–9). Nursing and Midwifery Board of Australia.

Nursing and Midwifery Council. (2019). *Standards of Proficiency for Midwives.* Nursing and Midwifery Council. Retrieved June 19, 2007 from https://www.nmc.org.uk/globalassets/sitedocuments/standards/2024/standards-of-proficiency-for-midwives.pdf

Rooke, N. (2014). An evaluation of nursing and midwifery sign off mentors, new mentors and nurse lecturers' understanding of the sign off mentor role. *Nurse Education in Practice, 14*(1), 43–48. https://doi.org/10.1016/j.nepr.2013.04.015

Sandall, J., Soltani, H., Gates, S., Shennan, A., & Devane, D. (2015). Midwife-led continuity models versus other models of care for childbearing women. *Cochrane Database of Systematic Reviews, 4*(4), CD004667. https://doi.org/10.1002/14651858.CD004667.pub6

Sheehan, A., Elmir, R., Hammond, A., Schmied, V., Coulton, S., Soresen, K., Arundell, F., Keedle, H., Dahlen, H., & Burns, E. (2022). The midwife-student mentor relationship: Creating the virtuous circle. *Women and Birth, 35*, E512–E520. https://doi.org/10.1016/j.wombi.2021.10.007

Stephenson, S., Kemp, E., Kiraly-Alvarez, A., Costello, P., Lockmiller, C., & Parkhill, B. (2023). Self-assessments of mentoring skills in healthcare professions applicable to occupational therapy: A scoping review. *Occupational Therapy in Health Care, 37*(4), 606–626. https://doi.org/10.1080/07380577.2022.2053923

Willis, E. (1983). *Medical Dominance: The Division of Labour in Australian Health Care.* George Allen and Unwin.

Zolkefli, Z., Mumin, K., & Idris, D. (2020). Autonomy and its impact on midwifery practice. *British Journal of Midwifery, 28*(2), 120–129.

6

MENTORING AS A PROFESSIONAL SUPPORT STRATEGY

Lyn Ebert

Introduction

Last chapter we examined mentoring through the lens of four concepts that can impact mentoring capabilities in the healthcare environment. The concepts identified were professional, educational, personal (Hishinuma et al., 2016), and workplace environment. In this chapter, we will explore more closely the environment, or workplace culture, in which the midwife works, teaches, and mentors. We will consider the factors that impact midwives' ability to have a sense of professional autonomy, confidence, and belongingness, which in turn can impact their ability to mentor the next generation of midwives. Next, we will look at how these issues can hinder or enhance the midwifery workforce: staff retention rates, job satisfaction, organisational productivity, and health outcomes. Finally, we investigate mentoring, a strategy often recommended as a means to improve the issues negatively impacting the midwifery workplace culture that either encourages or discourages midwives from mentoring.

The Midwifery Workplace Culture and Ability to Mentor

Midwives are often viewed as the lead providers of care for women throughout the childbirth continuum and transition to parenthood. To provide woman-centred care and facilitate the woman's choice and control over their birthing care options, midwives need to be confident and competent in their practice (Bedwell et al., 2015). Deery and Fischer (2017) argue that woman-centred care is less likely to transpire in midwifery workplace contexts characterised by patriarchal traditions and technical

DOI: 10.4324/9781003533733-7

competencies. That is, environments where workplace culture and conflict exist both intra-and inter-professional and professional dissonance is present. Moreover, woman-centred care is conditional on relationships which are reciprocal and mutually respectful of all parties. Bedwell and colleagues' (2015) study reported on factors affecting midwives' confidence in intrapartum care. The authors found that a practitioner's confidence in their practice can be fragile and that an acrimonious workplace culture and conflict are critical factors in diminishing a midwife's confidence. Conversely, a sense of professional autonomy was found to enhance confidence, with the most influential factor affecting midwives' confidence being their colleagues.

Confidence in one's midwifery practice impacts clinical competence, decision-making, and capacity to share knowledge with, or mentor, others. One study (Abdelkader et al., 2021) exploring students' self-confidence and competence reported that confidence is one of the important determinants of successful learning and therefore capability to manage a clinical situation or provide care in an accurate, relevant, and efficient method. However, participants (students) in this study voiced that "*their clinical educators had a high level of teaching abilities, competencies, and personal traits. Moreover, significant positive relationships existed between self-confidence in learning and the clinical educators' characteristics*" (Abdelkader et al., 2021, p. 1). This finding was echoed in an earlier study by Hecimovich and Volet (2011) who maintained that the development of professional confidence is enhanced when clinical practice is guided or supported in the workplace context. In other words, one's ability to develop professional confidence is influenced by the person attempting to teach, or facilitate, clinical competence and professional confidence. If the mentor or teacher lacks professional self-confidence, they are unlikely to facilitate self-confidence in their mentee. As discussed above, the issues impacting a midwife's ability to develop confidence in their practice are multifactorial. The next section looks at midwives' ability to achieve a sense of professional belongingness and collegiality, essential for confidence, competence, and the capacity for mentoring.

Belongingness and Job Satisfaction

Belongingness is understood to be "*the experience of personal involvement in a system where an individual feels valued, needed, and in alignment with the values or goals of a larger social group*" (Silver et al., 2024). That the relationship within the group, or sense of belongingness, is greater than simple membership. Before we look more closely at the concept of Belongingness in the healthcare context we will discuss why Belongingness, or group membership, plays a role in job satisfaction, retention, and potentially improved workplace outcomes.

The inherent desire to be accepted as part of a group encourages those who wish to belong to conform to the stated (laws and policies) and unstated (cultural behaviours) rules of the group. The motivation to comply, or conform, with group rules ensures a higher chance of being accepted as same or included in the group, with rejection or acceptance psychologically powerful motivators. Furthermore, when one confirms to the group norms, their likelihood of gaining group approval, being accepted, building social connections, and increasing self-esteem and confidence is improved (McClunie-Trust et al., 2024). Job satisfaction, staff retention, and attrition rates directly correlate with employees' sense of belonging, the social climate, and workplace connections acquired within the workplace environment (Bilginoğlu & Yozgat, 2023). With a positive workplace culture, increased staff satisfaction and retention of experienced staff, organisational productivity, and the working towards beneficial organisational goals increases (Radu, 2023).

When viewing healthcare organisational goals, one would assume that their goals align with the provision of safe and quality care. Furthermore, the care provided would be efficient in terms of resources, evidence-based, and result in improved patient (women and baby) health outcomes and satisfaction with care. Organisational efficiency in relation to resources, includes human resources or employees. High turnover of staff or low staff morale, which decreases workplace productivity is both inefficient but also perpetuates low productivity (Reeves, 2024). Without experienced staff to mentor new staff and build workplace connections through socialisation, the cycle of low workplace morale and high attrition is likely to continue.

While the terms group socialisation, belongingness, and conformity have been discussed in other literature and contexts, it came to the forefront in health care, and specifically nursing, through the work of Levett-Jones et al. (2007). The work of Levett-Jones and colleagues reported similar findings to those in psychology, finance, and the manufacturing industries. That is, a sense of belonging within the healthcare team is critical to a positive and productive learning experience. The definition of Belongingness attributed to the nursing context was, *"the need to be and perception of being involved with others at differing interpersonal levels … which contributes to one's sense of connectedness (being part of, feeling accepted, and fitting in), and esteem (being cared about, valued and respected by others)"* (p. 163). This early work explored the experiences of students undertaking their work-integrated learning (WIL) placements, as part of their undergraduate nursing degree. The authors concluded that welcoming, accepting, and supportive workplace environments that foster connectedness and intra-professional relationships facilitate a perception of being valued and respected as a member of the group.

The extent to which students achieve a sense of professional belongingness correlates with their ability to learn, their level of motivation, their satisfaction with placement experience, and, potentially, their future career decisions. Although contextual factors and interpersonal dynamics in the workplace can impact a student's experience, and therefore, ability to make connections, and achieve a sense of belongingness, the provision of consistent, quality mentorship can positively facilitate the student's feeling of connectedness (Levett-Jones et al., 2007). The authors recommend all students be provided with one, if not two mentors, to support integration and professional socialisation into the healthcare team. While the authors imply challenges exist in providing mentorship, they do not identify the specific challenges. Later, in the chapter, challenges associated with mentoring are discussed.

Belongingness was also examined within the student midwife context some years later. McKenna et al. (2013) used a tool adapted by Levett-Jones et al. (2009), previously used with nursing students to measure belongingness. McKenna and colleagues surveyed sixty undergraduate midwifery students from two campuses at one Australian university and found similar findings to those of Levett-Jones and colleagues. That is, *"environments where midwifery students feel they belong and are valued, are necessary to facilitate effective clinical learning"* (2013, p. 881). These authors reported that students perceived they belonged when *"they received recognition, challenge, and support through mentoring by staff. Furthermore, it was only when students felt a sense of belonging that they could focus on learning"* (McKenna et al., 2013, p. 881)

Registered or accredited healthcare professionals also experience workplace stress, professional burnout, and a sense of being undervalued. These factors can lead to career disruption and/or early exiting from their career. In 2011, Sullivan et al. published the results of a study examining the factors that led midwives to stay or leave the profession. Data were obtained from 209 midwives employed in one health service in Australia. The authors found that midwives' motivation to stay in the profession was achieved through *"having a positive outlook, having job satisfaction, and having... a sense of belonging"* (2011, p. 331). Job satisfaction was achieved when midwives believed they had made a positive difference in the care women receive and experienced positive interactions with women. Sullivan and colleagues advocate that health services consider these issues and create the conditions that enable midwives to achieve job satisfaction. They suggest, *"addressing the way care is arranged and how staff are supported may lead to higher retention rates, thus reducing costs"* (2011, p. 335).

Findings from Sullivan et al.'s study in 2011 were reinforced in 2023 when a systematic review exploring midwives' job satisfaction and related factors reported similar outcomes. Moradali et al. (2023) reviewed 23 articles encompassing 3,352 midwives. The systematic review found that job satisfaction was higher in those environments outside, or removed from, the medicalised model often found in maternity settings in hospitals. Again, close relationships and connectedness with colleagues increased job satisfaction, while conflict in the workplace environment was associated with decreased job satisfaction. The authors recommended health services implement strategies that promote professional belongingness and occupational health, and optimise midwifery models of care, allowing midwives to work in ways that align with their professional values (Moradali et al., 2023).

It is not only midwives in the healthcare environment that experience decreased job satisfaction when they are unable to work to their full scope of practice and work in ways that align with their professional values. Agarwal et al. (2020) examined professional dissonance and burnout in 26 primary care practitioners (PCP) in the USA. The term burnout can be described as a work-related syndrome characterised by emotional exhaustion, depersonalisation, and a sense of reduced accomplishment, which negatively impacts the healthcare worker's physical and emotional wellbeing and productivity as well as patient care. Participants in this study expressed dissatisfaction that their jobs involved a reduced ability to work with their clients and increased administrative or task-type work. This resulted in professional dissonance between their professional philosophical values and the values of the organisation in which they were employed. Computer technology and data entry requirements seemed to pull the practitioners away from, what they saw as direct care. They saw their core work as being undervalued by the local organisation and the broader healthcare system. Participants voiced that high workload minimised their ability to undertake activities they perceived as critical to their professional identity and high-quality patient care. The authors concluded that reduced job satisfaction led to higher staff turnover and that strategies should be put in place to improve staff retention and job satisfaction, foster cultural change in the workplace, and create strong leadership.

Professional or Value Dissonance

Value dissonance as described by Buss and Arnold (2023) is the experienced conflict between divergent values. For midwifery, the conflict may occur between organisational values and the workplace culture, and the underpinning values of the midwifery profession (woman-centredness, mutual respect, the midwife–woman partnership, and the midwifery continuity of care model of practice). Buss and Arnold claim emotional distress can result when the workplace values and reality differ from professional values and undermines professional identity. The impact of value dissonance is greater when professional integrity and/or autonomy is compromised, occasioning "job dissatisfaction, burnout, and feelings of low levels of empowerment" (2023, p. 4).

A workplace environment where professional identity is dampened, and conflicting value systems exist hinders midwives' abilities to lead and support the professional development of self and others (Deery & Fisher, 2017). In

Maternity services, there is an increasing focus on *"quantifiable targets, efficiency savings and rationalisation of service delivery…[with] increased use of protocols, guidelines and directives"* (Deery & Fischer, 2017, p. 144). These authors assert that maternity care is becoming guideline-centred rather than woman-centred. This environment impacts midwives' ways of working and it is argued that practice-based leadership is required to mentor midwives to navigate the system and maintain professional or value cohesiveness. Deery and Fischer describe a practice-based leader as one who emanates their own professional values and beliefs, fostering positivity in the workplace, thus influencing the group's beliefs, values, and behaviours within the workforce. Regardless of the leadership model, maternity units require midwifery leaders, with effective clinical decision-making skills, critical thinking capabilities, and competent reflective practitioners to ensure the midwifery workplace culture, regardless of the setting, remains woman-centred and technologically competent. Leadership and mentoring are discussed further in Chapter 3 while reflective practice and its application to mentoring is discussed in earlier chapters.

As integrated maternity services grow with the aim of providing cohesive maternity care for women with either low- or high-risk pregnancies, strong midwifery leadership may be even more crucial in supporting midwifery models of care and facilitating quality woman-centred care. Kristienne McFarland et al. (2020) undertook a qualitative meta-synthesis of the literature exploring the effect on the midwifery processes of care in integrated maternity settings and the experiences of midwives. The authors concluded that *"increasing medicalisation occurring in integrated maternity practices minimizes the profession of midwifery, and the ability to provide evidence-based quality midwifery care"* (p. 1) resulting in professional dissonance. These findings were comparable to those of Curtin et al. (2022) who undertook a meta-synthesis of the experiences of healthcare professionals (HCPs) on the humanisation of childbirth. Curtin and colleagues' review involved 14 studies and 197 participants, including clinical midwives, midwifery managers, midwifery academics, student midwives, nurse–midwives, nurses, obstetric–nurses, birth attendants, obstetricians, doctors, paediatricians, an anaesthetist, and healthcare administrator. The settings ranged from birth centres through to highly specialised university-affiliated hospitals. Curtin et al. reported that healthcare professionals wanted to build relationships with birthing women where the women were central to decision-making and had a choice and a voice. However, this was not always possible, especially when technology and/or interventions were thought to be required to provide a safe birth. The *"use of technology as an intervention was thought to remove women from the focus of care, shifting the focus HCPs and their ability to provide task-oriented care"* (p. 375). This resulted in professional dissonance for those whose professional ideologies aligned with a humanistic birth approach. The three defining attributes of the term humanism (in the context of childbirth) include Human Being Interaction, encompassing "communication, attentiveness, sensitivity, encouragement and collaboration" (Curtin et al., 2020, p. 1747); Benevolence, the desire to be kind and or do good for others; and Being a Protagonist, that is, someone who advocates for the woman so she can maintain a level of control and decision-making throughout her birth (Curtin et al., 2020). Curtin and colleagues argue that humanisation of childbirth should not be considered in opposition to the biomedical model of childbirth, and it supports the practice of care that focuses on the interactions between the woman and her healthcare provider(s) regardless of the level of care required. While midwives may recognise the needs of the woman, it can be difficult to respond to those needs in the presence of a techno-medicalised workplace culture, giving rise to 'professional dissonance'.

REFLECTIVE ACTIVITY 1 MIDWIFERY WORKPLACE CULTURE AND VALUE DISSONANCE

Reflect on the midwifery setting in which you currently work, and answer the following questions:

1 Is your midwifery workplace woman-centred or guideline-centred?
2 How are clinical decisions made in your unit? Is the woman involved?
3 Are you practising midwifery the way you the envisioned when you were a student?
4 Have you changed your views on 'midwifery work' and being 'with-woman' since entering the midwifery workforce? If so, why?
5 Do you believe you experience professional dissonance? (provide rationale)

Mentoring As a Strategy

Not only is mentoring portrayed as supporting the individual midwife's professional development, career projection, and capacity to learn in the workplace environment, but it is also understood to improve maternal health outcomes. Renfew (2021) reports that investing in and valuing the professional development of staff will retain highly experienced and skilled midwives, reducing maternal and neonatal deaths. As discussed in the next section, the term 'mentoring' and the elements of the mentoring relationship or role can vary in different healthcare models and healthcare contexts. Wissemann et al. (2022) describe mentoring as a relationship that involves an educated/experienced health professional who is assisting another, with less education or experience.

In New South Wales (NSW), Australia, a pilot study was undertaken to implement and evaluate a program titled: Mentoring in Midwifery (MIM) (Lennon et al., 2023). The MIM program was aimed at developing reciprocal learning relationships to expand the opportunities for connection, learning, growth, and support for midwifery students and midwives working in NSW maternity services. The findings from the study determined that mentoring relationships had the potential to rejuvenate, and nurture both mentors and mentees. The mentors and mentees developed a stronger sense of belonging, safety, and professional accomplishment. The authors propose that mentoring can support the retention of a strong, confident, and skilled midwifery workforce. For more information on the MIM program, see Section III *Mentoring, Leadership and Education in Practice*: Australia Chapters 24 and 25. Another study undertaken in Australia (Sheehan et al., 2023), evaluating the implementation of a midwifery mentoring program concluded that the *"mentoring program increased midwives' mentoring skills and was beneficial to their professional growth and leadership skills. Students equally reported positive outcomes, including someone to talk to, emotional support and a sense of belonging"* (p. 2).

A small study, involving five mentors from one health service in the United Kingdom (UK) (Moran & Banks, 2016), explored what value midwifery mentors place on their role as a mentor, and their perceived value of mentorship in midwifery practice. In this study, the mentors were designated 'sign-off' mentors. The sign-off midwife is responsible for the formal assessment and clinical progression of students throughout their midwifery program. While the sign-off mentors' role may vary from other models of mentoring, their experiences were similar. The mentors in this study *"appreciated their role and knew that it was an essential one. They expressed enjoyment from being part of the students' educational program, and ...felt valued by other mentors who understood the role and its attached responsibilities"* (p. 54). Like other studies, however, the mentors voiced they did not always feel valued by the mentees (students) or management. They also voiced a lack of appropriate mentoring training programs resulted in a lower number of mentors to support students. This combined with often high workloads and a stressful work environment negatively impacted their experience of, and ability to mentor.

From the mentee or students' perspective, mentorship, specifically continuity of the mentor–mentee relationship was found to enhance learning and clinical practice experiences (Hallam & Choucri, 2019). This literature review exploring student midwives' experiences of continuity of mentorship on the labour ward included eight articles originating from studies undertaken in Norway (n = 1), Australia (n = 1), and the UK (n = 6). Findings revealed that *"students who received continuity were likely to experience a sense of 'belonging' and 'connectedness' to the clinical area and this was thought to be necessary for an optimal learning experience"* (Hallam & Choucri, 2019,

p. 116). Conversely, a lack of continuity during initial placements results in a failure to connect with the placement area and potentially effects student progression in their studies. Although the literature review focused on student midwives' perspectives, the authors included data from midwifery mentors as well. Mentors voiced similar experiences as others in saying mentoring can be demanding on time and emotional resources. These midwives recommended team mentoring and peer support as a strategy to ensure sustainability (Hallam & Choucri, 2019).

Midwife mentors suggested team mentoring, where the student has a small number of mentors would maintain the students' sense of belonging, expose the students to other members of the multidisciplinary team, enhance team dynamics and cohesion, and enable mentors to have a break from the intensity associated with mentoring students.

While studies discuss the challenges faced with implementing and sustaining mentoring programs in the midwifery context, findings report, participants overwhelmingly espouse the values of mentoring. A study in one regional university in Australia, involving 39 third-year Bachelor of midwifery students and 39 registered midwives, providing clinical supervision, reported on what is valued and considered important within the mentoring relationship (Jefford et al., 2021). Findings from this study demonstrated that what is important for mentoring to reach its full potential is for both the mentee and mentor to express **goals and attributes** that "*demonstrate passion and enthusiasm, promote a sense of self-worth and mutual respect, be receptive and act as active participants in a reciprocal interaction*" (p. 3). Caring conversations and use of respectful and considered language within the interactions will **inspire communication**, facilitating effectual learning experience. When effective listening and interpretation and observation, with appropriate and timely responses, occur, a sense of self-worth and mutual respect is fostered. This supports a workplace culture where a **sense of safety and belonging** can exist. For these values to be embedded within the mentee–mentor relationship as well as the midwifery culture time is required (see Figure 6.1), that is, time to trust the process, each other, and feel safe with the outcomes. The authors concluded the development of trust was facilitated by having continuity of mentor/mentee. This supported the scaffolding of safe learning where mistakes could be made without loss of self-worth or a sense of professional belonging.

"*Learning to be a midwife, irrespective of where one is located around the world involves complex relational processes pertaining to professional and organisational socialisation*" (Jefford et al., 2021, p. 6). This process is best achieved through mentoring (or support) by midwives who demonstrate passion for the profession, enthusiasm, and receptiveness to shared learning, and promote mutually respectful interactions. Sustaining these characteristics can, however, be difficult in the maternity care environment. The barriers and facilitators to maintaining a workplace culture that values mentoring is discussed next.

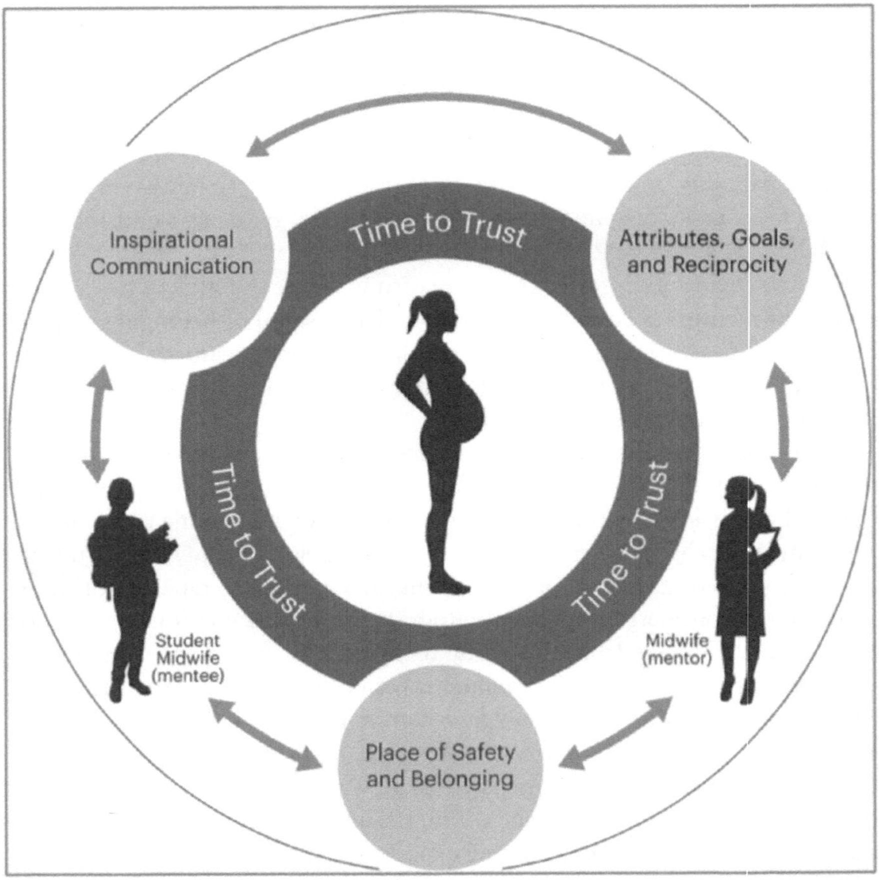

FIGURE 6.1 Requirements for positive mentoring relationship. Source: Jefford et al. (2021)

Barriers and Facilitators to Mentoring

Lack of job satisfaction, stress, burnout, and limited managerial support contributes to midwifery workforce attrition and the ongoing global shortage of midwives with mentoring portrayed as one way to improve staff retention, job satisfaction, and reduce burnout. Although the benefits of mentoring have been publicised (Hallam & Choucri, 2019; Lennon et al., 2023; Moran & Banks, 2016; Sheehan et al., 2023), less is known about the midwife mentors' perspectives and challenges they may perceive as hindering their ability to support new and less experienced midwives. In 2022, Wissemann et al. published an integrative review with the aim to understand midwives' perspectives of mentoring programs to influence the development of future midwifery-specific mentoring programs. With a clear understanding of what midwives need in relation to mentoring programs, the strategy mentoring is more likely to achieve its proposed benefits, that is, improved staff retention, job satisfaction, and increased workplace professional congruence.

For this review, the authors agreed the term 'mentoring' would encompass other frequently used terms, such as supervising, coaching, precepting, assessing, and guiding, which refer to *"the nature of an educated/experienced health professional who is assisting a midwife who has less education or experience"* (p. 2). The review included eight studies from which four themes were developed, relevant to mentoring in midwifery:

1 **Mentoring in midwifery facilitates effective learning and development.** Mentoring achieves this through providing the mentee with learning moments occurring by means of "relational and action processes and through feedback gleaned through reflection and debriefing" (p. 3). It has been claimed that capitalising on education and retention of highly proficient and experienced midwives could avert maternal and neonatal deaths globally (World Health Organisation [WHO], 2019).
2 **Mentoring positively impacts clinical and organisational outcomes.** Mentoring can realise this goal through providing a conductive climate to engage and ask questions, leading to the improvements in clinical practice. This in turn supports health service outcomes and productivity.
3 **Positive mentoring experiences are dependent on the relationships built between the mentee, mentor, and the organisation.** This theme highlighted the inability to choose one's own mentor, conflicts of interest when the mentor was the midwife in charge, and lack of accessibility to their mentor, when needed, impacted the relationship and therefore the capability for relational learning. Consequently, the positive impacts of mentoring, effective learning, and improved clinical and organisational outcomes are negated.
4 **Mentoring is not prioritised by midwives or their workplaces.** This finding highlighted the same issues that mentoring is championed as a cure for. That is, "toxic workplace culture, workplace shortages and increasing workloads" (p. 9) similarly prevent midwives from being able to implement and sustain mentoring. Additionally, lack of managerial support and lack of appropriate mentors further hindered the ability to create a midwifery workforce, supported through mentoring. In three of the included studies, midwives voiced that, "they had no time to undertake the process [of mentoring], viewing it as another commitment alongside increasing demands from the workplace" (p. 9).

The review emphasised that although clear benefits to mentoring exist, there are challenges that need to be addressed before mentoring programs are sustainable and seen as truly beneficial for all, including midwifery mentors.

For this to happen, organisations will need to value the midwifery workforce and strategies, such as mentoring, aimed at supporting midwives' learning, teaching, and professional development, as well as their clinical competencies. An approach to mentoring that may facilitate relationships is ensuring midwives can choose their own mentors. The authors concluded that *"midwives' ability to choose their own mentor outside the workplace reduced the issue of conflict of interest, highlighting that professional power can be detrimental to the mentor–mentee relationship"* (p. 9). A conflict of interest, or values, referred to in the context of midwifery mentoring may denote value incongruence or dissonance; when the mentor's values are aligned with the organisation (organisation-centred care) and the mentees are aligned with the woman or midwifery philosophy (woman-centred care).

Conclusion

In this chapter, we explored the environment, or workplace culture, in which the midwife works, teaches, and mentors. We examined the factors that impact midwives' sense of professional autonomy, confidence, and belongingness, which in turn impacts their ability to mentor the next generation of midwives. It became clear that the global shortage of midwives can be attributed, in part, to a lack of job satisfaction, stress, burnout, and limited managerial support. While many organisations, reports, and studies portray mentoring as a strategy to alleviate the negative issues impacting the midwifery workplace, there is a lot to be done in the way of supporting midwives to become a mentor. Value must be ascribed to mentoring programs through adequate education, resources, time, and recognition of midwives undertaking the role. Midwifery professional and accrediting bodies, healthcare organisations and services, as well as midwifery management must prioritise mentoring. Until mentoring is valued within the midwifery workplace, with adequate resources and recognition of the midwives undertaking the role, the implementation of mentoring programs is at risk of failing.

Further Readings

Fiabane, E., Dordoni, P., Setti, I., Cacciatori, I., Grossi, C., Pistarini, C., & Argentero, P. (2019). Emotional dissonance and exhaustion among healthcare professionals: The role of the perceived quality of care. *International Journal of Occupational Medicine & Environmental Health*, 32(6), 841–851. https://doi-org.ezproxy.scu.edu.au/10.13075/ijomeh.1896.01388

McNamara, M. S., Fealy, G. M., Casey, M., et al. (2014). Mentoring, coaching and action learning: Interventions in a national clinical leadership development programme. *Journal of Clinical Nursing*, 23(17–18), 2533–2541.

Roseghini, M., & Olson, S. (2015). What do midwives think about midwifery supervision? *British Journal of Midwifery*, 23(9), 660–664.

Silver, M. A. (2024). PCP's call to action: Addressing professional dissonance in primary care. *Journal of General Internal Medicine, 39*, 318–319. https://doi-org. ezproxy.scu.edu.au/10.1007/s11606-023-08368-0

Swain, M. S., Gliedt, J. A., de Luca, K., Newell, D., & Holmes, M. (2021). Chiropractic students' cognitive dissonance to statements about professional identity, role, setting and future: International perspectives from a secondary analysis of pooled data. *Chiropractic & Manual Therapies, 29*(1), 1–10. https://doi-org.ezproxy.scu. edu.au/10.1186/s12998-021-00365-6

References

Abdelkader, A., Saad, N., & Abdelrahman, S. (2021). The relationship between self-confidence in learning and clinical educators' characteristics by nursing students. *International Journal of Nursing Education, 13*, 1. https://doi.org/10.37506/ijone. v13i2.14614

Agarwal, S. D., Pabo, E., Rozenblum, R., & Sherritt, K. M. (2020). Professional dissonance and burnout in primary care: A qualitative study. *JAMA Internal Medicine, 180*(3), 395–401. https://doi-org.ezproxy.scu.edu.au/10.1001/jamainternmed.2019.6326

Bedwell, C., McGowan, L., & Lavender, D. T. (2015). Factors affecting midwives× confidence in intrapartum care: A phenomenological study. *Midwifery, 31*(1), 170–176. https://doi.org/10.1016/j.midw.2014.08.004

Bilginoğlu, E., & Yozgat, U. (2023). Retaining employees through organizational social climate, sense of belonging and workplace friendship: A research in the financial sector. *Istanbul Business Research, 52*(1), 67–85. https://doi.org/10.26650/ ibr.2023.52.806695

Buss, J., & Arnold, D. (2023). Communicative action, a path through the dissonance between nursing and corporate healthcare values. *Nursing Inquiry, 30*(4), 1–8. https://doi-org.ezproxy.scu.edu.au/10.1111/nin.12581

Curtin. (2022). A meta-synthesis of the perspectives and experiences of healthcare professionals on the humanisation of childbirth using a meta-ethnographic approach. *Women and Birth, 35*(4), e369–e378. https://doi.org/10.1016/j.wombi.2021.07.002

Curtin, M., Savage, E., & Leahy-Warren, P. (2020). Humanisation in pregnancy and childbirth: A concept analysis. *Journal of Clinical Nursing, 29*(9–10), 1744–1757. https://doi.org/10.1111/jocn.15152

Deery, R., & Fisher, P. (2017). Professionalism and person-centredness: Developing a practice-based approach to leadership within NHS maternity services in the UK. *Health Sociology Review, 26*(2), 143–159. https://doi.org/10.1080/14461242. 2016.1159525

Hallam, E., & Choucri, L. (2019). A literature review exploring student midwives' experiences of continuity of mentorship on the labour ward. *British Journal of Midwifery, 27*(2), 115–119. https://doi-org.ezproxy.scu.edu.au/10.12968/ bjom.2019.27.2.115

Hecimovich, M., & Volet, S. (2011). Development of professional confidence in health education: Research evidence of the impact of guided practice into the profession. *Health Education, 111*(3), 177–197. DOI: 10.1108/09654281111123475.

Hishinuma, Y., Horiuchi, S., & Yanai, H. (2016). Factors defining the mentoring competencies of clinical midwives: An exploratory quantitative research study in Japan. *Nurse Education Today, 36*, 330–336. https://doi.org/10.1016/j.nedt.2015.08.024

Jefford, E., Nolan, S., Munn, J., & Ebert, L. (2021). What matters, what is valued and what is important in mentorship through the appreciative inquiry process of co-created knowledge. *Nurse Education Today, 99*, N.PAG. https://doi-org.ezproxy. scu.edu.au/10.1016/j.nedt.2021.104791

Kristienne McFarland, A., Jones, J., Luchsinger, J., Kissler, K., & Smith, D. C. (2020). The experiences of midwives in integrated maternity care: A qualitative meta-synthesis. *Midwifery*, *80*, N.PAG. https://doi-org.ezproxy.scu.edu.au/10.1016/j.midw.2019.102544

Lennon, M. K., Tierney, M. O., Cook, M. M., & Roddy, E. (2023). O37 – The meaningful magic of mentoring: Evaluation findings from NSW health mentoring in midwifery program...Australian College of Midwives National Conference – Be the Change, September 12–14, 2023, Adelaide, South Australia. *Women & Birth*, *36*, S15. https://doi-org.ezproxy.scu.edu.au/10.1016/j.wombi.2023.07.039

Levett-Jones, T., Lathlean, J., Higgins, I., & McMillan, M. (2009). Development and psychometric testing of the belongingness scale – Clinical placement experience: An international comparative study. *Collegian*, *16*(3), 153–162.

Levett-Jones, T., Lathlean, J., McMillan, M., & Higgins, I. (2007). Belongingness: A montage of nursing students' stories of their clinical placement experiences. *Contemporary Nurse: A Journal for the Australian Nursing Profession*, 24(2), 162–174. https://doi-org.ezproxy.scu.edu.au/10.5172/conu.2007.24.2.162

McClunie-Trust, P., Jarden, R., Marriott, P., Winnington, R., Dewar, J., Shannon, K., Jones, S., Jones, V., Turner, R., Cochrane, L., & Macdiarmid, R. (2024). Graduate entry nursing students' development of professional nursing self: A scoping review. *International Journal of Nursing Studies*, *151*, 104670–104670. https://doi.org/10.1016/j.ijnurstu.2023.104670

McKenna, L., Gilmour, C., Biro, M. A., McIntyre, M., Bailey, C., Jones, J., Miles, M., Hall, H., & McLelland, G. (2013). Undergraduate midwifery students' sense of belongingness in clinical practice. *Nurse Education Today*, *33*(8), 880–883. https://doi-org.ezproxy.scu.edu.au/10.1016/j.nedt.2012.09.009

Moradali, M. R., Hajian, S., Majd, H. A., Rahbar, M., & Entezarmahdi, R. (2023). Job satisfaction and its related factors in midwives working in the health services system in Iran: A systematic review. *Journal of Midwifery & Reproductive Health*, *11*(2), 3650–3662. https://doi-org.ezproxy.scu.edu.au/10.22038/JMRH.2023.64824.1890

Moran, M., & Banks, D. (2016). An exploration of the value of the role of the mentor and mentoring in midwifery. *Nurse Education Today*, *40*, 52–56. ISSN 0260-6917. https://doi.org/10.1016/j.nedt.2016.02.010

Radu, C. (2023). *Fostering a Positive Workplace Culture: Impacts on Performance and Agility*. In A. A. V. Boas. (Ed.). Human Resource Management - An Update. https://doi.org/10.5772/intechopen.111166. Accessed July 10, 2024.

Reeves, M. (2024). *Impact of Staff Turnover on Organizational Culture: A Guide for L&D*. Available from: https://www.togetherplatform.com/. Accessed July 10, 2024.

Renfew, M. J. (2021). Scaling up care by midwives must now be a global priority. *Lancet Global Health*, *9*(1), e2–e3.

Sheehan, A., Dahlen, H. G., Elmir, R., Burns, E., Coulton, S., Sorensen, K., Duff, M., Arundell, F., Keedle, H., & Schmied, V. (2023). The implementation and evaluation of a mentoring program for bachelor of midwifery students in the clinical practice environment. *Nurse Education in Practice*, *70*, N.PAG. https://doi-org.ezproxy.scu.edu.au/10.1016/j.nepr.2023.103687

Silver, J. K., Fleming, T. K., Ellinas, E. H., Silver, E. M., Verduzco-Gutierrez, M., Bryan, K. M., Flores, L. E., & Sarno, D. L. (2024). Individual, organizational, and policy strategies to enhance the retention and a sense of belonging for health care professionals in rehabilitation medicine. PM & R. https://doi.org/10.1002/pmrj.13152

Sullivan, K., Lock, L., & Homer, C. S. E. (2011). Factors that contribute to midwives staying in midwifery: A study in one area health service in New South Wales, Australia. *Midwifery*, *27*(3), 331–335. https://doi.org/10.1016/j.midw.2011.01.007

Wissemann, K., Bloxsome, D., De Leo, A., & Bayes, S. (2022). What are the benefits and challenges of mentoring in midwifery? An integrative review. *Women's Health, 18,* 174550572211101–17455057221110141.

World Health Organisation (WHO), United Nations International Children's Emergency Fund International (UNICEF) Confederation of Midwives (ICM), United Nations Population Fund (UNFPA). (2019). *Strengthening Quality Midwifery Education for Universal Health Coverage 2030: Framework for Action.* Licence: CC BY-NC-SA 3.0 IGO. Available from: https://www.who.int/publications/i/item/9789241515849 Accessed July 16, 2024.

7

MENTORSHIP AS AN INCLUSIVE METHOD FOR PROFESSIONAL LEARNING AND DEVELOPMENT

Riza Kadilar

What Is the European Mentoring and Coaching Council (EMCC)

EMCC Global is a leading international professional body dedicated to advancing excellence in mentoring, coaching, and supervision. In an era characterised by digital transformation, shifting workplace dynamics, and evolving societal needs, EMCC Global aspires to be the go-to organisation, shaping a future where these practices significantly contribute to personal development and corporate success. Since 1992, EMCC Global has expanded from its European roots to become a globally recognised organisation with a strong presence in over 140 countries. Through our extensive network of Country and Region Affiliated Boards, we have provided high-standard accredited education and training programmes to over 60,000 graduates, which are esteemed worldwide. Our mission is to cultivate thriving environments for individuals and organisations by prioritising well-being, leadership, continuous learning, distributive leadership, and reflective practices. This commitment ensures that our members are well-equipped to excel in an ever-changing landscape marked by tech-driven change, dynamic work shifts, and new societal needs.

In an era of rapid change and unprecedented challenges, leadership, mentoring, coaching, and supervision have never been more essential in fostering societal resilience, adaptability, and innovation. EMCC Global, therefore, aims to ignite transformative change by harnessing the collective expertise and our forward-thinking vision together with every member of our community and with policymakers, professionals, and partners from around the globe. Our journey is central to cultivating excellence and transforming futures. We embrace the complexities of modern challenges through strategic alignment

DOI: 10.4324/9781003533733-8

and proactive action. In that respect, EMCC Global calls upon international policymakers and stakeholders to support and reinforce the frameworks that underpin our areas of expertise. By advocating for improved policies and frameworks, we can continue to shape a future where leadership, mentoring, coaching, and supervision are acknowledged as foundational to a dynamic, informed, and thriving human-centred society. Every leader's participation and partnership are critical in this effort, paving the way towards a future where professional development and societal advancement are seamlessly intertwined. We can begin an era marked by profound professional impact and widespread mental well-being.

The role and vision of EMCC are discussed in more detail later in the chapter.

The Meaning of Mentoring

The power of mentoring lies in the transfer of knowledge and skills and in cultivating personal effectiveness. One's position or authority does not solely determine effective leadership; it is a product of self-awareness, emotional intelligence, and the ability to inspire and empower others. Mentoring offers a unique platform for honing these essential qualities, equipping individuals with the tools to thrive as leaders in our rapidly changing world.

As per EMCC Global,

> Mentoring is a learning relationship involving the sharing of skills, knowledge, and expertise between a mentor and mentee through developmental conversations, experience sharing, and role modelling. The relationship may cover various contexts and is an inclusive two-way partnership for mutual learning that values differences.
>
> *(2025a)*

Through the mentor's non-judgemental stance and contextual wisdom-sharing dialogue, individuals are exposed to diverse perspectives, enabling them to broaden their horizons and challenge their assumptions. Mentoring fosters a deep curiosity, encouraging mentees to explore uncharted territories and embrace innovation. In this dynamic relationship, mentors provide a safe space for mentees to experiment, learn from their failures, and develop resilience. Furthermore, mentoring transcends traditional boundaries, reaching beyond the confines of hierarchical structures. It thrives in shared humanity, where wisdom flows both ways, creating a mutually beneficial exchange of knowledge and experience. Mentoring ignites a flame of compassion, empathy, and connection, bridging the gaps between generations, cultures, and backgrounds. Through these meaningful connections, mentoring catalyses personal and professional growth, profoundly transforming lives Kadilar and Balkan 2016).

Mentoring: A Conceptual and Practical Framework

Mentoring is a developmental relationship that facilitates sharing skills, knowledge, and expertise between a mentor and a mentee through developmental conversations, experience sharing, and role modelling.

This relationship is characterised by:

- Valuing Differences: Respecting and leveraging the unique backgrounds and perspectives of the mentor and mentee.
- Mutual Learning: Fostering a two-way exchange of knowledge and insights.
- Contextual Adaptability: Encompassing various situational contexts to address individual needs.
- Inclusivity: Creating a partnership that values and integrates diverse perspectives.

Notably, mentoring refrains from debate, negotiation, or argument. Instead, it fosters a non-judgemental dialogue in which the aim is not persuasion but shared understanding (Clutterbuck and Megginson 1999).

The Role of Dialogue in Mentoring

Mentoring is a unique form of interaction that relies heavily on dialogue: a process that fosters understanding, growth, and collaboration. It stands apart from debate or discussion, offering a more inclusive and transformative approach to communication.

While often used interchangeably, debate, discussion, and dialogue hold distinct meanings and outcomes:

1 **Debate** involves holding a fixed point of view and attempting to convince others of its correctness. This approach often entrenches existing beliefs, creating resistance to change rather than openness to new perspectives.
2 **Discussion** entails having an outcome in mind while being willing to consider and accept other viewpoints. While discussion may lead to modest shifts in perception and compromise, it rarely fosters profound change or mutual commitment.
3 **Dialogue,** by contrast, is characterised by an open-minded approach to issues. It aims to understand diverse perspectives and potentially co-create new ways of thinking. Dialogue often results in a more profound commitment and a genuine willingness to embrace change.

Mentoring employs dialogue at a higher level than almost any other workplace activity. This emphasis on dialogue fosters a reflective and inclusive environment where both mentor and mentee can engage meaningfully. To truly embody the spirit of dialogue in mentoring, the following principles are essential:

- **Create a supportive environment:** Begin with a setting that encourages calm, thoughtful, and creative engagement. A safe and non-judgemental atmosphere sets the tone for productive conversations.
- **Practice active listening:** Prioritise understanding the other person's thoughts and perspectives over formulating your own responses. This level of attentiveness builds trust and encourages openness.
- **Respect differing viewpoints:** Seek to uncover the reasoning and experiences underlying someone else's perspective, even if it differs from your own.
- **Be open to learning:** Expect every conversation to offer valuable insights and opportunities for growth.
- **Challenge assumptions:** Be willing to examine your thinking as rigorously as you would challenge others. This self-reflective approach ensures that dialogue remains balanced and respectful.
- **Allow for reflection:** Embrace moments of pause during conversations to give yourself and others time to reflect. Silence can often lead to greater clarity and deeper understanding.

Dialogue serves as the foundation for meaningful connections and transformative learning experiences in mentoring. It shifts the focus from persuading or winning to fostering mutual understanding, collaboration, and growth. By practising authentic dialogue, mentoring becomes a powerful personal and professional development tool.

Historical Perspective of Mentoring

As a concept, mentoring has evolved significantly over the centuries, shaped by cultural, social, and historical contexts which are discussed in Chapter 1, so what follows is a brief summary. The origins of the term "mentor" can be traced back to Homer's The Odyssey, where the mentor was entrusted with guiding Telemachus during Odysseus' absence. Despite modern interpretations that depict the mentor as nurturing and developmental, scholars such as Garvey (2017) argue that the original story was more a narrative of violence and vengeance than care and learning. Athene, the goddess of wisdom, ultimately took on the mentor role to prepare Telemachus for a violent confrontation, underscoring the aggressive undertones of the original tale.

In the medieval period, mentoring was often associated with the relationships between knights, squires, craftspersons, and apprentices. Unlike today's perspective, historical accounts reveal that these systems were frequently exploitative and characterised by harsh conditions and rigid hierarchies.

Apprentices, for instance, were often legally bound to their master's and subjected to considerable abuse, undermining this era's idealised notions of mentorship.

The evolution of mentoring took a more structured and developmental turn in the eighteenth century, mainly through the work of François Fénelon. His book, *Les Adventures de Télémaque*, introduced principles that resonate with modern mentoring practices, such as learning through practical experiences, reflective dialogue, and positive feedback. Fénelon's work influenced prominent thinkers like Rousseau and Montesquieu, embedding mentoring within educational and leadership development frameworks. The term "mentor" entered the French and English languages during this period, symbolising guidance, and personal growth.

According to Garvey, mentoring gained prominence in literature and organisational structures in the nineteenth and early twentieth centuries. For example, Lord Chesterfield referenced mentoring in his letters, and the Mentor Association was established in the United States in 1912 to promote knowledge-sharing among men. Around the same time, Ernest Coulter founded the Big Brothers mentoring organisation to support boys transitioning out of the justice system. This model evolved into Big Brothers Big Sisters of America by 1977. These developments laid the groundwork for mentoring as a structured practice aimed at personal and professional development.

The late twentieth century saw a significant expansion of mentoring, particularly in organisational and academic contexts. Research such as Levinson's Seasons of a Man's Life (1978) highlighted mentoring's role in accelerating personal development. Similarly, David Clutterbuck's Everyone Needs a Mentor (1985) brought mentoring into the UK, distinguishing between the US model of career sponsorship and the European focus on learning and development. Over time, mentoring practices diversified across sectors and regions, reflecting cultural variations in their application. For instance, mentoring in China emphasises the "passing on of wisdom" while aligning with Soviet-era professional supervision practices in Eastern Europe.

Mentoring has also become integral to the health and social care sectors. In health, mentoring programs such as the United Kingdom's National Institute for Health and Care Research (NIHR) initiatives provide structured professional and leadership development support. Participants report outcomes such as increased confidence, improved decision-making, and enhanced work-life balance. These programs demonstrate mentoring's capacity to address complex social challenges while promoting personal growth. Modern mentoring programs share several common principles, including clear purpose definition, rigorous evaluation, and structured training for mentors. Matching mentors and mentees based on compatibility and shared goals is also critical to their success. Additionally, ongoing support for mentors helps maintain the quality and impact of these relationships. Many mentoring arrangements emphasise voluntarism, reflecting a commitment to the intrinsic value of mentorship rather than its commodification.

Principles of Mentoring

Mentoring operates on several foundational principles:

1 **Reflective Practice:** Reflective practice is a cornerstone of effective mentoring, emphasising not just the events that occur but the lasting impact these events have on an individual's emotions, cognition, and actions. This practice involves creating a safe space for the mentee to explore and articulate the internal shifts triggered by their experiences. Through reflective dialogue, mentees gain deeper insights into the "residues" left by these experiences – the emotions, thoughts, and realisations that influence their future decisions. Reflective practice also encourages a forward-looking approach, asking mentees to consider how their reflections can inform their future actions. This approach helps mentees identify patterns, uncover hidden assumptions, and cultivate greater self-awareness. The mentor's role in reflective practice is to facilitate this exploration through open-ended questions and empathetic listening, guiding the mentee to articulate their thoughts and feelings without imposing judgement or solutions. Furthermore, reflective practice integrates the concept of the "paradox of change," which suggests that meaningful transformation occurs when individuals fully acknowledge and accept their current state. By honouring the resistance to change as a natural part of the growth process, reflective practice helps mentees navigate transitions with greater resilience and clarity. It is not about fixing problems immediately but understanding their roots and implications, enabling mentees to approach their challenges confidently and purposefully.
2 **Active Agency:** Mentoring aims to empower mentees to transition from passive observers to active agents of their own lives. This involves fostering a mindset where the mentee takes responsibility for their reactions and approaches to circumstances rather than attributing outcomes to external factors.
3 **Empathy and Non-Judgement:** Mentoring distinguishes between emotional and cognitive empathy. While emotional empathy may lead to biases, cognitive empathy involves understanding another's perspective without judgement. For instance, in challenging situations, the mentor supports the mentee by metaphorically "sitting in the dark" with them rather than attempting to immediately "turn on the light."
4 **Present-Centred Focus:** Mentoring prioritises the present moment over unresolved past issues or uncertain future concerns. The emphasis is on how past and future influences shape the mentee's actions.

5 **Issue-Oriented Guidance:** The mentor's role is to guide the mentee in gaining clarity and new perspectives on their issues. The focus is not on solving the mentee as a person or prescribing solutions to their challenges.

6 **Avoidance of Direct Advice:** Mentoring discourages the mentor from offering advice to which they may become personally attached. Instead, if advice is deemed necessary, it is shared with permission and framed to inspire rather than dictate actions. For instance, a mentor might preface advice: "This may resonate differently for you, but here is an idea to consider…"

Situational Roles of a Mentor

A mentor may assume various roles based on the mentee's needs:

- Coach: Poses questions that encourage new perspectives.
- Storyteller: Shares anecdotes to inspire and guide.
- Discussion Partner: Engages in dialogues that challenge the mentee and provide constructive feedback.
- Advisor: Offers professional insights without imposing personal ownership of the solutions.
- Knowledge Sharer: Provides access to relevant expertise as required.
- Network Builder: Assists the mentee in creating and leveraging professional connections.
- Guardian: Offers career guidance and strategic advice.
- Encourager: Motivates and supports the mentee through challenges Kadilar and Balkan (2016).

Evolving EMCC Mentoring Competencies

EMCC Global (EMCC 2025a) identifies eight key competencies essential for effective mentoring and coaching:

1 Understanding Self: Awareness of personal strengths, limitations, and areas for development.
2 Commitment to Self-Development: Continuous learning and professional growth.
3 Managing the Contract: Establishing clear agreements about the mentoring/coaching process and expectations.
4 Building the Relationship: Creating a trust-based, collaborative relationship with the mentee.
5 Enabling Insight and Learning: Facilitating the mentee's ability to gain new perspectives and understanding.
6 Outcome and Action Orientation: Helping the mentee focus on achieving specific goals and actions.

7 Use of Models and Techniques: Employing appropriate frameworks, tools, and methodologies.
8 Evaluation: Continuously assessing the effectiveness of the mentoring/coaching relationship and outcomes.

A recent comprehensive unpublished study by EMCC Global has collected substantial evidence based on feedback from various leading practitioners and academicians. It has been suggested the addition of two new competencies, based on observed gaps in current practices.

Being a Role Model

This competency emphasises the mentor's intentionality in using their behaviour, experiences, and authenticity to positively influence the mentee. It includes demonstrating humility and acknowledging the two-way learning journey inherent in mentoring. Acknowledging the role of power dynamics in the mentor–mentee relationship and ensuring that the mentor avoids creating replicas of themselves.

Use of One's Professional Experience

This competency combines the skills of experience sharing and contextual understanding. Mentors are encouraged to use their professional wisdom to guide mentees in navigating specific ecosystems, understanding power structures, and addressing implicit cultural dynamics. The ability to judge when and how to offer contextual information (e.g., models, anecdotes, or observations) enriches the mentee's reflective process and decision-making abilities.

Rationale for the New Competencies

The suggested additions are rooted in the understanding that mentoring is distinct from coaching primarily because it relies on the mentor's ability to draw on personal experiences and contextual insights. These competencies recognise that:

• Role Modelling: Mentors influence mentees through context sharing and embodying behaviours and attitudes that mentees can observe and adapt. Authenticity, coupled with humility, fosters deeper connections and learning opportunities.
• Contextual Application of Experience: Sharing professional knowledge appropriately and tailoring it to the mentee's context enables more meaningful, actionable mentoring. This competency ensures that the mentoring process adapts to diverse challenges and environments, enhancing its relevance.

Both competencies enrich the mentoring process by incorporating elements that enhance mutual learning, provide practical insights, and adapt to mentees' evolving needs. These recommendations distinguish further mentoring from coaching while maintaining EMCC's commitment to evidence-based practices (EMCC 2025b).

Mentoring and Inclusive Leadership in a Transforming World

Leadership practices are profoundly transforming in a world characterised by rapid change, emerging technologies, and evolving paradigms. Evidence suggests that inclusive leadership, underpinned by collaboration, empathy, and systemic thinking, is essential for navigating the complexities of modern organisational environments. By fostering trust and inclusion, leaders can enable their teams to adapt to challenges and seize opportunities for growth and innovation.

Historically, leadership has often been associated with command-and-control models that prioritise hierarchical decision-making. However, research by Dhiman (2017) indicates a shift towards more holistic, human-centric approaches. This evolution is particularly evident in leadership development frameworks that emphasise reflective practices, emotional intelligence, and collaborative strategies. The transition from transactional leadership to transformational paradigms highlights the importance of engaging stakeholders across diverse organisational contexts. Kadilar and Balkan (2016) have also demonstrated the significant role of mentoring and coaching in fostering leadership development. When aligned with human-centric models such as Gestalt and positive psychology, these practices provide actionable insights for addressing resistance to change and promoting a growth mindset. Such frameworks encourage leaders to approach challenges as opportunities for innovation and learning.

The modern business environment is shaped by constant disruptions, new business models, and emerging technologies. This landscape necessitates a paradigm shift in leadership. Strategy and research (PricewaterhouseCoopers (PwC) 2025) identifies six paradoxes of leadership, illustrating the dual expectations placed on contemporary leaders. For instance, leaders must balance humility with heroism, adopt a strategic yet executor mindset, and integrate technological proficiency with humanistic values. These paradoxes suggest that leadership today demands navigating both ends of a spectrum. The transition from linear to systemic thinking underscores the growing importance of addressing interconnected challenges. Questions such as "What does the world of tomorrow expect from leadership today?" and "Whose voices are not being heard?" frame the evolving expectations of leadership in addressing global issues.

The Role of Inclusion in Organisational Dynamics

Kadilar (2024) highlights the critical role of inclusion in shaping team dynamics and overall organisational performance. Inclusive environments are those where individuals feel valued, respected, and safe to express themselves. Kadilar (2024) has shown that fostering such conditions leads to enhanced motivation, higher productivity, and more substantial organisational commitment. Inclusion also aligns with contemporary perspectives on workplace collaboration. It is recognised that collaboration involves not only sharing resources but also co-creating visions, power, and accountability. Organisations can create mutual learning and growth spaces by prioritising non-judgemental dialogue and developmental mentoring programs. EMCC Global believes developmental mentoring as an inclusive partnership that facilitates sharing knowledge, skills, and expertise through reflective conversations and role modelling.

Overcoming Barriers to Inclusion

Despite the recognised benefits, barriers to inclusion persist in many organisational contexts. Kadilar (2024) identifies unconscious biases, privileges, and systemic inequalities as primary obstacles. For example, privileges often manifest in design choices, workplace norms, and access to opportunities favouring certain groups. Recognising and addressing these barriers is a critical step toward fostering inclusive environments. One practical approach to overcoming these challenges is through curiosity-driven inquiry. By cultivating an attitude of curiosity, individuals can challenge their biases and adopt a growth mindset. This perspective not only supports the dismantling of systemic barriers but also enhances organisational resilience and adaptability.

Practical Strategies for Building Inclusive Cultures

Building an inclusive culture requires deliberate action and sustained effort. It could be suggested the following strategies are particularly effective:

1 Empowering Dialogue: Establishing open and non-judgemental communication channels encourages trust and collaboration among team members.
2 Implementing Mentoring Programs: Structured mentoring initiatives provide opportunities for mutual learning and reinforce the principles of inclusivity.
3 Aligning Organisational Goals: Focusing on shared objectives fosters a sense of unity and purpose among diverse stakeholders.
4 Promoting Empathy: Cognitive empathy, which involves understanding others' perspectives, has strengthened team cohesion and collaboration.
5 Facilitating Co-Creation: Involving employees in decision-making ensures that diverse voices are heard and valued.

Embedding Inclusivity into Organisational Values

Emerging technologies, such as artificial intelligence and digital platforms, present challenges and opportunities for inclusive leadership. While these tools enable personalisation, global reach, and accessibility, they also risk perpetuating biases if not thoughtfully implemented. The importance of incorporating diverse perspectives into the design and application of technological solutions to ensure inclusivity is warranted. Furthermore, inclusive leadership practices must evolve to address the ethical implications of technology. This involves fostering digital literacy, questioning potential biases, and leveraging AI-driven insights to expand access and equity within organisations. Leaders can amplify their impact by approaching technology as a collaborator rather than a replacement for human effort.

It must move beyond superficial measures to ensure that inclusivity becomes integral to organisational culture. It is important to note the pitfalls of performative inclusivity, which focuses on outward appearances rather than meaningful change. Instead, organisations must embed inclusivity into their core values and practices. This requires mechanisms to align values across teams, integrate new cultural perspectives, and foster a sense of belonging. In this context, leadership is less about directing individuals and more about nurturing relationships within the system. Leaders can create environments that reflect true inclusivity by listening to organisational dynamics and empowering individuals to take action.

The Role and Vision of EMCC Global

The goal of building a human-centred society can be achieved by fostering an environment in which individuals and organisations can thrive. EMCC actions are grounded in the following core beliefs:

1 **Empowering Well-being and Leadership:** We prioritise comprehensive individual growth, integrating mental well-being and leadership development to empower individuals at all levels. We provide opportunities for personal growth, emotional resilience, and leadership capabilities.
2 **Championing Upskilling and Reskilling:** We acknowledge shifting work dynamics and societal changes and commit ourselves to lifelong learning. Our educational and training programmes endorse ongoing workforce upskilling and reskilling efforts.
3 **Integrating Human-Centred Practices:** We commit to a human-centred society by embracing diversity and inclusivity, recognising the importance of personal connections, and appreciating each individual's unique contributions.

4 **Fostering a Reflective and Resilient Society:** We envision a society where individuals are not only equipped to face the complexities of the modern world but are also empowered to reflect, learn, and grow from their experiences.

Challenges arise as frequently as opportunities in the dynamic landscape of leadership, mentoring, coaching, and supervision. EMCC Global views each challenge not as a barrier but as a catalyst for innovation and success. Here is how we transform potential obstacles into compelling opportunities for growth and development:

- Digital Transformation as a Pathway to Accessibility: Embracing technology allows us to develop new, flexible modes of engagement and learning, ensuring our practices are more adaptable, ethical, accessible, and impactful.
- Globalisation and Cultural Diversity as a Foundation for Richer Learning: By engaging with diverse perspectives, practices, and approaches, we deepen our understanding, enhance empathy, and foster a more holistic approach to leadership, mentoring, coaching, and supervision.
- The Evolving Nature of Work as an Opportunity for Continuous Development: By focusing on upskilling and reskilling, we prepare our community to meet future demands, ensuring resilience, adaptability, and continued relevance in a changing world.
- Environmental and Social Challenges as Catalysts for Ethical Leadership: Our commitment to ethical practice positions us to contribute meaningfully to sustainability and equity.
- Mental and Emotional Wellness as Priorities for a Supportive Community: EMCC Global sees this as an opportunity to prioritise mental well-being, integrate these considerations into our practice, and offer support beyond professional development.

EMCC Global continues exploring new teaching forms and assessing experiential learning specific to work-based contexts and collaborations with industry partners. Our international standards (EMCC 2025a and 2025b) for organisations set a global benchmark for Excellence, ensuring our commitment to quality and innovation in professional development is recognised worldwide. EMCC Global's commitment to lifelong learning is in line with the objectives of the European Commission's Pact for Skills. We catalyse the development of a robust global network of over 400 education and training providers worldwide, including leading universities, business schools, and corporate academies. Through these partnerships, EMCC Global embraced bespoke programs, micro-credentials, and individual learning accounts, facilitating countless opportunities for upskilling, reskilling, and personal growth.

This prepares individuals and organisations for future challenges and opportunities. Our dedication to supporting evidence-based research and innovation is evident in the substantial investment in research development grants. These initiatives have spurred advancements in leadership, mentoring, coaching, and supervision methodologies, enhancing effectiveness and cutting-edge practices.

EMCC Global extends its influence beyond the professional realm, addressing critical societal issues such as mental health, workplace well-being, and social equity. Through advocacy and outreach, we encourage organisations to adopt more inclusive, equitable, and sustainable practices. We call upon international policymakers and stakeholders to recognise and support leadership, coaching, mentoring, and supervision in fostering a resilient, adaptive, and innovative society. Our professional practice addresses key challenges, including digital transformation, workplace well-being, and lifelong learning. By backing our policy recommendations, policymakers and stakeholders can ensure this practice thrives and contributes positively to society and the global economy. The policy recommendations and actions of EMCC Global can, therefore, be summarised as follows.

Enhanced Support for Lifelong Learning

We urge policymakers to bolster programs and funding for lifelong learning, increasing access to personalised education and training pathways. These align with EMCC Global's commitment to continuous growth, adaptability, and work-based learning experiences.

Recognition of Professional Standards

Policymakers should formally acknowledge EMCC Global Accreditation Professional Practice Frameworks as benchmarks for excellence in leadership, mentoring, coaching, and supervision. This recognition harmonises quality and empowers practitioners globally.

Investment in Skills Development

Rapid digital transformation demands significant investment in skills development. We advocate for policy funds to support EMCC-aligned programs, which prepare the workforce for AI integration and dynamic shifts in the professional landscape.

Promotion of Mental Well-Being

Integrating leadership, mentoring, and supervision into workplace strategies cultivates environments that support mental and emotional wellness, enhancing societal engagement and productivity.

Support for Innovation in Professional Practice

Policymakers should incentivise partnerships that pioneer new methodologies, tools, and approaches to keep professional practices at the forefront of global innovation.

The support of international policymakers and stakeholders is critical in realising our vision for a society empowered by leadership and mentoring excellence. We can collectively foster a more resilient, inclusive, and thriving society by aligning efforts with global policy frameworks.

EMCC and Midwifery

Although started as a mentoring body, over time EMCC Global has also evolved in coaching and supervision. Having an inclusive stakeholder perspective by keeping a good balance between evidence-based researchers, practitioners, and beneficiaries of mentoring and coaching services, EMCC Global has witnessed remarkable growth and global reach during the last decade. During the same time, our community have witnessed a surge of mentoring initiatives all over the world including within midwifery. Although this is good news and encouraging, more and more questions have emerged around quality, ethical practice, and governance. As a solution to this growing concern, EMCC Global has developed standards that can be used across programmes to establish good practice and benchmarking between different programmes.

In that regard, the ISMCP (International Standards for Mentoring and Coaching Programmes, EMCC 2025b) accreditation adds both substance and credibility to programmes and bolsters internal business cases for individual development. The framework ensures (midwifery) programmes are designed to align with participant and business objectives under the professional umbrella of the EMCC Global standards and the Global Code of Ethics.

ISMCP offers a benchmarking tool for anyone who is willing to design and execute a midwifery-related mentoring programme. It's an independent accreditation awarded to organisations that design, deliver, and evaluate mentoring and/or coaching programmes in-house or externally. It is an integral and essential step to establishing the professional credibility and status of good (midwifery) mentoring and/or coaching programme management, ensuring programmes are thoughtfully designed and systematically managed. In that regard, ISMCP significantly contributes to the development of participants, strategic drivers of the organisation, and broader stakeholder objectives. Organisations applying the ISMCP framework also promote ethical standards. For example, governance can be supported by having identified a programme manager. EMCC Global offers a dedicated accreditation for programme managers as well. PMQA (Programme Managers Quality Award) and PMIA (Programme Managers Individual Accreditation) aimed to ensure the highest quality standards in the execution of (midwifery) mentoring programmes.

Another area where EMCC Global could offer a meaningful contribution to midwifery is continuous professional development for mentors. EMCC Global has developed standards of supervision for mentors. The definition offered by EMCC Global emphasises the role of supervision as encouraging the shared practice of reflection as an aid to learning. The aim is to determine what is working well and how different results can be achieved through reviewing and evaluating alternative approaches that improve the mentor's offering and safeguard their well-being. There are a number of successful examples in that regard – for instance, the U.K. National Institute for Health and Care Research. NIHR aims to develop a highly skilled academic research workforce capable of advancing the best research, which improves health and benefits for society and the economy in England and beyond. The NIHR provides postdoctoral Academy Members with career development support through its mentoring programme. The programme supports postdoctoral researchers from a broad range of professional and disciplinary contexts across our diverse health and social care communities to mentor others and to seek a mentor. For their mentoring programme framework, NIHR adopted the EMCC Global ISMCP as an overarching framework for the programme's design, implementation, and evaluation.

Another impressive example is Médecins Sans Frontières (MSF), referred to in English as Doctors Without Borders. MSF is an international humanitarian medical non-governmental organisation. Staff work in extraordinary circumstances within varying contexts, performing functions within roles that often stretch them personally and professionally. As part of the HR Development Strategy, back in 2011, they introduced their mentoring programme. MSF adopted the EMCC Global ISMCP as their programme framework and subsequently was accredited at the gold standard level.

Conclusion

In an era where change is the only constant, we are confronted with an ever-evolving landscape of challenges, opportunities, and complexities. Change has never been so fast and will never be so slow ever again in the future. The pace of technological advancements, global interconnectedness, and societal shifts is unprecedented. As we strive to adapt and thrive, the value of mentoring becomes increasingly apparent. It is a beacon of guidance, providing a trustworthy source of wisdom and support amidst turbulence.

When rooted in reflective practices, inclusivity, and a structured yet adaptable framework, mentoring emerges as a powerful personal and professional development tool. By valuing diversity, fostering empathy, and maintaining a present-centred focus, mentoring empowers individuals to navigate challenges and unlock their potential. These principles and competencies define effective mentoring relationships and offer a roadmap for fostering growth and innovation across diverse contexts.

The future of leadership is expected to be defined by convergence – the intersection of technology, humanity, and purpose. Leadership will increasingly prioritise collaboration, systemic thinking, and sustainability. Evidence points to the growing importance of curiosity, empathy, and resilience as foundational attributes for navigating the complexities of the modern world. As organisations adapt to emerging challenges, mentoring and inclusive leadership will play a pivotal role in fostering innovation, building trust, and creating sustainable value. By aligning leadership practices with broader societal goals, leaders can contribute to a future that is both equitable and transformative.

In the future, mentoring will continue evolving in response to societal needs. One emerging trend is blending mentoring and coaching practices, focusing on facilitating dialogue and sharing experiences. Group mentoring models are also gaining traction, expanding the scope of traditional dyadic relationships. While debates around the professionalisation and potential payment of mentors persist, the essence of mentoring remains rooted in its historical foundations of learning, development, and mutual support.

References

Cloverpop. Hacking Diversity with Inclusion Decision- Making. Sage.

Clutterbuck, D. (1985). Everyone Needs a Mentor. IPM.

Clutterbuck, D., & Megginson, D. (1999). Mentoring Executives and Directors. Butterworth-Heinemann.

Dhiman, S. (2017). Holistic Leadership: A New Paradigm for Today's Leaders. Palgrave Macmillan.

European Mentoring and Coaching Council. (2025a). Mentoring. Accessed January 2025. https://www.emccglobal.org/leadership-development/leadership-development-mentoring/

European Mentoring and Coaching Council. (2025b). International Standards for Mentoring and Coaching Programmes (ISMCP). Accessed 20 January 2025. https://www.emccglobal.org/accreditation/ismcp/

European Commission: Pact for Skills. Accessed 20 January 2024. https://employment-social-affairs.ec.europa.eu/policies-and-activities/skills-and-qualifications/working-together/pact-skills_en

Garvey, B. (2017). Philosophical origins of mentoring: The critical narrative analysis. In D. A. Clutterbuck, F. K. Kochan, L. G. Lunsford, B. Smith, N. Dominguez, & J. Haddock-Millar (Eds.) The SAGE Handbook of Mentoring (pp. 15–33). Sage. https://doi.org/10.4135/9781526402011.n2

Kadilar, R. (2024). The Contemporary Leader: The Value of Inclusion in Successful Leadership. Wiley.

Kadilar, R. & Balkan, O. (2016). Mentorluk: Birlik ve Bilgelik Sanatı. Kerasus.

Kochan, F., Lunsford, L. G., Smith, B., Dominguez, N., & Haddock-Millar, J. (Eds.) The SAGE Handbook of Mentoring (pp. 15–33). Sage.

PricewaterhouseCoopers (PwC). (2025). Six paradoxes of leadership defined. Accessed 28 January 2025. https://www.pwc.com/gx/en/issues/succeeding-in-uncertainty/six-paradoxes-of-leadership.html

8

MIDWIFERY MENTORSHIP IN ABU DHABI, UNITED ARAB EMIRATES

Maeve O'Connell

Background

The United Arab Emirates is experiencing a critical shortage of midwives (DoH, 2020; O'Connell & Sosa, 2023). According to the World Health Organisation (2024), the country reported a density of just 6.4 nurses and midwives per 1,000 residents in 2020. This figure falls below the threshold required to ensure effective healthcare delivery, as highlighted by the Abu Dhabi Health Authority (2010). Obstetric care in the UAE mirrors a similar system to that of the USA, with services largely shaped by its unique historical and demographical context. Founded just over 50 years ago following the discovery of oil, the UAE united the Trucial States of Arabia into a state of tolerance. Today, the UAE comprises seven emirates, with Dubai being the most well-known and Abu Dhabi serving as the capital city. A notable feature of the UAE is its predominantly expatriate population – over 11 million residents, compared to just over one million Emiratis. While Arabic is the official language, English is widely spoken due to the diverse demographic. As a Muslim-majority country, Shariah law governs Muslims, whereas non-Muslims adhere to their home country laws. Muslim men are allowed to practise polygamy and marry up to four wives. While the age of an Adult is 21 years old, the age of sexual consent is 18 years old and women may marry with the permission of their father or closest male relative (brother). Social policies, such as the marriage grant for Emiratis and mandatory premarital screening, aim to preserve cultural values and promote public health. These screenings test for genetic and communicable diseases, including HIV and Beta-Thalassemia, ensuring compatibility and health among prospective

DOI: 10.4324/9781003533733-9

couples. Recent reforms, such as the 2023 amendment to abortion laws, have increased women's autonomy and safeguarded their rights to make informed decisions by removing the 120-day limit, protecting the pregnant woman's life.

Historically, childbirth in the UAE was overseen by local women known as the *Qabila* or *Daya*, who used traditional practices like herbal remedies and Quranic readings. However, these unassisted births often led to complications, contributing to poor maternal and neonatal outcomes. The shift to hospital-based care, driven by healthcare privatisation and modernisation, dramatically improved maternal and newborn mortality rates – from 6:100,000 in 2020 to 3:100,000 in 2022 – placing the UAE among the world's leaders in maternal health.

This transformation was fuelled by visionary leadership, particularly Her Highness Sheikha Fatima bint Mubarak, the 'Mother of the Nation'. Her Highness has been a steadfast advocate for women's health and empowerment, authoring the Strategy for Motherhood and Early Childhood (2017), which emphasises the vital role of midwifery. This strategy integrates cultural sensitivity with international best practices, promoting education, professional recognition, and holistic care for women and newborns (Childhood, 2017).

Sheikha Fatima's leadership has been instrumental in developing the Strategy for Motherhood and Early Childhood (2017), a comprehensive framework that emphasises the importance of midwifery in achieving optimal maternal and child health outcomes. This vision has not only elevated the role of midwives but also nurtured a holistic approach to care, integrating cultural sensitivity with international best practices. By advocating for enhanced education, training, and professional recognition for midwives, Her Highness has paved the way for a robust and sustainable healthcare model that continues to benefit generations of mothers and children across the UAE.

Despite these advancements, maternity care in the UAE predominantly follows a biomedical model, where obstetric nurses and midwives operate under the supervision of obstetricians (O'Connell & Sosa, 2023). This model risks iatrogenic harm due to the extremes of 'too much, too soon' and 'too little, too late', as overmedicalisation can lead to adverse outcomes (Miller et al., 2016). High-quality evidence supports the critical role of midwifery in improving more than 50 health-related outcomes (Cummins & Symon, 2023; Renfrew et al., 2014). Recognising this, the UAE has prioritised expanding its midwifery workforce as part of its Emiratisation strategy to support families during this transformative time (DoH, 2020). Moreover, in the UAE, 96% of healthcare professionals are expatriates, with a significant proportion of the workforce in neighbouring Gulf countries also consisting of expatriates. This reliance often results in higher turnover rates, highlighting the need for locally trained graduates (Mohammad & Al-Hmaimat, 2024).

Introduction to Midwifery Education and Practice

To address the country's healthcare needs, the UAE has made high-quality midwifery education a national priority. Historically, there was a small cohort of UAE midwifery graduates from a postgraduate midwifery program offered in 2010. However, following this initial effort, there was a prolonged period during which no UAE midwifery graduates entered the workforce.

A postgraduate two-year Master of Science in Midwifery program began in 2020 in Ras Al Khaimah with 12 midwifery graduates to date as of 2024. In 2022, the UAE launched its first four-year Bachelor of Midwifery Direct-Entry Program, marking a significant milestone in midwifery education. The program received full accreditation in 2023, and the inaugural cohort of seven graduates is expected to qualify in July 2025. Another similar Direct-Entry Program was approved in 2023 and commenced in 2024. The UAE defines a registered midwife as someone who has successfully completed an accredited academic educational program at minimum of bachelor level in midwifery (Authority, 2022). This program must be based on ICM Essential Competencies for Basic Midwifery Practice (ICM, 2024) and the ICM Global Standards for Midwifery Education (ICM, 2021) and must also be registered and licensed as 'Registered Midwife' by National Health Regulatory Bodies in United Arab Emirates, in accordance with the national professional qualification requirements (PQR) (Ministry of Health and Prevention) (MOHAP); Department of Health Abu Dhabi (DoH); Dubai Health Authority; Sharjah Health Authority, 2022). Only recognised midwifery professionals by the Professional Qualification Requirements (PQR) are eligible to provide care in the field of midwifery (Department of Health Abu Dhabi (DOH) 2023; Ministry of Health and Prevention (MOHAP); Department of Health Abu Dhabi (DoH); Dubai Health Authority; Sharjah Health Authority, 2022).

Given the relatively recent reintroduction of midwifery education, the concept of midwifery mentorship in the UAE is still in its early stages and continues to evolve to meet the demands of this developing profession. While the growth of midwifery programs has been gradual, the increasing number of midwifery students may present challenges in securing sufficient clinical placements, given that mentorship is a critical component of their training. Furthermore, it is essential to ensure that midwifery graduates have opportunities for employment and can practice as qualified midwives. Implementing a structured preceptorship program would support their transition into the workforce, fostering confidence and competence as newly qualified midwives and should be considered moving forward. The midwifery profession in accordance with the International Confederation of Midwives (ICM), 2017) is defined in the UAE Scope of Practice (2024) which applies to midwives practising in the Emirate of Dubai as:

> an approach to care of women and their newborn infants whereby midwives: optimise the normal biological, psychological, social processes of childbirth and early life of the newborn; work in partnership with women, respecting the individual circumstances and views of each woman; promote women's personal capabilities to care for themselves and their families; collaborate with midwives and other health professionals as necessary to provide holistic care that meets each woman's individual needs.
>
> *(Dubai Health Authority (DHA), Ministry of Health and Prevention, (MOHAP) UAE (2024, p. 4)*

Whereas the scope of midwifery applying to midwives practising in the Emirate of Abu Dhabi defines midwifery as:

> skilled, knowledgeable and compassionate care for childbearing women, newborn infants and families across the continuum from pre-pregnancy, pregnancy, birth, postpartum and the early weeks of life.
>
> *(Adopted from WHO, 2019; Department of Health Abu Dhabi (DOH), 2023, p. 3)*

Midwifery academics have endeavoured to involve the education managers and key stakeholders, including student midwives as members of the Midwifery Advisory Board for the program to encourage positive engagement of the organisations and hear the student voice (O'Connell, 2025). Updates of student progress and experience in the clinical areas are provided regularly with student feedback collected by survey at the end of each placement and fed back. Since each midwifery student has specific competency and skill requirements to achieve for each course, it is vital that they are given opportunities to practice 'hands-on' in clinical. The students use a clinical competency document requiring sign-off by a mentor and midwifery academic which was based on the ICM Essential Competencies for Midwifery (ICM, 2024) and the Baby-Friendly Hospital Initiative (BFHI) breastfeeding competencies World Health Organization and the United Nations Children's Fund (UNICEF) (2020). In accordance with EU Directives (Union, 2005; Vermeulen et al., 2018), midwifery students here, like in other countries, must achieve a range of competencies, including attending 40 births, conducting 100 antenatal and 100 postnatal assessments, performing 100 newborn checks, managing 40 complex cases, supporting breastfeeding assessments, and demonstrating medication knowledge, among other requirements.

Prior to commencing the program, the midwifery academics consulted the midwifery management, clinical education teams and key midwifery staff to ensure the required learning outcomes could be met on the placement using a standardised education audit tool from the college. The WHO Midwifery Assessment Tool for Europe (MATE) was useful in navigating these conversations with a midwifery lens (WHO, 2020). This self-assessment tool encouraged self-reflection in each unit as to how midwifery students would interact as part of the team and whether available midwifery support would be adequate for students. Members of staff needed to be aware that midwifery students may need to be prioritised over other student professions at times. For example, a nursing student objective on the labour ward may be to observe or witness birth, whereas a midwifery student needs to lead under direct supervision 40 births as per the EU Directive stipulated in our requirements to graduate (European Parliament and the Council of the European Union, 2005). In addition, attendance of clinical placement is mandatory with any days missed being made up before completion of each course. Ensuring that clinical practice is completed allows enough time for the required competencies to be achieved. During our audits, the organisations highlighted a preference for student midwives to engage in clinical placement blocks, promoting shift work to help them integrate into the team dynamic and gain valuable experience with long shifts and night shifts, where normal births frequently occur. In other models of learning, students may do two 8-hour shifts per week over a 16-week Semester. In practice, the students may benefit from the onsite presence of the midwifery academic course lead on a daily basis and in certain instances where midwifery mentorship is not available, and care is led by obstetrics and nurses, the midwifery academics have been able to attend a birth alongside the student to ensure there is appropriate midwifery guidance. But, with growing student cohorts, this may not be feasible. The aim would be that our midwifery students will be able to cascade the mentorship as they become employed after graduation.

Midwifery education programs which lead to midwifery licensure require graduates to achieve clinical, academic, and professional competence (Folkvord & Risa, 2023). Therefore, clinical placement comprises a large part of the work expected to be completed which is under the direct supervision of a licensed midwife (Folkvord & Risa, 2023). In the current curriculum where I work, clinical placement comprises more than half (56%). Midwifery students learn to become a midwife under this supervision which is a reciprocal relationship of teaching and learning facilitating the transfer of knowledge, skills, and behaviours expected of a professional midwife. Recognising the value of continuity of care, we encourage our students to engage in a limited number of continuity cases each year, wherever feasible. Those who have embraced this opportunity consistently report positive experiences and valuable learning outcomes. To further enhance their development, the students' competency documentation includes a dedicated section for service user feedback, providing an additional perspective on their practice. Ensuring a positive culture of learning is a vital aspect which needs to be nurtured in clinical areas accepting midwifery students for mentorship.

Preparation for Clinical Placement

Students may experience anxiety before commencing any clinical placement, so ensuring adequate preparation by enhancing confidence in their capability for clinical placement is vital for success (Folkvord & Risa, 2023). We use simulation in our midwifery labs as well as various innovative teaching and learning strategies such as Case-Based Learning to help prepare midwifery students in advance. A strong theoretical foundation is vital in preparation to deliver Evidence-Based Practice in learning situations. The opportunity to practice hand-on skills before being 'hands-on' is important and helps build confidence in their capabilities (Folkvord & Risa, 2023).

REFLECTIVE ACTIVITY 1 NAVIGATING CULTURAL SENSITIVITY IN MENTORSHIP

Amira, a senior midwife, mentors a group of student midwives at a government hospital. She notices that some new students hesitate to perform intimate procedures such as assisting with personal hygiene, citing cultural discomfort. While the student was prepared in simulation, the reality of the situation is a different experience. Additionally, Amira struggles to align the hospital's standardised mentorship protocols with the culturally diverse backgrounds of the students and patients.

Reflective Activity:

1 How does cultural sensitivity impact the mentorship process in Abu Dhabi's multicultural healthcare setting?
2 What specific actions can mentors take to address cultural barriers while maintaining professional standards?
3 How can mentorship programs incorporate cultural awareness training to better prepare students and mentors?

Undergraduate Mentorship

According to a systematic review examining factors that enhance the self-efficacy of student midwives during placements (Folkvord & Risa, 2023, p. 10), 'gaining access to and belonging to an enabling educational and working culture' is pivotal for student midwives to thrive. Therefore, when designing clinical placements, the engagement and commitment of the clinical area are essential. Each site must be fully invested in mentoring students and ensuring service users or women are comfortable with students practising on them. The colleges offering the new bachelor's midwifery degree programs already provide clinical placements for various other professions, including nursing, physiotherapy, radiography, paramedicine, and pharmacy, benefiting from established links with clinical sites willing to accept midwifery students. However, key challenges in the UAE include the predominance of privatised healthcare over a teaching hospital culture. Service users may not fully understand the teaching and learning dynamic and practising doctors and midwives may not view teaching as part of their role.

Additionally, the limited number of licensed midwives poses a significant barrier to effective mentorship. As a result, midwifery academics have had to adopt flexible and adaptive approaches to student supervision, ensuring that care practices are interpreted and delivered through a distinctly 'midwifery' lens. Reflective practice is a pivotal component in fostering critical thinking. This may be structured using a model or unstructured using more creativity such as a poem or art. For instance, in a given scenario, students can reflect on what occurred, why it happened, and how physiological processes might have been optimised. Clear and constructive feedback is essential to support students' progression and learning (Folkvord & Risa, 2023). Evidence demonstrates that debriefing – discussing or reflecting immediately after an event – enhances critical thinking and sharpens the focus of learning. Providing a safe and supportive space for debriefing is crucial, and midwifery academics have prioritised creating such environments to support the development of student midwives. Written reflections may help a student to self-assess and recognise their strengths, weaknesses and where they need to develop (Folkvord & Risa, 2023).

Other types of mentorships described in midwifery include 'peer to peer (midwife student to midwife student),' 'midwife to student', and 'midwife to new graduate' (Bradford et al., 2022). The notion of mentoring between students may also be beneficial; however, in this capacity, the senior learner should not have any influence on the junior learner's academic progression (Bradford et al., 2022). When engaged in midwife student to midwife student mentorship, it may boost student self-esteem, reduce anxiety, and role transformation.

In October 2024, the UAE revised its Scope of Midwifery Practice to align with international standards, emphasising the importance of midwives in optimising childbirth processes and supporting women in individualised care (Dubai Health Authority (DHA), Ministry of Health and Prevention, (MOHAP) UAE, 2024; ICM, 2024). This scope adheres to the International Confederation of Midwives (ICM) standards and defines midwifery as a partnership with women, focusing on holistic and culturally sensitive care (ICM, 2021). To be recognised as a midwife in the UAE, individuals must complete an accredited bachelor-level program in midwifery that meets ICM standards and be licensed by national regulatory bodies (ICM, 2021). Mentorship is a cornerstone of the updated scope, underscored in domains such as Professional, Ethical, and Legal Practice, as well as Communication and Leadership. Midwives are expected to guide students, support professional development, and provide clear guidance in complex clinical situations (Dubai Health Authority (DHA), Ministry of Health and Prevention, (MOHAP) UAE, 2024). Although mentorship is outlined in the UAE scope of practice, there are no formalised standards or official training programs in place. With numerous hospitals and healthcare corporations operating independently, each organisation is responsible for its own staff training. While many institutions require mandatory mentorship or preceptorship training, the lack of standardisation across the UAE leads to significant variability in the experiences of midwifery students who may be under the supervision of a midwife, nurse, or doctor while on placement. In the UAE, the term 'mentorship' may be used when referring to the support of student midwives, whereas 'preceptorship' is commonly used for graduate programs also referred to as 'residency programs' which support the transition to newly qualified. However, there may be confusion as the term 'preceptorship' has been used in undergraduate nursing programs referring to support of student nurses (Williams et al., 2021). So, it is possible that the two terms may be used interchangeably. Mentorship for midwives is highlighted in two key domains in the Scope of Practice:

- Domain 1: Professional, Ethical, and Legal, item 1.16 emphasises contributing to mentoring, peer support and the learning experiences and professional development of others. Item 1.20 highlights the importance of supporting orientation and ongoing education programs, and guiding students to meet their learning needs and objectives.
- Domain 5: Communication, Leadership, and Relationship Management, item 5.16 focuses on the mentor and preceptor's role in providing clear guidance, supporting clinical decision-making, problem-solving, and managing complex situations while also offering constructive feedback (Ministry of Health and Prevention (MOHAP), 2024).

REFLECTIVE ACTIVITY 2 SUPPORTING CLINICAL COMPETENCY IN DIVERSE SETTINGS

Fatima is a final-year midwifery student enrolled in the newly launched Bachelor of Midwifery program. During her placement at a private hospital in Abu Dhabi, she observes that her mentor, Sarah, a licensed expatriate midwife, is often unavailable due to high patient loads. Fatima is expected to perform clinical tasks but struggles with gaining hands-on experience because the nurses and doctors prioritise patient safety over student learning. Fatima worries about meeting her graduation requirements, such as conducting 40 births and supporting 100 postnatal assessments.

Reflective Activity:

What challenges are evident in Fatima's mentorship experience, and how do they reflect broader issues in Abu Dhabi's healthcare system?

How can clinical sites balance patient safety with educational needs for midwifery students?

1 Propose strategies that Sarah and the hospital management could adopt to enhance the mentorship experience for students like Fatima?

Mentorship in Abu Dhabi Post-Registration

One way to improve the retention of midwives may be through wider organisational support including mentorship or preceptorship support and guidance which can reduce attrition through structured mentorship programs (Wissemann et al., 2022). At present, there is no specific midwifery preceptorship program in the UAE. However, some UAE hospitals have developed nursing residency programs (NRPs) (Mohammad & Al-Hmaimat, 2024; Williams et al., 2021). The main barrier to residency programs has been reported as cost since they may be expensive. However, Mohammad and Al-Hmaimat (2024) argue that participation in NRPs may reduce staff turnover in the first year which may occur due to immigration where graduate nurses see overseas opportunities to countries with perceived better opportunities and support such as New Zealand which offers an immediate residency pathway. This global movement of the medical workforce is often described as a 'brain drain' (Mohammad & Al-Hmaimat, 2024). The findings of their systematic review of nurse residency programs recommended the establishment of structured twelve-month NRPs in the UAE with clearly defined quality standards and performance indicators (Mohammad & Al-Hmaimat, 2024). In addition, the review recommends the integration of NRPs into the organisation's strategic plan as a workforce development and retention strategy (Mohammad & Al-Hmaimat, 2024).

REFLECTIVE ACTIVITY 3

SWOT Analysis: What barriers to effective mentorship exist in the UAE (e.g., limited midwifery workforce, privatised healthcare system), and how could these be overcome?

Cultural Sensitivity: How can mentorship programs integrate cultural awareness and respect for Emirati traditions while adhering to international midwifery standards?

In small groups, discuss your reflections and propose strategies to address the following:

- Building an enabling educational culture in clinical areas.
- Promoting mentorship roles among licensed midwives while managing workload pressures.
- Ensuring mentees meet ICM Essential Competencies for Basic Midwifery Practice.

Future of Midwifery Mentorship in the UAE Every Midwife Is A Leader

To progress the midwifery profession, thereby improving care experiences and outcomes, every midwife must be viewed as a leader. In an editorial for Women and Birth Journal (Medway & Rehayem, 2024) about Midwifery Leadership, Midwifery is championed as a key strategy for high-quality maternity care. Engaging in mentorship is highlighted as a vital strategy, with Professor Caroline Homer referring to 'holding the ladder' for those coming up behind you (Medway & Rehayem, 2024). Mentorship should be viewed as an important element of professional development, growing the profession by passing on critical midwifery skills and professional behaviours. Midwives at all career stages, contexts and settings should engage in leadership activities and assume leadership roles. Our midwifery curriculum in Abu Dhabi has woven the concept of leadership throughout the program and a Leadership and Management Theory and Clinical Course in the fourth year. Our senior midwifery students already show leadership characteristics through their behaviours and participation in various national activities such as the Emirates Nursing and Midwifery Association. Being an active member in a country professional association is a keyway to demonstrate leadership (Medway & Rehayem, 2024).

Conclusion

Mentorship and leadership are inseparable pillars of midwifery practice, essential for advancing the profession and improving maternal and newborn outcomes. By cultivating leadership skills through education, mentorship, and professional engagement, midwives are empowered to take initiative, inspire change, and uphold the highest standards of care. The integration of leadership concepts into the midwifery curriculum in Abu Dhabi, alongside active participation in professional associations, reflects a commitment to shaping future midwifery leaders who will drive the profession forward and make a lasting impact on healthcare in the UAE.

Country-Specific Resources

To provide additional guidance, participants can explore the following UAE-specific resources:

1 **Abu Dhabi Health Workforce Plan** (DoH, 2020)
2 **UAE Scope of Midwifery Practice** Dubai Health Authority (DHA), Ministry of Health and Prevention (MOHAP), UAE (2024).

References

https://www.who.int/europe/publications/i/item/WHO-EURO-2020-5577-45342-64887. Accessed 12 January 2025.

Abu Dhabi Health Authority. (2010). *Emiratisation of Health Care Present and Future Report*. Abu Dhabi Health Authority.

Bradford, H., Hines, H. F., Labko, Y., Peasley, A., Valentin-Welch, M., & Breedlove, G. (2022). Midwives mentoring midwives: A review of the evidence and best practice recommendations. *Journal of Midwifery & Women's Health*, 67(1), 21–30.

Cummins, A., & Symon, A. (2023). Transforming the quality maternal newborn care framework into an index to measure the quality of maternity care. *Birth*, *50*(1), 192–204.

Department of Health Abu Dhabi (DOH). (2023). *Scope of Practice for Midwives (DOH/SoP/HCWS/Midwives/V1/2023)*. DOH. https://www.doh.gov.ae/en/resources/scope-of-practice. Accessed 11 June 2025.

Department of Health (DOH). (2020). *Abu Dhabi Health Workforce Plan*.

Dubai Health Authority (DHA), Ministry of Health and Prevention, (MOHAP) UAE. (2024). *Ministerial Resolution No. 208 Regarding: National Scope of Practice Standards – Registered Midwives*. https://dha.gov.ae/en/circulars/details/CIR-2024-00000181. Accessed online 16 January 2025.

European Parliament and the Council of the European Union. (2005). Directive 2005/36/EC of the European parliament and of the council of 7 September 2005 (English). *Official Journal of the European Union*, 48, 22–142. https://eur-lex.europa.eu/eli/dir/2005/36/oj/eng

Folkvord, S. E., & Risa, C. F. (2023). Factors that enhance midwifery students' learning and development of self-efficacy in clinical placement: A systematic qualitative review. *Nurse Education in Practice*, 66, 103510.

International Confederation of Midwives (ICM). (2017). *International Definition of a Midwife [Core Document]*.

International Confederation of Midwives (ICM). (2021). *Global Standards for Midwifery Education (Revised 2021) [Core Document]*. The Hague Netherlands. https://internationalmidwives.org/resources/global-standards-for-midwifery-education/. Accessed 11 June 2025.

International Confederation of Midwives (ICM). (2024). *Essential Competencies for Midwifery Practice*.

Medway, P., & Rehayem, A. (2024). Midwifery leadership. *Women and Birth*, 37(1), 4–5.

Miller, S., Abalos, E., Chamillard, M., Ciapponi, A., Colaci, D., Comandé, D., Diaz, V., Geller, S., Hanson, C., & Langer, A. (2016). Beyond too little, too late and too much, too soon: A pathway towards evidence-based, respectful maternity care worldwide. *The Lancet*, *388*(10056), 2176–2192.

Ministry of Health and Prevention (MOHAP); Department of Health Abu Dhabi (DoH); Dubai Health Authority; Sharjah Health Authority. (2022). *Unified Healthcare Professional Qualification Requirement (PQR)*. https://www.doh.gov.ae/en/pqr. Accessed online16 January 2025.

Mohammad, Z., & Al-Hmaimat, N. (2024). The effectiveness of nurse residency programs on new graduate nurses' retention: Systematic review. *Heliyon*.

O'Connell, M. (2025). Nurturing future midwives in Abu Dhabi. *The Practising Midwife Advance* [For publication in March 2025]. 28(2), 17–21. https://doi.org/10.55975/OHBU3621

O'Connell, M., & Sosa, G. (2023). Midwifery in Abu Dhabi: A survey of midwives. *Women and Birth*, 36(4), 439–444. https://doi.org/10.1016/j.wombi.2023.02.002

Renfrew, M. J., McFadden, A., Bastos, M. H., Campbell, J., Channon, A. A., Cheung, N. F., Silva, D. R. A. D., Downe, S., Kennedy, H. P., & McCormick, F. (2014). Midwifery and quality care: Findings from a new evidence-informed framework for maternal and newborn care. *The Lancet*, 384(9948), 1129–1145.

The Supreme Council for Motherhood and Early Childhood. (2017). *National Strategy for Motherhood and Early Childhood 2017–2021*.

Vermeulen, J., Luyben, A., Jokinen, M., Matintupa, E., O'Connell, R., & Bick, D. (2018). Establishing a Europe-wide foundation for high quality midwifery education: The role of the european midwives association (EMA). *Midwifery*, 64, 128–131.

Williams, G., Al Hmaimat, N., AlMekkawi, M., Melhem, O., & Mohamed, Z. (2021). Implementing dedicated nursing clinical education unit: Nursing students' and preceptors' perspectives. *Journal of Professional Nursing*, 37(3), 673–681.

Wissemann, K., Bloxsome, D., De Leo, A., & Bayes, S. (2022). What are the benefits and challenges of mentoring in midwifery? An integrative review. *Women's Health*, 18, 17455057221110141.

World Health Organisation. (2019). *Midwifery Education and Care. Maternal Health Unit*. https://www.who.int/teams/maternal-newborn-child-adolescent-health-and-ageing/maternal-health/midwifery. Accessed online 16 January 2025.

World Health Organisation (WHO). (2020). *Midwifery Assessment Tool for Education*. WHO.

World Health Organization and the United Nations Children's Fund (UNICEF). (2020). *Competency Verification Toolkit Ensuring Competency of Direct Care Providers to Implement the Baby-Friendly Hospital Initiative*. https://iris.who.int/bitstream/handle/10665/333689/9789240009417-eng.pdf. Accessed online 16 January 2025.

9

MIDWIFERY MENTORSHIP IN BANGLADESH

Jennifer Stevens and Rondi Anderson

Background

Bangladesh sits in South Asia with India wrapped around it to the West, North, and East and Myanmar to the Southeast. It is the eighth most populated country in the world. The national language is Bangla, yet college and university education is taught in English. As a flat delta, the country is susceptible to flooding and the impact of global warming. Natural disasters, including earthquakes, tsunami's, cyclones, and droughts, are regular occurrences. Culturally, Bangladesh is considered a conservative yet tolerant Muslim majority country. Current gender inequity in Bangladesh is partly the result of deeply embedded social norms, with child marriage rates being the fourth highest in the world (CIA.gov, 2024). Economically, Bangladesh has made enormous advances in part through the growing garment industry. Identified as a least developed country, Bangladesh is now on at the crossroads to graduate from least developed country status (World Bank, 2024). An overview of demographics in Bangladesh are noted in Table 9.1.

The health system, as in many low- and middle-income countries, is structured around a large, generally free public health system, and a much smaller number of private facilities. Public hospitals are organised around the level of acuity available in the facility with the highest being the Medical Teaching Colleges and Specialist Hospitals, District Hospitals, then Upazila Health Complex (UHC). The UHCs were developed to provide community-based primary healthcare, including birth services, increasing access to facilities for rural communities. Finally, there are community-based clinics including Family Welfare Centers, Union Health & Family Welfare Centers, Union Subcenters and Community Clinics generally focused on family planning and antenatal care.

DOI: 10.4324/9781003533733-10

TABLE 9.1 Bangladesh National Demographics

	National Rate
Land mass	130,170 sq km (slightly larger than the US state of Pennsylvania), on a delta of large rivers flowing from the Himalayas
Population	165,650,475 (2022 est)
Language	Bangla
Birth Rate	17.69 births/1,000 population (2022 est)
Maternal mortality ratio	173 deaths/100,000 live births (2017 est)
Population below the poverty line	5% (2022 est) (Based on the international poverty line of $2.15 USD a day)
Literacy	74.9% (2020)
Child marriage	Women married by 15yo – 15.5%, Women married by 18yo – 51.4%
Improved sanitation (flush, pour, or pit latrine)	78% (2020 est)
Healthcare worker density (Doctors, nurses, midwives)	11.7 HCW/10,000 population (WHO global median of 48.6 per 10,000)[1]

There is a severe shortage of healthcare providers with Bangladesh reporting 11.7 providers per 10,000 population (CIA.gov, 2024). The World Health Organization's (WHO) minimum recommendation for healthcare providers (doctors, nurses, and midwives) is 44.5 providers per 10,000 population, and the global median is 48.6 providers per 10,000 population. The wealthy, who can attend higher education, tends to become doctors, so the nursing and midwifery shortage is even more severe. Additionally, healthcare providers are poorly distributed, with a heavy concentration in the urban areas and many posts, over 24% remaining unfilled especially in rural areas (WHO, 2017).

Bangladesh fell short of its Millenium Development Goal (MDG) to reduce the maternal mortality ration (MMR) from 574 to 143 by 2017 (Rajia, 2019). Bangladesh's most recent WHO MMR estimate from 2017 was 173 (CIA.gov, 2024). Nevertheless, maternity care is a priority for the Government of Bangladesh with universal access to antenatal and birth services at low or no cost at all public maternal and child health facilities. Yet, many women choose to give birth at home without a skilled birth provider. The government trains community skilled birth attendants (CSBAs) to support safe birth at home and increase referrals to facilities as needed. Unfortunately, because of perceived poor quality and experience of care in facilities, many women refuse or delay referral and can be turned away when they do present (Mahumud, 2019). In facilities, the majority of maternity care is provided by nurses with specialised maternity training called 'nurse–midwives'.

TABLE 9.2 Facility-Based Birth in Bangladesh 2007 (NIPORT, 2016) to 2017 (DHS, 2019)

Place of birth	2007	2007 Proportion of facility births by caesarean	2017	2017 Proportion of facility births by caesarean
Public	8%	34.6%	14.3%	36%
Private	8.6%	67.3%	31.5%	84%
Other	0.4%		0.3%	
Home	83%		50%	
National caesarean section rate	9% of all births		32.7% of all births	67% of facility deliveries

Source: Bangladesh Demographic and Health Survey 2007 & 2017–2018.

The current facility-based birth rate in Bangladesh from 2019 is approximately 53.4% (MoHFW, 2019). The Bangladeshi government has used various programs to increase facility-based birth with some success. This increase occurred primarily in private facilities, who provide caesarean sections (NIPORT, 2016). The small improvement in public facility-based birth occurred almost exclusively in the district hospitals that also offer caesarean sections, with little increase in the community-based Upazila Health Complex (UHC) health facilities. Bangladesh reports a national caesarean rate of 32.7% (NIPORT, icddr,b, MEASURE Evaluation, 2017) (Table 9.2). With almost 50% of women birthing at home, the caesarean rate is shockingly high. In 2016, of all facility-based births, 67% were delivered by caesarean. Poor women aren't getting care, and the upper middle class are getting too much, medically inappropriate care.

Additionally, care quality is a serious concern. A recent report by NIPORT, a Bangla research group, found that 26% of women in Bangladesh lacked even one antenatal care visit, while the current recommendation from the WHO is eight visits (NIPORT, 2016; WHO, 2016). More importantly, the quality of the visits is poor, and inconsistent, for example, only 39.7% of women report receiving information on signs of potential pregnancy complications, yet 80.2% receive an ultrasound. This interesting point here is, an ultrasound is a billable procedure (NIPORT, 2016).

The Introduction of Professional Midwifery in Bangladesh

In 2008, in response to the Prime Minister, a new cadre of professional midwives was called for in Bangladesh. The goal of this cadre was to improve the quality and availability of comprehensive sexual, reproductive, maternal, and newborn health care. At that time, generalist nurses (termed nurse–midwives) were serving in the role of midwife. Significant gaps in skills and knowledge were found. After the Prime Minister's commitment of 3,000 midwives by 2015, multi-stakeholder discussions moved the education and deployment of professional midwives forward. The Ministry of Health and Family Welfare (MOHFW) created the legal framework and 3,000 midwife posts. The Ministry also determined where the midwives would be educated and subsequently deployed. Development of the regulatory system consisted of establishing a Bangladesh code of ethics and scope of practice, as well as licensing, registration, and practice guidelines, and the needed administration for education programs. The scope of practice was developed to include all aspects of International Confederation of Midwives (ICM) standard competencies, such as independent antenatal care (ANC), labour care, postnatal care, initial stabilisation of emergencies (including administration of medicines), contraceptive provision, cervical cancer screening and treatment, clinical management of rape, and first line management of common sexually transmitted infections (STIs). The national curriculum also aligned with some international countries' minimum number of clinical experiences such as 40 births, 100 ANC visits, and 100 PNC.

The first class of professional midwives educated in the direct entry; three-year diploma program graduated in 2015. As of 2024, there are 120 midwifery educational programs throughout the country providing the three-year diploma program in midwifery and four providing a BSc program in midwifery, with the MSc planned to begin in 2026. Currently, 2,556 midwives serve in 667 government health facilities with more working in nongovernmental organisations and the private sector. Midwives are deployed in 95% of all government sub-district hospitals (UHC). Of these, 50% are fully staffed with four or more midwives. Within the hospitals, midwives oversee 90% of the maternity wards and attend over 75% of the births.

To assist the reader understand the uniqueness of Bangladesh's education and cadres called midwife, a summary is presented in Table 9.3.

To support the introduction of professional midwives, midwifery-led care (MLC) units were introduced by the Directorate General of Nursing and Midwifery (Zaman & Sabur, 2019). The MLC units provide antenatal care in a designated 'midwifery corner' in government-run UHCs and some hospitals, as well as space in the birth room. Midwives, nurses, and doctors are posted to the healthcare facilities and work in the MLC, but midwives are the only health professional who do not rotate outside the MLC.

Initially, the physical space was enabled to support midwifery. Walls were painted pink, the colour for midwifery in Bangladesh, to promote the new profession, and supplies for normal birth such as birth balls and squat chairs were provided. But resistance to change in healthcare delivery is ubiquitous. Resistance is generally motivated by a desire for control, entrenched habits, the perception of increased workload, and/or patient demand for existing

TABLE 9.3 Education of Cadres Called 'Midwife' in Bangladesh

	Education required for admission	*Length of program*	*Scope of practice & primary place of practice.*
Nurse midwives	12 years of general education (Equivalent to US high school)	3 years of basic nursing, then additional 12 months in midwifery (Do NOT meet ICM standard).	SOP regulated. Were licensed as nurse and midwife (**additional 12-month program no longer exists**), now licensed only as nurse. Work in all health care facilities.
New **professional midwives:** Registered midwives	12 years of general education (Equivalent to US high school)	3 years in midwifery (meets ICM standard)	SOP regulated. Licensed as a midwife. Currently working in the UHCs and Union sub-centres. Also in the private institutions, humanitarian and marginalised community settings.
Certified midwives	3 years of general nursing and 1 year of midwifery	Additional 6 months in midwifery (for total of 18 months in midwifery-meets ICM standards	1600 trained (**this program is no longer active**), met ICM standards, **no regulation**
Community skilled birth attendants (CSBAs)	8 years of general education (Equivalent to US grade school education)	12 months (Do NOT meet ICM standards)	Work in the community, **no regulation**
Family Welfare Visitors (FWVs)	10 years of general education (Equivalent to US middle school education)	18 months (Do NOT meet ICM standards)	Work in community-based facilities, **no regulation**
Junior midwives	10 years of general education (Equivalent to US middle school education)	18 months (Do NOT meet ICM standards)	Work in private hospitals as a midwife, **no regulation**

practices (Mittman, 1992). Alenchery et al. (2018) found that staff in India resisted immediate mother/baby skin-to-skin contact due to a perceived increased demand on their time. Likewise, Payne et al. (2021) found resistance to delayed cord clamping in a multi-country study, despite the availability of guidelines, due to entrenched habits.

As a new profession in Bangladesh, midwifery has faced many challenges (Zaman & Sabur, 2019). The term *'midwife'* was used by many to mean *'provides care at birth'*, so there was confusion over what education the new midwives needed, what services they could provide, and what is unique and different about a midwifery-specific profession. Midwives were introduced to make unprecedented changes throughout the existing care systems, yet nurses, doctors, and managers who it could be suggested were not across the philosophy of midwifery care provision were in positions of leadership (Bogren, 2018; Pappu et al., 2023). Consequently, as the new midwives were deployed, outdated and harmful practices (e.g., supine birth, routine episiotomy, antibiotics, and manual exploration of the uterus) were commonly performed. Evidence-based practices (e.g., delayed umbilical cord clamping, skin-to-skin contact) were not routinely followed. Additionally, hesitance to manage obstetric emergencies at rural facilities was common (Afsana, 2004). Once deployed, midwives were often placed in generalist nursing roles, while nurses remained posted on maternity wards. Even when placed in maternity care roles, midwives' provision of emergency obstetric care, particularly for those coming from the community in critical condition, was often discouraged by supervisors. Nurses felt midwives were 'too young' to lead care provision including the use of medicines and evidence-based midwifery (Anderson, 2022). Nurses and managers attributed their resistance to a lack of familiarity, inadequate time, and women's preference. Managers indicated that nurses may feel competitive with the midwives in part due to the potential loss of tips provided by patients, which is a common practice and often bolsters nurses' pay. Furthermore, there was pushback against the midwives' scope of practice that included independent autonomous use of emergency medications to stabilise a woman's condition during an emergency, without requiring consultation or supervision that would delay care. The healthcare environment added a layer of challenge towards the new midwives, with the routine practices of over-medicalisation, lack of evidenced-based care, and a lack of respectful care embedded throughout the system.

Mentorship in Bangladesh

Mentorship is part of the vision of the Ministry and the health directorates, integrating this model into government systems and their work plans. Mentorship is a term used by the Bangladeshi government for *someone providing on-site capacity building*.

The work done to support the development of midwives in Bangladesh, and mentoring programs was initiated and coordinated by the Bangladeshi government, supported by the United Nations Population Fund (UNFPA). UNFPA is a UN agency focused on three priorities:

1 No gender-based violence,
2 No unmet need for family planning, and
3 No maternal mortality.

All UN agencies support work done through the government in any country they are working in. This allows for sustainability of projects and national coordination. Additionally, work to support the education and strengthening of the health work force is done pre-service (the initial education given prior to licensure and working in the health system) and in-service (any education or training done after a cadre is working in the health system), thus 'in-service'.

As the profession of midwifery was created and introduced throughout Bangladesh, many barriers were encountered. Initial mentoring projects were more likely to use external mentors, both nationals and internationals, funded through the United Nations (UN) to strengthening government systems. Quickly the national surplus of young female doctors was identified as ideal mentors with additional training on mentorship, midwifery, and quality of care standards. These mentors were trained to support evidence-based care, the midwifery profession, and the midwifery model of care. The mentors received a one-week orientation on the role of midwives, midwifery model of care, and the latest World Health Organization (WHO) quality maternity care guidelines. After this initial training, they receive semi-annual multi-day training updates and ongoing access to midwifery experts. In addition to this training, government staff, such as peer faculty, obstetric–gynaecology doctors, midwives, and paediatricians at tertiary-level facilities, and public health nurses who take on the role of mentor receive additional training on their responsibilities and duties specific to the role. These mentors were used throughout the entire system, supporting midwives during their initial education, when deployed in practice, and when working in humanitarian settings. This enabled the new midwives to practice respectful, evidence-based care to the extent of their scope of practice – including the independent stabilisation of obstetrical emergencies – increasing access to high-quality midwifery care throughout the country. Given the wide range of mentoring needs, several on-site and virtual mentoring projects were implemented over a period of 5 years.

Over time, mentorship was shifted to the government and monitoring was expanded. Currently the district SRH officers have largely taken over the role of facility mentors, focusing on enabling environment for midwifery to flourish. Clinical experience of students – including monitoring of experiences, and OSCEs prior to initiating clinical experience – remains supported by midwifery faculty who continue to be mentored. However, international faculty mentors were not given additional training beyond their midwifery and midwifery faculty expertise, although there were ongoing discussions and program evaluations to refine the process.

Mentoring Projects:

In Bangladesh, midwifery was introduced to change the maternal healthcare system, but there were no experienced midwives. To fully integrate the new profession of midwifery and support midwives to practice the midwifery model of care, three areas were identified for mentoring support:

1 **Initial education pre-service (education mentors)** Supporting and strengthening non-midwife faculty to teach midwifery.

   - Weekly virtual mentoring of nursing faculty, who were functioning as midwifery faculty, through international academic institutions.
   - Bi-monthly faculty mentoring at educational institutions by nationally trained doctors.
   - A certificate program for government faculty peer mentors, conducted by an international academic program, followed by those faculty mentoring peer faculty at least monthly.

2 **In the practice setting, in-service (facility mentors at midwifery practice sites)** Enabling the culture shift needed for high-quality, evidence-based, midwifery model of care to become the standard.

   - Bi-monthly mentoring by nationally trained doctors, at midwife deployment sites. Over time this was integrated into the government system.
   - Daily mentoring by nationally trained obstetrics–gynaecology doctors at two tertiary-level hospitals.

3 **Humanitarian response (clinical mentors in humanitarian settings)** To enable midwives to provide SRH in the ever-changing humanitarian setting.

   - Daily mentoring by government obstetrics–gynaecology doctors, midwives, paediatricians, and international mentors to support new professional midwives deployed to the Rohingya refugee camp.

Initial Education Pre-Service

Upon the establishment of professional midwifery education, nursing faculty moved into the role of midwife educators. To prepare them, they received a one-month orientation covering midwifery model of care, the curriculum, evidence-based care, and the skills to be practised within a clinical skills lab. Yet, as anticipated gaps in their understanding of midwives and midwifery including both didactic knowledge and skills remained.

In pre-service education, education mentors focused on faculty development including classroom teaching, simulation labs, and clinical sites. One mentor covered 3–5 midwifery educational institutions and would visit each a minimum of monthly. During that visit, she would monitor activities in the classroom, the institution, and the clinical education site. She provided skills lab training for the faculty, management support for the principals, technical guidance in the classroom, and monitoring of students' clinical experiences.

In the Practice Setting, In-Service

Midwives require an enabling environment to achieve optimal outcomes (Sandall et al., 2016; Turkmani, 2013). Initially, strong regulation was felt to be adequate to enable the effective implementation of quality MLC. However, it became clear the new midwives would need on-site post-deployment support to succeed in improving sexual, reproductive, maternal, and newborn healthcare quality and availability (Alenshery, 2018; Billah, 2019; Meadows, 2011).

Once graduated and deployed to UHCs, facility mentors were introduced to support the implementation of evidenced-based care and the midwifery model by the new midwifery graduates by creating an enabling environment. The mentors encouraged the sites to provide evidence-based care such as activity and liberal food and water during labour, upright birth, newborn–mother skin-to-skin contact after birth, delayed cord clamping, breastfeeding in the first hour, and a labour and birth companion for the mother. Additionally, these young female doctors were to support the environmental, cultural, and philosophical changes needed for the new midwives to succeed. This occurred by focusing on managers, maternity staff, and equipment to support the practice of midwifery. To this end, one facility mentor, a female medical doctor, was placed full-time at each site where midwives were practising. The facility mentors received regular coaching from an international midwifery specialist with the United Nations. The facility mentor's tasks including establishing a supportive relationship with the maternity ward department heads to counter resistance from doctors and nurses to the midwives and WHO-guided quality maternity care.

As a result of the understandings gained from the mentor, the department heads encouraged acceptance of the midwives among the maternity ward managers, staff, and other students who were all largely unfamiliar with midwifery and many aspects of quality maternity care. Mentors provided regular on-the-spot feedback and education to all managers, staff, and interns, and held weekly monitoring meetings to review progress and conduct mini-practical sessions on key skills and/or new guidelines (Khatun, 2022). Across key targeted behaviours of non-supine positions for labour and birth, no episiotomy, no oxytocin augmentation, no manual exploration of the uterus, skin-to-skin contact immediately following birth, and delayed cord clamping, a pattern was observed in which the use of evidence-based practices increased significantly immediately following the introduction of midwives and continued more gradually over time. In essence, there was a significant effect of midwives and mentoring on the use of evidence-based birth practices both immediately and over time.

Creating an Enabling Environment and Culture

Mentors were young female doctors trained to champion midwives within their workplaces. They visited each facility twice per month. Mentor visits included observations of care, as well as education and support for needed changes. An evidence-based low-dose, high-frequency mentoring approach was used (Jhpiego, 2016). These mentors played a crucial role in changing the culture in the health facilities to one of quality and team care. Because midwifery was a new profession, doctors were chosen as mentors because their professional status drew respect from hospital managers, other doctors, and nurses. This respect allowed the mentors to form peer relationships with management and advocate for the value of the midwives, midwifery model of care, and quality improvements. This resulted in midwives and midwifery model of care being seen as one more element of evidence-based care.

In a study from Bangladesh comparing 19 hospitals with and without midwives, and those with and without mentors, midwives improved quality of care, but those who had midwives and mentors performed better (Anderson et al., 2023). Key practices were followed including the use of an antenatal cards during outpatient visits, companionship of midwifery, upright positions during labour and birth, delayed cord clamping, immediate skin-to-skin contact, use of a partograph, and active management of the third stage of labour. Of these evidence-based maternity practices, greater use was observed in hospitals with mentors creating an enabling environment by assuaging nurses' and doctors' concerns about midwives' competencies and navigating solutions to resistance.

Qualitative research in the same project found midwives and maternity staff report greater positive experiences with quality improvement when midwives were supported by mentors. In settings with mentoring, maternity staff stated availability and quality of care was improving with doctors, nurses, and midwives expressing comfort with quality improvements and providing emergency care. Managers explained the mentors facilitated positive relationships between midwives and nurses and supported enabling environments for midwifery care. In addition, maternity staff spoke about midwives providing autonomous care and expressed that maternity wards now had expert staff. Nurses specifically talked about midwives' specialised education and gave examples of midwives expanding services, including counselling and education for women, and the promotion of vaginal birth over caesarean section. Nurses also stated the antenatal care that midwives provide is 'correct'. Nurses in mentored hospitals were less concerned about the midwives' youth. Rather, they referred to them as being young but mature and 'not inferior' in knowledge. Supervisors described feeling midwives provide better maternity care than nurses and expressed that midwives have more expertise. Nurses and managers shared stories of midwives motivating nurses to improve quality. Staff and managers at the mentored facilities were the most likely to state they manage obstetric emergencies and some shared that this was relatively new. Most of the non-midwife maternity staff talked about midwives providing initial stabilisation of emergencies. When maternity staff were asked what helped them make changes to more evidence-based care in their units, they described both the introduction of the new midwives and the importance of mentoring.

Existing district public health nurses added midwifery oversight to their duties and began tracking progress in care quality and midwives' ability to practise autonomously. Of the 64 facilities monitored by district public health nurses, the maternity wards in 62 facilities (97%) are run by midwives, births are managed independently by midwives in 63 facilities (98%), and at least 75% of women give birth upright or laterally in 57 facilities (89%) (REF 49).

Teaching Hospitals

To support high-quality midwifery education, in August of 2019, midwifery services, inclusive of mentorship, commenced at two major government teaching hospitals in Dhaka, the capital of Bangladesh. The midwifery services were supported by the physician's Obstetrical and Gynecological Society of Bangladesh (OGSB) organisation. These tertiary-level teaching hospitals in Bangladesh provide the highest acuity of care nationally.

Both hospitals serve over 1,000 pregnant women monthly with over 40,000 births/year. Both hospitals have large numbers of maternity staff with approximately 100 doctors including interns and residents and over 40 nurses. Every three months, 70 medical students, 50 midwife students, and 30 nursing students rotate through each maternity ward. The hospitals are also clinical sites for obstetrician–gynaecologist interns and residents. Between these two hospitals, over 1,200 healthcare provider students are taught annually. After the introduction of midwifery and mentoring at the teaching hospitals, the proportion of vaginal births attended by midwives increased from 0% prior to the initiation of the intervention to 86% at the end; the highest level was 95%, six months after the onset of COVID-19. Additionally, evidence-based practice improved immediately with the introduction of midwives and mentoring, and those improvements continued, notably not just for midwives but also for doctors and nurses in the maternity area.

It was an encouraging finding that the increase in use of WHO recommended maternity practices occurred not just among births attended by midwives, but also among births attended by midwife, medical, and nursing students on clinical rotation. This demonstrates that placement of midwives in a teaching hospital setting with facility mentorship can lead to improved quality practices by existing clinicians as well as students. As described by Anderson et al. (2023), mentors' work to establish commitment for midwifery care, and paved the way for midwives to lead and role model high-quality, midwifery model of care. This is a critical finding, as midwifery care quality in clinical education settings, and the impact of mentors in clinical education in the literature is sparse, despite WHO recommendations (WHO, 2019) and ICM (ICM, 2019) describing the importance of enabling environments.

Smartphones are widely available in Bangladesh and social media popular. Social media was used iteratively over time to guide midwives regarding new quality-of-care practices. Facebook groups were formed and became a platform to mentor new midwives through peer and leadership interaction and images of quality care. They also provide a platform for problem-solving, allowing midwives to interact with leadership, and promote the midwives' quality care. More than 5,000 midwives, hundreds of midwife faculty and international midwifery experts participate in these Facebook groups, posting comments on quality midwifery care practices, including managing postpartum haemorrhage and eclampsia.

Humanitarian Response

Bangladesh has some of the most frequent and severe humanitarian crises globally, including natural disasters, refugees, and pandemics. Using the above discussed mentoring model of 'enabling environment', both the natural disasters and refugee crises have been met by midwives and mentors supporting them. Professional midwives have been a critical provider of care in the humanitarian setting (Kemp, 2021). A few examples of the midwife's role in in the humanitarian setting are:

- Midwives were initially deployed for cyclone response through projects where they expanded sexual and reproductive health (SRH) and prenatal service availability, increasing access and use (Begum, 2023). Soon after this, a large refugee influx created an opportunity for the new midwives to make a significant contribution. For example, in 2015, over 300 midwives were deployed to the refugee camps of Cox's Bazar and the nearby host communities. This response benefited the midwifery profession as many gained significant professional experience through training, mentoring, and experience and later brought it to their government posts, including an emphasis on comprehensive sexual and reproductive health and rights.

- After the identification of the first COVID-19 case in Bangladesh, maternity service availability dramatically declined due to staff absence, being overwhelmed, and fear (Ainul, 2020; Data for Impact, 2023). More than 200 midwives were deployed to medical college, district, and sub-district hospitals. In many cases, midwives and mentors led the introduction of COVID-19 safety protocols for hospital triage systems and for establishing separate rooms for COVID-19 symptomatic mothers to receive ANC and give birth (Anderson et al., 2023). Before and after the pandemic, surveys of 91 hospitals with midwives showed significant improvements across all measures of COVID-19 readiness thanks to the midwives partnered with mentors.

- In a flood response in 2022 in north-eastern Bangladesh, midwives were deployed to remote rural flood-affected primary health centres, to provide quality SRHR services with a focus on labour, birth, initial management of obstetric and newborn emergencies, and referral. A total of 29 community health facilities and 20 referral sub-district hospitals were selected. Before the intervention, the community facilities were staffed with either a community health worker, or a midwife, most of them only providing outpatient care. These facilities had supervision and mentoring provided by a national project doctor and social media groups aimed to support them. During the flood response, over 28,729 women received sexual, reproductive, maternal, and newborn health services from the community health facilities. These services included antenatal care, postnatal care, normal vaginal births, family planning services, response to gender-based violence, and referral support. Over 3,323 vaginal births were conducted. The midwives demonstrated a steep learning curve and were able to perform their clinical and counselling tasks remarkably well over time. Although these midwives had completed the nationally accredited 3-year professional midwifery diploma, it was evident that they required close mentoring in the initial stages, as they became proficient in their role as independent practitioners. Deploying midwives with mentors as a response to climate-induced natural disasters was successful in establishing quality sexual and reproductive health services.

In these humanitarian response projects, international midwives were sometimes used as mentors. Despite certain disadvantages (e.g., language, culture), international mentors are a high-impact investment and aided in enabling new midwives to independently implement the reproductive health minimum initial service package (MISP) used in humanitarian response. As the midwives in humanitarian settings matured, some have themselves moved into mentoring roles. In part, because of mentorship, midwives have significantly improved quality, availability, access and use of sexual and reproductive health services.

Mentorship and Leadership in <u>Bangladesh</u>

Currently, formalised leadership roles for midwives are nascent. With a maximum of 6 years of experience, professional midwives have only recently entered the prerequisite higher education needed. Four midwives have recently been deployed to the Director General of Nursing and Midwifery (DGNM) to lead the profession. Midwives who have moved into the role of mentors will have an advantage to become leaders, and many have been selected to move forward into the recently formed BSc programs. The national midwifery Bachelor of Science and Master of Science programs were developed to create pathways for professional growth. The Bachelor of Science program in midwifery started in July 2022 with 76 students enrolled in four education institutions. The Master of Science program plans to start in 2024 and will be led by doctoral candidates once they have completed their program (BMS, 2023). As this new cadre of professional midwives receives higher education, they will move into more leadership roles. Although there is no mentorship currently for those roles, their experience with mentors and as mentors will enable strong leadership.

Bangladesh's Future

The creation of a profession of midwifery, their education, and eventual practice in Bangladesh is seen as a huge success. Regionally, Bangladesh has led the introduction of professional midwives. The use of mentors was key in overcoming hurdles such as non-evidence-based maternity care, lack of midwifery leadership, lack of enabling culture for midwifery, and a lack of power in the workplace. The government, committed to the success of the midwives, wisely adopted the mentoring model as key whenever midwifery care is introduced. Looking forward, the development of midwifery mentors to replace the physician mentors and midwifery leadership will continue to support midwifery throughout the country.

References

Afsana K. (2004). The tremendous cost of seeking hospital obstetric care in Bangladesh. Reprod Health Matters. 12(24):171–180.

Ainul S, Hossain M, Bhuiyan M, et al. (2020). Trends in Maternal Health Services in Bangladesh Before, During and After COVID-19 Lockdowns: Evidence from National Routine Service Data. COVID-19 Research Brief. Population Council. https://doi.org/10.31899/rh14.1037

Alenchery AJ, Thoppil J, Britto CD, de Onis JV, Fernandez L, Suman Rao PN. (2018). Barriers and enablers to skin-to-skin contact at birth in healthy neonates – a qualitative study. BMC Pediatrics. 18(1):48.

Andaleeb SS. (2007). Patient satisfaction with health services in Bangladesh. Health Policy Plan. 263–273.

Anderson R. (2022). The Impact and Experience of Introducing Professional Mid-wives into Rural Government Hospitals in Bangladesh, a Mixed-Methods Study. Lancaster University. Accessed October 15, 2022. https://www.proquest.com/openview/f74cfc00d8d7e72dd8a7a5846618e9dc/1?pq-origsite=gscholar&cbl=20 26366&diss=y

Anderson R, Williams A, Emdadul Hoque DM, et al. (2023). Implementing mid-wifery services in public tertiary medical college hospitals in Bangladesh: a longitudinal study. Women Birth. 36(3):299–304. https://doi.org/10.1016/j.wombi.2022.09.006

Anderson R, Zaman SB, Limmer M. (2023). The impact of introducing midwives and also mentoring on the quality of sexual, reproductive, maternal, newborn, And adolescent health services in low- and middle-income countries: an integrative review protocol. Methods and Protocols. 6:48.

Bangladesh Midwifery Society (BMS);World Health Organization (WHO). (2022). At a Glance the Journey of Midwifery in Bangladesh. BMS/WHO. Accessed September 22, 2023. https://pmc.ncbi.nlm.nih.gov/articles/PMC10615233/

Begum F, Ara R, Islam A, Marriott S, Williams A, Anderson R. (2023). Health system strengthening through professional midwifery in Bangladesh: best practices, chal-lenges and successes. Global Health: Science and Practice. 11(5):1–18. https://doi.org/10.9745/GHSP-D-23-00081

Billah SM, Chowdhury MAK, Khan, ANS, et al. (2019). Quality of care during child-birth at public health facilities in Bangladesh: a cross-sectional study using WHO/UNICEF 'Every mother every newborn (EMEN)' standards. BMJ Open Quality. 8(3):e000596.

Bogren M, Erlandsson K, Byrskog U, Members of the Midwifery Faculty Master's degree holders in Sexual and Reproductive Health and Rights. (2018). What pre-vents midwifery quality care in Bangladesh? A focus group enquiry with midwifery students. BMC Health Services and Research. 18(1):639. https://doi.org/10.1186/s12913-018-3447-5

CIA.gov. (2024, Dec 1). 2022. The World Factbook. Retrieved from https://www.cia.gov/the-world-factbook/about/archives/2022/countries/. Accessed 11 June 2025

Data for Impact. Estimating the Effect of COVID-19 on Total Utilization of Health Services in Bangladesh. (2021) Data for Impact. Accessed September 22, 2023. https://www.data4impactproject.org/wp-content/uploads/2021/02/Estimating-the-effect-of-COVID-19-on-utilization-of-health-services-in-Bangladesh_FS-20-513_D4I.pdf

DHS. (2019). UNFPA Sexual and Reproductive Health Working Group Bulleting Jan-Dec 2021, 1–7. Government of Bangladesh. https://bangladesh.unfpa.org/sites/default/files/pub-pdf/srh_working_group_annual_bulletin_2021.pdf

ICM. (2019). Essential Competencies for Midwifery Practice: International Con-federation of Midwives. https://www.internationalmidwives.org/asse ts/files/general-files/2019/02/icm-competencies_english_final_jan-2019-update_final-web_v1.0.pdf

Jhpiego. (2016). Low Dose, High Frequency: A Learning Approach to Improve Health Workforce Competence, Confidence, and Performance. Jhpiego. Accessed September 22, 2023. https://hms.jhpiego.org/wp-content/uploads/2016/08/LDHF_briefer.pdf

Kemp J, Maclean GD, Moyo N. (2021). Global Midwifery: Principles, Policy and Practice. Springer. https://link.springer.com/book/10.1007/978-3-030-46765-4

Khatun M, Akter P, Yunus S, Alam K, Pedersen C, Byrskog U, et al. (2022). Chal-lenges to implement evidence-based midwifery care in Bangladesh. An interview study with medical doctors mentoring health care providers. Sexual & Reproduc-tive Healthcare. 31:100692. https://doi.org/10.1016/j.srhc.2021.100692

Mahumud RE. (2019). Women's preferences for maternal healthcare services in Bangladesh: evidence from a discrete choice experiment. Journal of Clinical Medicine. 8(2):132. https://doi.org/10.3390/jcm8020132

Meadows KA (2011). Patient-reported outcome measures: an overview. British Journal of Community Nursing. 16(3):146–151.

Mittman BS, Tonesk X, Jacobson PD. (1992). Implementing clinical practice guidelines: social influence strategies and practitioner behavior change. QRB Quality Review Bulletin. 18(12):413–422. https://doi.org/10.1016/S0097-5990(16)30567-X

MoHFW. (2019). Government of Bangladesh HRH Data Sheet 2019. HSD.

NIPORT. (2016). Bangladesh Demographic and Health Survey 2014. Bangladesh NIPORT Associates, M and International ICF.

NIPORT, icddr,b, MEASURE Evaluation. (2017). Bangladesh Maternal Mortality and Health Care Survey (BMMS) 2016: Final Report. MEASURE Evaluation. https://www.measureevaluation.org/resources/publications/tr-18-297.html

Pappu NI, Öberg I, Byrskog U, et al. (2023). The commitment to a midwifery centre care model in Bangladesh: an interview study with midwives, educators and students. PLoS One. 18(4):e0271867. https://doi.org/10.1371/journal.pone.0271867

Payne L, Walker KF, Mitchell EJ. (2021). Timing of umbilical cord clamping for preterm infants in low-and middle-income countries: a survey of current practice. European Journal of Obstetrics & Gynecology and Reproductive Biology. 264:15–20.

Rajia SS. (2019). Trends and future of maternal and child health in Bangladesh. PLoS ONE. 14(3):e0211875. https://doi.org/10.1371/journal.pone.0211875.

Sandall J, Soltani H, Gates S, Shennan A, Devane D. (2016). Midwife-led continuity models of care compared with other models of care for women during pregnancy, birth and early parenting. Cochrane Database of Systematic Reviews. 4:CD004667. https://doi.org/10.1002/14651858.CD004667.pub6

Turkmani S, Currie S, Mungia J, Assefi N, Rahmanzai AJ, Azfar P, et al. (2013). 'Midwives are the backbone of our health system': lessons from Afghanistan to guide expansion of midwifery in challenging settings. Midwifery. 29:1166–72.

WHO. (2016). WHO Recommendations on Antenatal Care for a Positive Pregnancy Experience. WHO. https://doi.org/10.1016/j.midw.2013.06.015

WHO. (2016). Standards for Improving Quality of Maternal and Newborn Care in Health Facilities. World Health Organization.

WHO. (2017). Bangladesh Workforce. WHO.

WHO. (2018). WHO Recommendations Intrapartum Care for a Positive Childbirth Experience. World Health Organization. https://www.who.int/publications/i/item/9789241550215.

WHO. (2019). Strengthening Quality Midwifery Education for Universal Health Coverage 2030: Framework for Action. World Health Organization. https://www.who.int/publications/i/item/9789241515849

World Bank. (2024). Bangladesh Overview. Retrieved from World Bank Group. https://www.worldbank.org/en/country/bangladesh/overview

Zaman R, Sabur M. (2019). Research on the Long-Term Impacts of Trained Midwives on Health Outcomes in Bangladesh: Key Findings from the Baseline Study. Oxford Policy Management. https://www.opml.co.uk/projects/assessing-long-term-impacts-of-trained-midwives-on-health-outcomes

10

MIDWIFERY MENTORSHIP IN BELGIUM

Mieke Embo

Section 1: Midwifery in Belgium

Belgium and Midwifery Care

Belgium is a country in Western Europe, bordered by the Netherlands, Germany, Luxembourg, and France. Its political organisation is complex and structured on both regional and linguistic grounds. It is divided into three highly autonomous communities and regions: Flemish Region (Dutch-speaking), Walloon Region (French-speaking), and the Brussels-Capital Region (bilingual) (Vermeulen et al., 2021). Belgium has a population of 11,697,557 (2023), with 113,739 births in 2020 (Belgian Government, 2024).

The midwifery profession, as well as the professional title, qualification, training and practice, is included in the Coordinated Law of 10 May 2015, on the practice of healthcare professions (FOD Volksgezondheid, 2015). The law distinguishes between activities performed by midwives with complete autonomy and those that require medical supervision. Autonomous midwifery activities are listed in the law and include pregnancy diagnosis, follow-up of low-risk pregnancies (maternal and child risk assessment, birth preparation, and parent education), normal vaginal births without any complications (including amniotomy, episiotomy, and perineal suturing), postnatal care, care of healthy newborns, preventive measures, and emergency procedures. Midwives also have the right to prescribe a limited number of drugs listed in the law. The management of fertility problems, high-risk pregnancies, high-risk deliveries, and newborns with life-threatening conditions are out of scope of an autonomous midwife. In such cases, midwives are required to work under medical supervision or refer clients to obstetric care. In addition, the

DOI: 10.4324/9781003533733-11

law describes procedures that are explicitly prohibited for midwives, namely: artificial dilation of the cervix, use of forceps and vacuum, administration of anaesthesia (except local anaesthesia for performing or suturing episiotomy), and inducing abortion. Except in emergencies, midwives are also prohibited from performing the following procedures: internal version, breech extraction, manual removal of the placenta, and manual exploration of the uterus (Benahmed et al., 2023).

In Belgium, the healthcare system allows women the freedom to choose their healthcare providers. Women can choose a midwife, but they have also the ability to consult directly with doctors (obstetrician, gynaecologist, and general practitioner) without needing a referral. The number of births per service ranges from 120 to 3,500. The number also varies between regions: the median number of births per maternity service is 2,172 in Brussels against 790 in Flanders and 786 in Wallonia (Lefevre et al., 2020). The average length of postnatal hospital stay after vaginal birth has decreased from 5 days in 2000 to 3.1 days in 2016. This reduction had an impact on the midwifery workforce, and a shift to primary care has been noted (Benahmed et al., 2016; Vermeulen et al., 2021).

Practising midwives in Belgium have responsibilities in four professional domains: obstetrics, reproductive medicine, gynaecology, and neonatology. In 2019, 12,088 people were licensed to practise using the title of a midwife (Benahmed et al., 2023; Planning Unit for Health Professional Supply, 2022), of whom 57% worked in the healthcare sector (7 175 FTEs) (Durand et al., 2022). With more than 9 out of 10 births taking place in hospitals (Leroy & Van Leeuw, 2022; Van Leeuw & Leroy, 2022), most of the midwifery activity took place in hospitals. As a result, less than 10% of the midwives worked in an outpatient setting (Benahmed et al., 2023; Durand et al., 2022). It is estimated the demand for midwifery care in Belgium will increase from 11.4% to 17.4%, between 2016 and 2026. This increase is mainly due to the expected rise in postnatal outpatient care activities (Benahmed et al., 2019; Vermeulen et al., 2021).

Belgium and Midwifery Education

In Belgium, midwifery education is provided through either a) a direct-entry bachelor's programme consisting of a specific full-time training as a midwife compromising at least three years of theoretical and practical study or b) a specific full-time training as a midwife of 18 months' duration after training of nurses responsible for general care. These programmes are aligned with the European Directive, which ensures that midwives acquire the essential knowledge and skills outlined in Directive 2005/36/EC to competently practise the profession (Article 21, Article 40) (European Parliament Council of the European Union, 2013). Education, however, is managed at the regional level, with separate Ministers of Education for each region. Each minister is responsible for the education system within their respective region, including higher education. In Flanders, bachelor's in nursing and/or midwifery can follow a Master in Nursing and Midwifery programme, but it is not necessary to practise midwifery.

Midwifery education is provided in 12 Higher Education Institutions in Flanders and in nine in the French Community (Embo & Valcke, 2016). Although the minimum content requirements for midwifery training are outlined in the Belgian Coordinated Law of 10 May 2015, each linguistic community may determine the duration of training necessary to meet the required competencies, leading to a three-year program in Flanders (180 ECTS) and a four-year program in the French Community (Walloon and Brussels-Capital Region, 240 ECTS) (Benahmed et al., 2016, 2023). Midwifery schools have the freedom to organise their programme individually if they follow the legal requirements (European Parliament Council of the European Union, 2013; FOD Volksgezondheid, 2015). Belgium also has a professional competency profile (Federale overheidsdienst Volksgezondheid, 2016) that results in distinctive educational profiles for Flanders and the French Community. In 2014, the twelve midwifery schools in Flanders developed a competency-based educational profile (Flemish Education Council, 2014) which was recently revised and is currently awaiting approval from The Flemish Agency for Higher Education. This profile challenged the available curricula and especially stressed the need to reconsider workplace learning and assessment during midwifery practice. It was the catalyst to standardise education, to introduce a workplace learning model based on current socio-cultural learning theories and to put an end to adopting too many different assessment instruments and criteria (Embo & Valcke, 2016).

Midwifery Practical and Clinical Training

Directive 2005/36/EC (European Parliament Council of the European Union, 2013) regulates the requirements for midwifery training and establishes common standards. This is important because it enables qualified midwives to work freely across European Union (EU) member states without the need for additional exams or training. By setting uniform training standards, the directive ensures midwives throughout Europe possess a similar baseline of knowledge and skills, which is crucial for patient safety and quality of care.

The directive consists of two parts, and it mandates that theoretical and technical training (part 1) must be balanced and coordinated with clinical training (part 2) to ensure that the necessary knowledge and experience outlined in the Directive are acquired effectively. The directive allows for a degree of flexibility when developing the curriculum, including the balance between simulation-based education at the university and clinical education at the workplace. There are differences in the choice of disciplines, length of internships, innovative modes (such as the learning workplace where students take over the ward), and workplace programmes. Some schools build and align their practical programme on competencies, with a few schools introducing the theory of Entrustable Professional Activities (Moore et al., 2024; Shorey et al., 2019; ten Cate & Schumacher, 2022). To ensure graduating students are competent to enter the midwifery workforce, the directive contains a list of essential practical tasks and clinical skills that must be achieved.

REFLECTIVE ACTIVITY 1

Read: Moore, J., Chan, T., Doucette, J., Lipps, T. and Slager, D. (2024). Defining nurse practitioner core entrustable professional activities: essential step toward competency-based education. *Nurse Educator, 49*(5), 235–240, DOI: 10.1097/NNE.0000000000001673

After reading this article:

- Reflect on your work unit and what you consider to be essential midwifery discipline Entrustable Professional Activities, and
- Briefly outline how Entrustable Professional Activities align with patient safety and quality care.

Section 2: Midwifery Mentorship in Belgium

Mentorship

Belgium lacks national legislation regulating mentorship and thus follows the European Directive, stating:

> Clinical instruction shall take the form of supervised in-service training in hospital departments or other health services approved by the competent authorities or bodies. As part of this training, student midwives shall participate in the activities of the departments concerned in so far as those activities contribute to their training. They shall be taught the responsibilities involved in the activities of midwives.
> *(European Parliament Council of the European Union, 2013)*

As a result, there are no national guidelines regarding mentorship concepts, definitions, or roles. Each organisation is free to define its own terms (e.g., supervisor, teacher, mentor, preceptor, coach) and to formulate its own role descriptions. This leads to conceptional diffusion, where a mentor in one organisation may be considered a teacher in another. Nevertheless, in general, most Flemish midwifery programmes work with the following roles: 1) student, 2) mentor (workplace), 3) supervisor (school), and 4) internship coordinator (school). Sometimes, a fifth role is defined, the 'learning coach' (school). Since 2000, hospitals also have a 'support nurse [Begeleidingsverpleegkundige]' to organise internships and support mentors. We describe the identified roles within the Belgium midwifery education context in Table 10.1.

TABLE 10.1 Roles within Belgium

Identified Position	Role within Midwifery Education Context
Student	A self-regulating learner undertaking a midwifery education programme.
Mentor Affiliated with the workplace	The role of the mentor varies according to the workplace unit and organisational structure. The role may be voluntary or a compulsory component of the midwife's responsibilities. The mentor's role is to guide the student's learning process during their placement by discussing learning goals, observing performances, reviewing reflections, and providing feedback.
Supervisor [stagebegeleider] Affiliated with the school and usually linked to specific placement site/s to foster professional relationships.	Role is to support both the mentor and the student, take responsibility for the final summative assessment score, and ensure continuity of guidance throughout the internship periods.
Internship coordinator Affiliated with the school	Responsible for all administrative aspects of clinical learning at the workplace such as planning, student contracts, and medical checks. They serve as the point of contact for the placement sites, providing students with information on all aspects of their internship, including the assigned placement and mentors.
Learning Coach Affiliated with the school	This is a teacher who supports the midwifery students throughout their entire programme and facilitates the meta-cognitive reflection on their learning process and the development of their midwifery identity. Support may be provided individually or in small groups, with peer review and supervision.
Support Nurse Affiliated with the hospital	Role includes welcoming and guiding students, new staff, and those returning to practice. Responsibilities also encompass coordinating placement planning, providing orientation, acting as a contact person for students and placement supervisors/educational institutions, and training and supporting mentors (Netwerk Verpleegkunde, 2024).

In Belgium, there is no required training programme for mentors, and often, no additional time is allocated for the role. In internships, with a one-to-one relationship between the student and midwife, such as in independent midwifery practices, the midwife clearly assumes the mentor role. This differs from internships where multiple midwives work together. In some settings, each student is assigned one formal mentor, while in others, two or more mentors may be assigned per student. This is important because students are sometimes on short placements, and mentors may not work full-time or may work in shifts. Unfortunately, there are also places where no formal mentor is assigned, and in such cases, the head of the department often takes on this role. The mentor's role is to guide the student's learning process during their placement. In principle, students have the right to expect this support, as mentoring is a key competency in the professional role of a midwife. Since mentors are tasked with providing feedback, they always play a role in formative assessments. In some schools, they also participate in summative assessments, though this is not always the case.

Although healthcare organisations are motivated to train students in the hope they will seek employment there after qualifying, numerous challenges persist in improving the quality of clinical education for midwives in Flanders (Embo, 2015; Embo & Valcke, 2016, 2019; Janssens et al., 2023). Some of these challenges include finding a balance between the number of students and the availability of meaningful learning experiences and adequate supervision. Students often rely on the willingness of midwives to supervise them, as this is an unpaid activity, and midwives frequently lack the time to provide supervision due to heavy workloads. The government is aware of these issues, and recommendations to improve the workplace culture have been reported. For further information on the recommendations, see:

- Vlaamse Vereniging van Studenten. (2024). *Standpunt stages in de zorgsector*. https://vvs.ac/standpunt/standpunt-stages-in-de-zorgsector

An Evidence-Based Mentorship Model

In the context of this chapter and midwifery in Belgium, we present a feasible and evidence-based methodology that has been developed to support learning, assessment, and supervision of midwives at the workplace, as illustrated in Figure 10.1 (Embo et al., 2015). It is a model that has been developed to tackle barriers to implement competency-based education in clinical practice such as: 1) divergent values among stakeholders, 2) discontinuous supervision, 3) inadequate guidance of developing reflective ability, 4) poor feedback quality, and 5) a lack of a consistent and programmatic approach. Initially, midwifery programmes relied on paper-based portfolios. However, almost all programmes now utilise digital portfolios (Janssens et al., 2022).

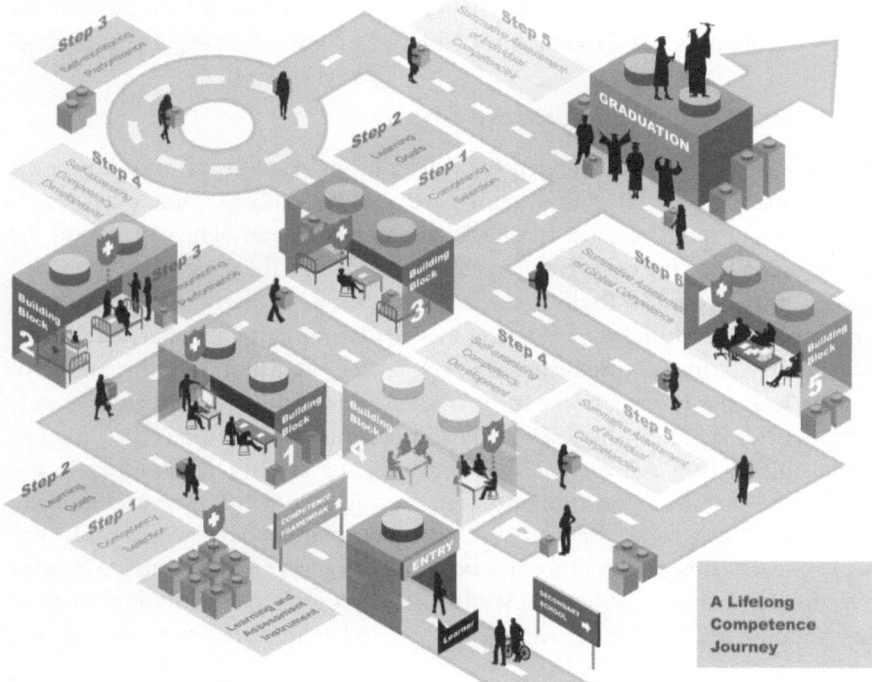

FIGURE 10.1   Integrated learning assessment and supervision competency framework (Embo et al., 2015)

Step 1: Mentoring Student Competency Selection

The midwifery competencies that are the basis of the workplace learning curriculum are clearly defined and each placement commences with the student identifying which competencies from the competency framework can be learned and assessed in the context of that workplace. This step emphasises the importance of context in workplace learning (Epstein & Hundert, 2002). The selection of competencies at the start of an internship constitutes an agreement between the student, the workplace, and the school. This step is aligned with the school (curriculum) and the workplace (learning environment) and clarifies mutual expectations (Harden, 2007b).

Step 2: Writing Learning Goals

After selecting relevant competencies, students formulate personal learning goals aligned to selected competencies (Dannefer, 2013; Embo et al., 2015; Harden, 2007). Students formulate the learning goals, linked to one or more competencies, according to the SMART principle (Specific, Measurable, Acceptable,

Realistic, and Time-bound). The learning goals are reviewed by their mentor and or supervisor and are used to monitor and assess clinical learning and progress.

Step 3: Mentoring and Self-Monitoring Performance

The third step involves an extensive learning phase, with self-monitoring of performances. The goal of this step is to document daily learning experiences and link them to reflections, feedback, and competencies. The instruction for 'reflection on learning experiences' is based on the STAR+R method (Situation, Task, Action, Result + Reflection on the result). This phase is important for promoting the continuity of learning in an environment characterised by discontinuity. All unstructured learning experiences (snapshots) can be collected, and the learning information can be organised by date, learning experiences, competencies, or internships. The collection of this information is the student's responsibility. In a self-regulated curriculum, the student is expected to actively seek learning opportunities, write meaningful reflections, and actively request feedback from the observer. Every workplace supervisor (observer, mentor, teacher) is expected to observe student's performances, critically read reflections to assess whether the student has a correct understanding of their performance, provide high-quality feedback, and validate this with a signature.

Step 4: Mentoring and Self-Assessing Competency Development

During the internship, the student is instructed to reflect on competency development to learn how to take a more objective and comprehensive view of their progress (Yuan et al., 2012). In this reflection, the student should not provide a detailed account of actions (step 3) but is asked to take a step back and view the learning process from a distance. Reflection on competency development is based on SWOT (Strengths, Weaknesses, Opportunities, and Threats). The student observes progress, identifies further learning needs, checks off achieved learning goals and formulates new ones, to write an action plan for the next learning period. The supervisor reads this reflection, provides feedback, and assessment is based on evaluation criteria that are discussed with the student. When this step is completed, at the end of an internship, the new learning goals immediately become step 2 for the next learning period, thereby promoting continuity across the different internships (Embo et al., 2014).

Step 5: Summative Assessment of Individual Competencies and Mentor Feedback

Step 5 focuses on the summative assessment of individual competencies, consisting of a preparatory phase and a dialogue. In preparation for the assessment meeting, the student self-assesses using the competency list with assessment criteria and further expands with assessment rubrics for each year (Embo et al., 2017). The mentor (workplace) also assesses the student using the same assessment list, but the student and mentor do not see each other's evaluations. The supervisor (school) organises an assessment meeting with the student and mentor to compare and discuss their evaluations. The supervisor (school) then records the conclusion on the same assessment list. The assessment is conducted and grades according to the following criteria: extremely weak, fail, pass, excellent, and not applicable (e.g., no learning opportunity).The conclusion should not surprise the student, as it is based on reflections and feedback from steps 3 and 4. This assessment meeting requires about an hour per student and is a crucial step in preparing the final assessment of 'professional competence'.

Step 6: Mentor's Summative Assessment of Professional Competence

The concept of 'professional competence' is defined as the reliable and judicious application of various competencies in daily practice (Epstein & Hundert, 2002). A positive assessment of professional competence means the assessor has confidence the student possesses all competencies and can also apply them in an integrated manner in new and unexpected situations. This step is important within the holistic view of competency-based education.

Summative assessment of professional competence takes place in school. The assessment school committee aggregates pass/fail judgements on individual competency level into a final judgement on professional competence (score from 1 to 20). Learners are informed of the score and can ask for feedback from the teachers. These teachers take part in the assessment meetings in the workplace and in the school committee, and this way, teachers can be seen as learning assistants, generating a unique 'competence fingerprint' for each student (Pijl-Zieber et al., 2014).

A pitfall of competency-based assessment is the tendency to calculate an arithmetic average of individual competencies, which could result in the student passing with a 10/20, while professionals may feel the student is not competent enough to progress to the next level of education. Therefore, we emphasise the importance of mentors and supervisors in correcting and supplementing the information collected in steps 3 and 4, if necessary. This ensures that a panel of experts from the school can make an objective yet 'subjective' decision.

What Happens Next?

In principle, these steps are repeated each learning period. The cycle can be completed one or more times per internship, but it is also entirely possible for one cycle to span multiple learning periods. Current literature in medical education refers to 'programmatic assessment' (Andreou et al., 2024; Van Der Vleuten et al., 2012, 2015) and shows that it is not necessary to apply the sixth step in every learning period.

What Are the Benefits and Challenges of This Model?

This model demonstrates numerous advantages such as the potential to capture experiences in several authentic situations; to collect and manage learning information according to the midwifery competencies; to share information with all the stakeholders involved with workplace learning; to measure competency development over time because of validated assessment checklists integrating competency components; and to support continuing professional development after graduation (Embo, 2018; Janssens et al., 2022; van Ostaeyen et al., 2023; Van Ostaeyen et al., 2022). In a recent study, Janssens et al. (2023) used this model to explore how students, mentors, and educators from different healthcare disciplines (among them also midwifery) perceived the implementation of competency-based education at the workplace. The results showed the model is valuable to support student learning and address weaknesses in current mentorship programmes.

There were, however, challenges around implementing the model, such as: 1) a gap between the educational programme and the workplace learning reality, 2) a lack of overview of predefined competencies, 3) an overemphasis on technical competencies at the expense of generic ones, 4) poorly formulated learning goals, 5) obstacles related to reflection, 6) poor feedback quality, and 7) perceived subjectivity in the assessment approach. Despite these challenges, authors in other healthcare domains have highlighted the model's strength in addressing the need for assessment tools that accurately reflect workplace performance (Busch et al., 2023). Other researchers have praised the comprehensive competency assessment, which includes direct observation of hands-on performance alongside other competencies such as communication competencies (Zechariah et al., 2022). Van Loon et al. (2019) emphasised the model's value in supporting feedback-seeking behaviour (Van Loon, 2019).

Mentoring, CPD, and the Midwifery Workforce

The European Directive 2013/55/EU (European Parliament Council of the European Union, 2013)(states in article 15 that CPD contributes to the safe and effective practice of professionals. CPD should cover professional, technical, scientific, regulatory, and ethical developments and motivate professionals to participate in lifelong learning relevant to their discipline.

In Belgium, two important laws regulate CPD. Midwives are required to continuously update their training to maintain their accreditation by completing at least 75 hours of continuing education every five years (Belgian Government, 2018). Furthermore, in 2022, Belgium enacted a Quality law stating that '*The healthcare practitioner provides only healthcare for which he/she has the necessary demonstrable competence and experience. It is the individual healthcare practitioners' responsibility to keep the necessary data/ evidence of competence and experience in a portfolio*' (article 8). A unique aspect of the current CPD requirements in Belgium is the absence of regulations concerning mentorship, accreditation, or mandatory membership in a professional organisation. CPD remains the individual practising midwife's responsibility.

Despite the voluntary nature of membership, many midwives choose to join a professional association. Belgium has three professional associations – one in Flanders and two in Wallonia – that are united under the Belgian Midwifery Association. This alliance allows them to be a member of the International Confederation of Midwives (ICM). These organisations stimulate midwives to continuously developing their professional competencies by organising professional learning activities such as webinars and conferences.

The Flemish Professional Organisation of midwives (https://www.vroed-vrouwen.be/) has introduced a quality label for midwives in Flanders to enhance and standardise midwifery care. This quality label aims to promote the professional identity of midwives and ensure they provide high-quality services aligned with established standards. The initiative is part of a broader effort to transition from obstetric- to midwifery-led care. The quality label encourages midwives to adhere to best practices and continuously improve their skills through professional development.

The implementation of mentoring programmes that educate and support experienced midwives to guide and support students, new staff, and those returning to practice can enhance their sense of well-being and job satisfaction. It has the potential to reduce attrition and turnover rates for mentors and mentees. For mentees, it can instil a sense of belonginess and professional identity, thus supporting the future midwifery workforce (Squire et al., 2024). Furthermore, it can foster group cohesion, improve team functioning, and ultimately enhance the quality of patient care (Gijbels, 2024).

References

Andreou, V., Peters, S., Eggermont, J., & Schoenmakers, B. (2024). A needs assessment for enhancing workplace-based assessment: A grounded theory study. *BMC Medical Education*, 24(1), 659. https://doi.org/10.1186/s12909-024-05636-3.

Belgian Government. (2018). *De erkenning en permanente vorming voor vroedvrouwen.* https://zorg-en-gezondheid.be/de-erkenning-en-permanente-opleiding-voor-vroedvrouwen

Belgian Government. (2024, September 20). *Statbel: België in cijfers.* https://statbel. fgov.be/en

Benahmed, N., Hendrickx, E., Adriaenssens, J., & Stordeur, S. (2016). *Planning van Gezondheidszorgpersoneel en Gegevens over Vroedvrouwen [Planning of Health Care Staff and Data on Midwives]; Belgian Health Care Knowledge Centre (KCE): Brussels, Belgium,* 2016. https://kce.fgov.be/nl/publicaties/alle-rapporten/ planning-van-gezondheidszorgpersoneel-en-gegevens-over-vroedvrouwen

Benahmed, N., Lefevre, M., Vinck, I., & Stordeur, S. (2019). *Alternative scenarios for the forecasting of the midwifery workforce: Horizon scanning and quantification model.*

Benahmed, N., Lefèvre, M., & Stordeur, S. (2023). Managing uncertainty in forecasting health workforce demand using the robust workforce planning framework: The example of midwives in Belgium. *Human Resources for Health, 21*(1), 75.

Busch, G., Rodríguez Borda, M. V., Morales, P. I., Weiss, M., Ciambrone, G., Costabel, J. P., Durante, E., Gelpi, R., & De Lima, A. E. A. (2023). Validation of a form for assessing the professional performance of residents in cardiology by nurses. *Journal of Education and Health Promotion, 12*(1), 127. https://doi.org/10.4103/ jehp.jehp_44_23

Dannefer, E. F. (2013). Beyond assessment of learning toward assessment for learning: Educating tomorrow's physicians. *Medical Teacher, 35,* 560–563.

Durand, C., Jouck, P., Miermans, P., Steinberg, P., & Vivet, V. (2022). *PlanCad Sages-femmes 2019, Cellule Planification des professions de soins de santé. Brussels: Division Heath Professions and professional practices - Health Care Department from Federal Public Service Health, Food chain safety and Environment. [Service Professions des soins de santé et pratique pro- fessionnelle, DG Soins de santé, Service Publique Fédéral Santé publique, Sécurité de la chaîne alimentaire et Environnement];* 2022.

Embo, M. (2015). *Integrating Workplace Learning, Assessment and Supervision in Health Care Education.* University of Maastricht. https://cris.maastrichtuniversity.nl/en/ publications/integrating-workplace-learning-assessment-and-supervision-in-heal

Embo, M. (2018). A competency-based midwifery e-workplace learning portfolio: Concept, theory and pedagogy. *Global Journal of Health Science & Nursing, 1*(1), 4. http://gslpublishers.org/journals/current-issue.php?title=global-journal-of-health-science-and-nursing

Embo, M., Driessen, E., Valcke, M., & van der Vleuten, C. P. M. (2014). A framework to facilitate self-directed learning, assessment and supervision in midwifery practice: A qualitative study of supervisors' perceptions. *Nurse Education in Practice, 14*(4), 441–446. https://doi.org/10.1016/j.nepr.2014.01.015

Embo, M., Driessen, E., Valcke, M., & van der Vleuten, C. P. M. (2015). Integrating learning assessment and supervision in a competency framework for clinical workplace education. *Nurse Education Today, 35*(2), 341–346. https://doi. org/10.1016/j.nedt.2014.11.022

Embo, M., Helsloot, K., Michels, N., & Valcke, M. (2017). A Delphi study to validate competency-based criteria to assess undergraduate midwifery students' competencies in the maternity ward. *Midwifery, 53,* 1–8.

Embo, M., & Valcke, M. (2016). Workplace learning in midwifery education in Flanders (Belgium). *Midwifery, 33,* 24–27. https://doi.org/10.1016/j. midw.2015.11.021

Embo, M., & Valcke, M. (2019). Improving student midwives' workplace learning by moving from self- to co-regulated learning! *Women and Birth, 32*(3). https://doi. org/10.1016/j.wombi.2018.08.004

Epstein, R. M., & Hundert, E. M. (2002). Defining and assessing professional competence. *JAMA, 287*(2), 226–235. http://www.ncbi.nlm.nih.gov/pubmed/11779266

European Parliament Council of the European Union. (2013). *Directive 2005/36/ EC of the European Parliament and of the Council of 7 September 2005 on the Recognition of Professional Qualifications and Regulation.* http://data.europa.eu/ eli/dir/2005/36/oj

Federale overheidsdienst Volksgezondheid, veiligheid van de voedselketen en leefmilieu. (2016). *Het beroeps- en competentieprofiel van de Belgische vroedvrouw* [The professional and competency profile of the Belgian midwife].

FOD Volksgezondheid. (2015). Gecoördineerde wet gezondheidszorgberoepen 10 mei 2015. In *Staatsblad.* http://www.ejustice.just.fgov.be/cgi_loi/change_lg.pl?lan guage=nl&la=N&cn=2015051006&table_name=wet

Gijbels, F. (2024). *Begeleidingsverpleegkundigen - schriftelijke vraag aan minister Vandenbroucke.* Begeleidingsverpleegkundigen - schriftelijke vraag aan minister Vandenbroucke [Mentoring nurses – written question to Minister Vandenbroucke]. https://www.friedagijbels.be/nieuws/begeleidingsverpleegkundigen-schriftelijke-vraag-aan-minister-vandenbroucke

Harden, R. M. (2007a). Learning outcomes as a tool to assess progression. *Medical Teacher, 29*(7), 678–682. https://doi.org/10.1080/01421590701729955

Harden, R. M. (2007b). Outcome-based education: The future is today. *Med Teach, 29,* 625–629.

Janssens, O., Embo, M., Valcke, M., & Haerens, L. (2023). When theory beats practice: The implementation of competency-based education at healthcare workplaces. *BMC Medical Education, 23*(1), 484. https://doi.org/10.1186/s12909-023-04446-3

Janssens, O., Haerens, L., Valcke, M., Beeckman, D., Pype, P., & Embo, M. (2022). The role of ePortfolios in supporting learning in eight healthcare disciplines: A scoping review. In *Nurse Education in Practice* (Vol. 63). Elsevier Ltd. https://doi.org/10.1016/j.nepr.2022.103418

Lefevre, M., Bouckaert, N., Camberlin, C., Devriese, S., Pincé, H., De Meester, C., Fricheteau, B., & Van de Voorde, C. (2020). *Organisation of Maternity Services in Belgium.* https://kce.fgov.be/en/organisation-of-maternity-services-in-belgium

Leroy, C., & Van Leeuw, V. (2022). *Santé périnatal en wallonie-Année 2021.* Centre d'Épidémiologie Périnatale.

Moore, J., Chan, T., Doucette, J., Lipps, T., & Slager, D. (2024). Defining nurse practitioner core entrustable professional activities: Essential step toward competency-based education. *Nurse Educator, 49*(5), 235–240. https://doi.org/10.1097/ NNE.0000000000001673

Netwerk Verpleegkunde. (2024). Begeleidingsverpleegkundigen. Begeleidingsverpleegkundigen

Pijl-Zieber, E. M., Barton, S., Konkin, J., Awosoga, O., & Caine, V. (2014). Competence and competency-based nursing education: Finding our way through the issues. *Nurse Education Today, 34*(5), 676–678. https://doi.org/http://dx.doi.org/10.1016/j.nedt.2013.09.007

Planning Unit for Health Professional Supply. (2022). *Statistiques annuelles des professionnels des soins de santé en Belgique - Nombre de profession- nels en droit d'exercer au 31/12/2021 et influx 2021.*

Shorey, S., Lau, T. C., Lau, S. T., & Ang, E. (2019). Entrustable professional activities in health care education: A scoping review. *Medical Education, 53*(8), 766–777. https://doi.org/10.1111/medu.13879

Squire, D., Gonzalez, L., & Shayan, C. (2024). Enhancing sense of belonging in nursing student clinical placements to advance learning and identity development. *Journal of Professional Nursing, 51,* 109–114.

ten Cate, O., & Schumacher, D. J. (2022). Entrustable professional activities versus competencies and skills: Exploring why different concepts are often conflated. *Advances in Health Sciences Education, 27*(2), 491–499. https://doi.org/10.1007/ s10459-022-10098-7

Van Der Vleuten, C. P. M., Schuwirth, L. W. T., Driessen, E. W., Dijkstra, J., Tigelaar, D., Baartman, L. K. J., & Van Tartwijk, J. (2012). A model for programmatic assessment fit for purpose. *Medical Teacher, 34*(3), 205–214. https://doi.org/10.3109/0142159X.2012.652239

Van Der Vleuten, C. P. M., Schuwirth, L. W. T., Driessen, E. W., Govaerts, M. J. B., & Heeneman, S. (2015). Twelve tips for programmatic assessment. *Medical Teacher, 37*(7), 641–646.

Van Leeuw, V., & Leroy, C. (2022). *Santé périnatale en Région bruxelloise–Année 2021.* [Perinatal health in the Brussels-Capital Region – year 2021]. Centre d'Épidémiologie Périnatale.

Van Loon, M. H. (2019.). *Self-Assessment and Self-Reflection to Measure and Improve Self-Regulated Learning in the Workplace.* In McGrath, S., Mulder, M., Papier, J. & Suart, R. (Eds.), *Handbook of Vocational Education and Training: Developments in the Changing World of Work* (pp. 1389–1408). Springer. https://doi.org/10.1007/978-3-319-94532-3_88

van Ostaeyen, S., Embo, M., Rotsaert, T., de Clercq, O., Schellens, T., & Valcke, M. (2023). A qualitative textual analysis of feedback comments in ePortfolios: Quality and alignment with the CanMEDS roles. *Perspectives on Medical Education, 12*(1), 584–593. https://doi.org/10.5334/pme.1050

Van Ostaeyen, S., Embo, M., Schellens, T., & Valcke, M. (2022). Training to support ePortfolio users during clinical placements: A scoping review. *Medical Science Educator.* https://doi.org/10.1007/s40670-022-01583-0

Vermeulen, J., Luyben, A., Buyl, R., Debonnet, S., Castiaux, G., Niset, A., Muyldermans, J., Fleming, V., & Fobelets, M. (2021). The state of professionalisation of midwifery in Belgium: A discussion paper. *Women and Birth, 34*(1), 7–13. https://doi.org/10.1016/J.WOMBI.2020.09.012

Yuan, H., Bin, Williams, B. A., Fang, J. B., & Pang, D. (2012). Chinese Baccalaureate nursing students' readiness for self-directed learning. *Nurse Education Today, 32*(4), 427–431. https://doi.org/http://dx.doi.org/10.1016/j.nedt.2011.03.005

Zechariah, S., Waller, J. L., Stallings, J., Gess, A. J., & Lehman, L. (2022). Inter-rater and intra-rater reliability of the INSPECT (Interactive nutrition specific physical exam competency tool) measured in multi-site acute care settings. *Healthcare (Switzerland), 10*(2). https://doi.org/10.3390/healthcare10020212

11

MIDWIFERY MENTORSHIP IN CANADA

Deepali Y. Upadhyaya

Canada: Setting the Scene

Canada is the second-largest country in the world by land area, following Russia. Despite its immense size, the population of around 37 million is relatively small, similar to the US state of California's population (Statistics Canada, 2024b). This places Canada 38th in global population rankings, while Russia holds the ninth position (Statistics Canada, 2024a; World Data, 2024). Canada consists of 10 provinces and three territories. The provinces exercise constitutional powers granted to them, while the territories operate under authority delegated by the Parliament of Canada (Government of Canada, 2024a). In the 2021 Canadian Census, approximately 23 million individuals reported English as their primary language spoken at home, followed by French at just over 7 million. Additionally, many Indigenous languages are spoken alongside those introduced by newcomers and diaspora communities, with roughly 3.6 million people immigrating to Canada between 1980 and 2021 (Statistics Canada, 2024b).

Long before European settlers arrived in the land now called Canada, Indigenous Peoples lived and flourished. The Royal Proclamation of 1763, issued by King George III, marked the establishment of British territories in North America and served as the basis for treaties made with Indigenous Nations during the 18th century (Statistics Canada, 2024c). While treaties are meant to be mutually beneficial agreements, "over many centuries, these relationships were eroded by colonial and paternalistic policies that were enacted into laws" (Government of Canada, 2024b). The history of this Indigenous cultural genocide included a century-long practice of forcibly removing

DOI: 10.4324/9781003533733-12

children from their families and placing them in residential schools. While official apologies have been issued, the long-lasting ramifications run deep and wide. The Calls to Action from the Truth and Reconciliation Commission of Canada (2015) were developed on information gathered from over 6500 residential school survivors (Government of Canada, 2024c). It is essential for the Calls to Action to remain active and at the forefront of all initiatives. The Canadian Constitution identifies three distinct Indigenous groups: First Nations, Inuit, and Métis (FNMI). These communities are rich in diversity and continue to grow, with the 2021 census recording the FNMI population at 1.8 million in Canada (Statistics Canada, 2024b).

Canada and Midwifery Care

In 1986, the establishment of the Inuulitsivik Midwifery Education Program and Birth Centre became a pivotal step in reclaiming birth practices and ending forced birth evacuations from rural and remote settings with limited healthcare. This initiative was designed to serve Inuit pregnant people and their families, offering culturally grounded care and education provided by and for the Inuit community (Pambrun et al., 2019; Van Wagner et al., 2007). In many other areas in Canada, midwifery originated from a grassroots social movement whereby apprenticeship training was the means of passing forward knowledge and skill (MacDonald & Bourgeault, 2009). These systems laid the tracks for midwifery within future regulatory and educational developments (Upadhyaya et al., 2022). Midwifery was first regulated in Ontario in 1991, with undergraduate midwifery educational programs accepting the first intake of students in 1993 (MacDonald & Bourgeault, 2009; Pambrun et al., 2019).

In current healthcare systems in Canada, registered midwives (RMs) typically work in a case management model of care that emphasises the following principles: professional autonomy, partnership with clients, continuity of care, informed choice, choice of birthplace, evidenced-informed decision-making, and collaborative care (Canadian Association of Midwives [CAM], 2015). With only approximately 2,000 registered midwives in Canada managing 13% of the births, many actively practising midwives also serve multiple roles in health authorities, professional associations, academia, and governmental regulatory bodies (CAM, 2023a).

Regulatory and Educational Frameworks for Mentorship in Canada

The Canadian Midwifery Regulators Council (CMRC) sets national competencies for RMs (Canadian Midwifery Regulators Council, n.d.a). The National Council of Indigenous Midwives (NCIM) sets the competencies for knowledge and skills for Indigenous midwifery (National Council of

Indigenous Midwives, n.d.). Individual provinces and territories regulate the midwifery profession, setting registration, supervision, and professional conduct standards in their respective jurisdictions. The term "midwife" may only be legally used by RMs, with provinces such as Ontario having additional exemption clauses where Indigenous midwives also legally use the term "midwife" (National Council of Indigenous Midwives, 2020a).

The Canadian Association for Midwifery Education (CAMEd) Accreditation Council sets the standards for the six undergraduate midwifery education programs (CAMEd, 2024). In Canada, six undergraduate midwifery education programs are offered across five provinces, located at McMaster University, Mount Royal University, Toronto Metropolitan University, the University of British Columbia, the University of Manitoba, and the Université du Québec à Trois-Rivières (Canadian Association of Midwives, 2023b). Canadian undergraduate midwifery education programs follow the International Confederation of Midwives (ICM) Global Standards for Midwifery Education and CAMEd accreditation standards, where at least 50% of curricula are based on experiential learning, and preceptors facilitate learners' meeting clinical competencies (Butler et al., 2016; CAMEd, 2024; ICM, 2021). Furthermore, the CAMEd accreditation standards stipulate that students gain knowledge and skill in full-scope midwifery, cultural safety, professionalism, interprofessional collaboration, evidenced-informed decision-making, and reflective practice (CAMEd, 2024). In order to become a registered midwife, a graduate will need to meet minimum clinical experience requirements as determined by the jurisdiction for which they apply. As an example, the College of Midwives of Alberta (CMA) registration requirements include attendance at a minimum of 60 births in the past five years of which 40 were in the primary midwife role, at least 10 were in the hospital, 10 were in out of hospital settings, and 30 included the provision of continuity of care (CMA, 2020). The CMA defines continuity of care to include a minimum of two antenatal visits, attendance at the birth, and two postnatal visits (CMA, 2019).

Educational program graduates in Canada and internationally educated midwives (IEMs) who meet the qualifications must complete a specified number of supervised clinical hours, experience requisite roles in perinatal care (information not publicly available), and write a national board examination regulated by the CMRC to be eligible for registration (Canadian Midwifery Regulators Council, n.d.b).

Mentorship in Midwifery in Canada

Mentorship is universally recognised as essential to professional development and midwifery education. Historically, facilitating midwifery students in Canada was community-driven long before regulation. Although midwifery preceptors provide mentorship, the term mentor is used more often to describe the clinical supervision of a student in an Indigenous community-based midwifery program, or an NR or newcomer to the profession in Canada.

Mentorship in midwifery education has become a cornerstone of curricula where learners receive essential guidance while gaining hands-on experience in clinical practicum. The complexity of healthcare systems has expanded the midwifery mentorship role, including navigating the interprofessional dynamics of perinatal teams. Additionally, mentorship has become essential in integrating Internationally Educated Midwife (IEMs) who face unique challenges when adapting to the Canadian healthcare environment (Upadhyaya et al., 2023).

REFLECTIVE ACTIVITY 1

Consider the scenario and answer the two questions:

A newly registered midwife begins their NR's year in a rural community where only one other Registered Midwife acts as their mentor.

- How can the NR continue to learn from a variety of individuals?
- How can virtual mentorship support their development, and what frameworks can enhance this process?

Mentorship in Indigenous Community-Based Midwifery Programs

Mentorship by experienced Indigenous midwives is integral in Indigenous midwifery education programs, as is the relationship between mentor and mentee (Pambrun et al., 2019). This mentorship also facilitates passing on cultural aspects of perinatal and newborn care, in addition to clinical competencies. Two long-standing Indigenous midwifery educational programs are as follows: The Tsi Non: we Ionnakeratstha Ona' Aboriginal Midwifery Training Program in Ontario and the Inuulitsivik Midwife Training Program in Nunavik, Quebec. Both programs emphasise mentorship from Indigenous midwives, teaching and practice based on community and culture, and are aligned with allopathic health practice (National Council of Indigenous Midwives, 2020b). The NCIM ethos, *"where there are services, there will be education"*, highlights the value *placed on sustaining Indigenous midwifery* (National Council of Indigenous Midwives, 2020b). NCIM is currently seeking Indigenous communities to collaborate in additional educational programming to increase opportunities for expanding midwifery (National Council of Indigenous Midwives, 2020b).

Preceptorship in Undergraduate Midwifery Education in Canada

In Canadian undergraduate education, a preceptor is usually a registered midwife (RM) paired with a pre-registration midwifery student in a clinical setting (CAMEd, 2024; Upadhyaya et al., 2021). Furthermore, a university liaison (i.e., midwifery clinical instructor or tutor) supports the experiential learning environment and may be involved when challenges arise within the preceptor–student dyad (Upadhyaya et al., 2023).

Even though RM preceptors are not typically institutional employees, they may hold academic appointments (e.g., clinical faculty) and may receive a nominal honorarium for their precepting role (University of British Columbia (UBC), n.d.a). While other health professionals may act as preceptors, mainly RMs guide students by instructing, evaluating, and supervising over placements that typically last a term (13 weeks) (Butler et al., 2016).

In Canada, there are no national initiatives or funding mechanisms to support midwifery preceptor training. Furthermore, midwifery regulations do not have mandates for registrants to support the next generation of midwives, although many feel obligated to complete this role (Upadhyaya et al., 2023). With the small number of practising RMs in Canada compared to other health professions, there is often a shortage of available and eligible midwives to precept students. Individual midwifery educational programs facilitate their preceptorship programs, including application processes and training for the role (McMaster University, 2024; Toronto Metropolitan University (TMU), n.d.a; UBC, n.d.a). However, midwifery regulatory bodies, such as the CMA, set further eligibility requirements for preceptors and stipulate that the midwifery education program is responsible for preliminary and continuing education and training of preceptors (CMA, 2022). These preceptor eligibility requirements include:

- Forty births as a Primary Midwife beyond their NR program,
- Met the requirements of the CMA Continuing Competence Program,
- Current liability insurance to cover student preceptorship,
- No findings of unprofessional conduct for any CMA Hearings or Investigations that have led to a cancellation or suspension of Practice Permit, in the past two years,
- Practice permit without conditions; current work as a full-scope midwife/ not be enrolled in the CMA Alternate Practice Program (unless deemed appropriate by the MEP and/or the CMA,

- Competence in CMA Restricted Activities to enable appropriate facilitation of undergraduate student education in these Entry-to-Practice areas,
- Approval by the student's education program, and
- Been sufficiently oriented and trained by the Midwifery Education Program (MEP) to mentor and evaluate students, according to a plan and criteria set by the appropriate MEP, and this policy (CMA, 2022).

Undoubtedly, midwifery preceptors play a significant role in students' experiences. A qualitative study with 31 undergraduate midwifery students in Canada identified challenges and opportunities related to the role (Neiterman et al., 2022). While supportive preceptors who actively encouraged students to gain skills improved confidence, the opposite was true within an imbalanced power dynamic with preceptors who belittled their mentees. Neiterman et al. (2022) went on to propose three main strategies to counterbalance the adverse effects within a preceptorship program: 1. enhanced training, 2. development of an impartial system to address injustices, and 3. careful preceptor selection. Similar solutions were identified in studies interviewing midwifery preceptors affiliated with Canadian undergraduate programs (Upadhyaya et al., 2023). Furthermore, professional accountability in the preceptor role ensures quality clinical care (Upadhyaya et al., 2021).

In some innovative programs, senior students acting as peers provide mentorship to junior students. These processes have shown improvements in the academic environment regarding student retention and community building (Neiterman et al., 2023). Having recently experienced the challenges and opportunities associated with midwifery education, senior peers provide timely and relevant support to promote success and leadership. It is also well known that preceptors also help nurture resilience and a commitment to the care model to ensure the sustainability of the profession (Upadhyaya et al., 2023).

The Preceptor's Role in Assessment of Undergraduate Midwifery Students

Canadian midwifery undergraduate preceptors play a pivotal role in evaluating clinical students. Each program employs a distinct assessment matrix with a grading schema to determine student progression. A shared feature across programs is skills-based evaluation, often conducted through Objective Structured Clinical Examinations (OSCEs), which simulate clinical scenarios to assess practical competencies. Clinical evaluation documents are typically designed to align with national and jurisdictional midwifery competencies. However, there has been a perceived lack of autonomy for preceptors in cases where their assessment of a midwifery student's progression suitability differs from the midwifery education program's determination (Upadhyaya, et al., 2023).

REFLECTIVE ACTIVITY 2

Midwifery preceptors complete the essential roles of instructing, supporting, assessing, guiding, and role modelling while concurrently practising in clinical environments. It is important to continually think of innovative measures to deal with challenges as they arise. Consider the following section of the scenario and reflective questions below.

A midwifery student is in the midterm of their first placement. The student, who began the program directly out of high school, struggles with time management. They have repeatedly arrived at the clinic 30 minutes late and have even missed a few births, having slept through the pager call. The preceptor has communicated the necessity of being on time and available for clinical events, but there has been little improvement.

- How can this dynamic affect learning, and how might it be improved?
- What steps will ensure that this challenge is addressed appropriately?
- Discuss some strategies to promote professionalism for the mentee.

Post-Registration Mentorship: Supporting Professional Growth

In Canada, midwifery graduates are called NRs in the year following the successful completion of their undergraduate program and the Canadian Midwifery Registration Exam. Individual jurisdictions facilitate this registration category and the eligibility criteria for their mentors/clinical supervisors. In one example, the CMA requires NRs to participate in monthly chart reviews with another general RM registrant and work with a supervisor approved by the Registrar and Registration Committee (CMA, 2023). Furthermore, CMA policies dictate that RM mentors to NRs provide individualised support for a full year, focusing on fostering informed decision-making in client interactions. Their role includes helping the NR adapt to midwifery practice, hospital systems, and community birth settings, ensuring they gain experience as the primary midwife. Mentors offer ongoing guidance, constructive feedback, and emotional support while being available around the clock. They assist with program requirements, participate in monthly case reviews, and arrange alternative mentorship if unavailable. Mentors also support the NR through the completion of the program and address any additional needs based on examination outcomes. In most jurisdictions, there is little monetary remuneration for this role.

International Midwives and Mentorship

Three universities in Canada have bridging programs for internationally educated midwives (IEMs): the International Midwifery Pre-registration Program at Toronto Metropolitan University, the Internationally Educated Midwives Bridging Program at the University of British Columbia, and the Certificat personnalisé en pratique sage-femme au Québec at the Université du Québec à Trois-Rivières (Canadian Association of Midwives, 2023b). These programs range in length from six to nine months; however, IEMs may also face registration conditions requiring clinical supervision despite completing available bridging programs (British Columbia College of Nurses and Midwives, 2024; College of Midwives of Ontario, 2024; TMU, n.d.b; UBC, n.d.b). Programs for IEMs typically comprise online tutorial learning, in-person lectures, and a clinical practicum where a preceptor would facilitate the learning similar to the undergraduate experiential curriculum model.

Benefits of Mentorship

Graduating from an undergraduate or Indigenous midwifery education program or entering the midwifery profession for the first time in a new country does not eliminate the need for mentorship. In fact, midwives at all career points benefit from purposeful guidance, as evidenced by the increasing popularity of executive coaching programs. Mentors develop strong relationships with their mentees by understanding individual needs and the context of the clinical practice environment. For example, a new graduate will have different learning objectives than an experienced midwife who is new to practising in Canada. While the former may need assistance with skills such as perineal suturing, the latter may need support understanding the healthcare infrastructure and the appropriate process when consulting obstetricians.

As RMs become more proficient in their professional roles, they will need further mentorship to acquire advanced skills and to take on leadership roles. Mentors, especially those with leadership experience, must pass on this knowledge to maintain and sustain the profession and respond to care recipients' changing needs and other healthcare complexities. The future of midwifery depends on succession planning that empowers others to advocate for systemic changes, especially for clients, families, communities, and colleagues negatively impacted by current processes. Effective mentorship promotes critical thinking to navigate challenges, promotes systems integration, and diversifies the professional workforce (Neiterman et al., 2022).

The Future of Supporting (Student) Midwives in Canada

Midwifery preceptors, mentors, and clinical supervisors are essential role models for students, new practitioners, and midwives educated in other countries. Midwives must be appropriately supported, trained, and remunerated to complete their mentorship roles. Technologies are vital tools to increase access to information sharing and support. Furthermore, RM mentors can provide invaluable support to rural and remote areas where physical access may be a limiting factor. Video and telehealth can provide real-time solutions for emergency care and decision-making when clients require care in higher-level facilities.

Conclusion

Midwifery mentorship and preceptorship in Canada is essential for developing individuals along the career continuum, from students to experienced professionals. It is a means to promote growth, preserve culture in Indigenous communities, and support internationally educated midwives. Mentors are key collaborators in the evolution of midwifery in Canada to meet the needs of care recipients and the profession itself. Yet, midwifery mentorship (and preceptorship) programs will need to respond effectively to the diversifying workforce and client populations (Neiterman et al., 2023). Various modalities must be developed to meet diverse needs beyond the one-to-one preceptor–student dyad, virtual platforms, and peer support. Mentors and preceptors should consistently reflect on the diverse needs of the individuals they teach and care for, considering each person's unique identity and background. Like many other resourced countries, Canada has heterogeneous populations and must consider whether current measures are evidence-informed. In the post-pandemic era, Canada has faced significant healthcare workforce shortages. Student midwives and RMs play a vital role in addressing these gaps by advancing the profession and stepping into expanded roles to help meet the growing demand for care. A responsive midwifery mentorship program that emphasises leadership will perhaps encourage a mentee in this network to step forward one day as Canada's first Chief Midwife Officer.

Resources

The following list identifies key midwifery mentorship and leadership resources in Canada:

- Canadian Association for Midwifery Education
  - https://camed-acfsf.ca/
  - Accreditation
    - https://camed-acfsf.ca/accreditation/
- Canadian Association of Midwives (CAM)
  - https://canadianmidwives.org/
- Canadian Midwifery Regulators Consortium (CMRC):
  - https://cmrc-ccosf.ca/
  - Information for Internationally Educated Midwives:
    - https://cmrc-ccosf.ca/internationally-educated-midwives
- National Council of Indigenous Midwives
  - https://indigenousmidwifery.ca/

Additional Reflective Questions to Ponder

- What are the core values that define your approach to mentorship?
- Reflect on a time when you struggled in a mentor or mentee role. How did that experience shape your understanding of effective mentorship?
- How do you navigate cultural differences in mentorship relationships, particularly in a diverse field like midwifery?
- Have you ever mentored or worked with someone whose identity or experiences differ from your own? How did you approach this, and what did you learn from the experience?
- In what ways do your personal or professional experiences shape your approach to high-risk versus low-risk birthing practices? How can mentorship help bridge gaps in understanding between these settings?

References

British Columbia College of Nurses and Midwives. (2024). *Internationally-Educated Midwives*. https://www.bccnm.ca/RM/Applications/how_to_apply/Pages/InternationalEM.aspx

Butler, M. M., Hutton, E. K., & McNiven, P. S. (2016). Midwifery education in Canada. *Midwifery, 33*, 28–30.

Canadian Association of Midwives. (2015). *The Canadian Model of Care Position Statement*. https://canadianmidwives.org/wp-content/uploads/2016/06/CAM-MoCPSFINAL-OCT2015-ENG-FINAL.pdf

Canadian Association for Midwifery Education. (2024). *Accreditation of Midwifery Baccalaureate Degree Programs in Canada*. https://camed-acfsf.ca/accreditation/

Canadian Association of Midwives. (2023a). *Discover Midwifery Across Canada*. https://canadianmidwives.org/about-midwifery/

Canadian Association of Midwives. (2023b). *How to Become a Midwife*. https://canadianmidwives.org/becoming-a-midwife/#programs-in-canada

Canadian Midwifery Regulators Council. (n.d.a). *About CMRC*. https://cmrc-ccosf.ca/about-cmrc

Canadian Midwifery Regulators Council. (n.d.b). *Registration Exam*. https://cmrc-ccosf.ca/registration-exam

College of Midwives of Alberta. (2019). *Position Statement on Continuity of Care (S4)*. https://www.albertamidwives.org/copy-of-college-policies

College of Midwives of Alberta. (2020). *Registration Policy*. https://www.albertamidwives.org/copy-of-college-policies

College of Midwives of Alberta. (2022). *Student and Clinical Placement Registration Policy (P5)*. https://www.albertamidwives.org/copy-of-college-policies

College of Midwives of Alberta. (2023). *New Registrant (New Graduate) Policy*. https://www.albertamidwives.org/copy-of-college-policies

College of Midwives of Ontario. (2024). *Internationally Educated Midwives*. https://cmo.on.ca/midwives/internationally-educated-midwives/

Government of Canada. (2024a). *Provinces and Territories*. https://www.canada.ca/en/intergovernmental-affairs/services/provinces-territories.html

Government of Canada. (2024b). *About Treaties*. https://www.rcaanc-cirnac.gc.ca/eng/1100100028574/1529354437231

Government of Canada. (2024c). *Truth and Reconciliation Commission of Canada*. https://www.rcaanc-cirnac.gc.ca/eng/1450124405592/1529106060525#chp2

International Confederation of Midwives. (2021). *ICM Global Standards for Midwifery Education*. https://internationalmidwives.org/resources/global-standards-for-midwifery-education/

MacDonald, M., & Bourgeault, I. (2009). 3. The Ontario midwifery model of care. In R. Davis-Floyd, L. Barclay, J. Tritten, & B. Daviss (Eds.), *Birth Models That Work* (pp. 89–118). University of California Press. https://doi.org/10.1525/9780520943339-005

McMaster University. (2024). *Faculty of Health Sciences Midwifery Undergraduate Program: Preceptors*. https://midwiferyundergrad.mcmaster.ca/preceptors/#tab-content-becoming-a-preceptor

Nathalie Pambrun, R. M., Karen Lawford, R. M., & Carol Couchie, R. M. (2019). Indigenous midwifery in Canada: An example of healthy relationships. *Journal of Obstetrics and Gynaecology Canada, 41*(S2), S259–S262. https://doi.org/10.1016/j.jogc.2019.09.004

National Council of Indigenous Midwives. (2019). *Indigenous Midwifery Knowledge and Skills: A Framework for Competencies*. https://indigenousmidwifery.ca/publications/

National Council of Indigenous Midwives. (2020a). *Reconciliation, Regulation, and Risk*. https://indigenousmidwifery.ca/reconciliation-regulation-risk/

National Council of Indigenous Midwives. (2020b). *Education*. https://indigenous-midwifery.ca/become-a-midwife/

Neiterman, E., Beggs, B., HakemZadeh, F., Zeytinoglu, I., Geraci, J., & Lobb, D. (2022). "They hold your fate in their hands": exploring the power dynamic in the midwifery student-preceptor relationship. *Midwifery, 112*, 103430. https://doi.org/10.1016/j.midw.2022.103430

Neiterman, E., Beggs, B., HakemZadeh, F., Zeytinoglu, I., Geraci, J., & Lobb, D. (2023). Can peers improve student retention? Exploring the roles peers play in midwifery education programmes in Canada. *Women and Birth, 36*(4), e453–e459. https://doi.org/10.1016/j.wombi.2023.02.004

Statistics Canada. (2024a). *Canada's Population Estimates, Second Quarter 2024*. https://www150.statcan.gc.ca/n1/daily-quotidien/240925/dq240925d-eng.htm?HPA=1&indid=4098-1&indgeo=0

Statistics Canada. (2024b). *Census of Population.* https://www12.statcan.gc.ca/census-recensement/index-eng.cfm?MM=1

Statistics Canada. (2024c). *Indigenous History in Canada.* https://www.rcaanc-cirnac.gc.ca/eng/1100100013778/1607903934135

Toronto Metropolitan University. (n.d.a). *Midwifery Education Program: For Preceptors.* https://www.torontomu.ca/midwifery/Clinical-Teaching-Learning/for-preceptors/#!accordion-1615404494478-placement-policies-and-information-for-preceptors

Toronto Metropolitan University. (n.d.b). *International Midwifery Pre-Registration Program.* https://continuing.torontomu.ca/contentManagement.do?method=load&code=CM000074

University of British Columbia. (n.d.a). *Clinical Faculty.* https://midwifery.ubc.ca/about/clinical-preceptors/

University of British Columbia. (n.d.b). *Internationally Educated Midwives Bridging Program.* https://iembp.midwifery.ubc.ca/

Upadhyaya, D., Beran, T., Maruschak-Love, S., Clancy, T., & Oddone Paolucci, E. (2022). Benefits, rewards, support, and commitment: a survey of midwifery preceptors in undergraduate education in Canada. *Canadian Journal of Midwifery Research and Practice, 21*(1), 48–62.

Upadhyaya, D., Haines-Saah, R., Clancy, T., Beran, T., & Oddone Paolucci, E. (2023). The precepting dilemma: a reflexive thematic analysis study of midwifery preceptors in undergraduate education in Canada. *Canadian Journal of Midwifery Research and Practice, 22*(1), 35–39. https://doi.org/10.22374/cjmrp.v22i1.2

Upadhyaya, D., Maruschak-Love, S., Beran, T., Clancy, T., & Oddone Paolucci, E. (2021). Facilitators and barriers for clinical preceptors in midwifery education: a scoping review of the published literature. *Canadian Journal of Midwifery Research and Practice, 20*(3), 37–42.

Van Wagner, V., Epoo, B., Nastapoka, J., & Harney, E. (2007). Reclaiming birth, health, and community: Midwifery in the Inuit Villages of Nunavik, Canada. *Journal of Midwifery & Women's Health, 52*(4), 384–391. https://doi.org/10.1016/j.jmwh.2007.03.025

World Data. (2024). *The Largest Countries of the World.* https://www.worlddata.info/the-largest-countries.php

12

MIDWIFERY MENTORSHIP IN THE UNITED KINGDOM

Sam Bassett

Background to Clinical Assessment in the UK

All nursing, midwifery and medical professions in the United Kingdom (UK) have required their trainees to be examined and certificated on successful completion of studies since the 19th century. Legislation commencing with *The Midwives Act* in 1902, followed by other healthcare professions in the 20th century, has led to a statutory requirement for professional registration based not only on completion of an accredited educational programme but also on trainees being able to successfully pass examinations or other forms of assessment set by their professional bodies.

Within the UK, nursing and midwifery professions are regulated by the Nursing and Midwifery Council (NMC), which came into being in 2002 following the Nurses and Midwives Order 2001 in April 2002 (NMC, 2001). Their primary mandate to safeguard the health and well-being of the public by keeping a register of all their registrants and ensuring they are fit to practise. To ensure this they are responsible for setting the standards for the education, training and conduct of those on the register. However, it is important to note they do not work in isolation but in collaboration with others, including statutory and professional bodies, education providers, employers and education commissioners.

IN 2002, the NMC published its first code of professional conduct now known as the Code: Professional Standards of Practice and Behaviour for nurses, midwives and nursing associates (NMC, 2018a) with safeguarding standards and principles of practice very much at the core. Standards then followed for education both in theory and practice with the premise that 50% of students' training should take place within the theoretical field and

DOI: 10.4324/9781003533733-13

50% within clinical practice. With the three-year direct entry being the predominant route into midwifery for most NMC-approved programmes, this equates to a minimum of 2,300-hour theory/2,300-hour practice. As such, there are few midwives who are not in some way involved in the training and supervision of students and such roles frequently form part of the contract of employment from NHS hospital Trusts.

NMC Education and Training Requirements

Three NMC standards for education and training currently govern midwifery education. Originally published in 2018, the standards were updated/amended in 2023

Part 1 – Standards Framework for Nursing and Midwifery Education (NMC, 2023a)

Provides a framework but allows approved education institutions (AEIs) and practice learning partners the flexibility to develop creative approaches to education. This means institutions delivering NMC-approved programmes are accountable to ensure delivery and management is in line with their programme standards.

Part 2 – Standards for Student Supervision and Assessment (SSSA) (NMC, 2023b)

Sets out the roles and responsibilities of practice supervisors and assessors, ensuring students receive high-quality learning, support, and supervision during their practice placements. They also set out the NMC expectations for the learning, support, and supervision of students in the practice environment as well as setting out how students are assessed for theory and practice learning.

Part 3 – Standards for Pre-Registration Midwifery Programmes (NMC, 2023c)

Set out the entry and practice learning requirements, curriculum, length of programme, methods of assessment and the level of award for NMC-approved programmes. They also set out the standards of proficiency required by all midwives (NMC, 2024)

In 2023, the NMC Commissioned the Nuffield Trust and Florence Nightingale Foundation to undertake a desk-based national and international evidence review and qualitative stakeholder engagement into nursing and midwifery students' practice learning requirements. Two main aims underpinned this commission. Firstly, to review NMC standards that still complied with the EU directives which ceased in legislation when the UK left the EU on 31 December 2020. Secondly, to ensure NMC standards continued to equip students with the knowledge and skills to deliver the best possible care in a range of diverse healthcare settings. What followed was comprehensive entailing workshops with UK policy leaders; focus groups with registered nurses and midwives, students, higher education staff, and members of the public; interviews with strategic leaders in health and social care both within the UK and internationally. These workshops resulted in gathering 6,266 views (Palmer et al., 2024).

Their first report was published in early December 2024; however, perhaps surprisingly overall there was limited evidence or consensus for change to the approach to midwifery and nursing education programmes. For midwifery, main points to note included expanding the variety of placement settings facilitating students gaining experience in a variety of services and settings, providing holistic care for the diversity of populations and helping ease pressure on securing placements. In contrast to nursing education, the counting of simulation towards practice hours is currently not permitted within midwifery education with the belief that some skills can only be fully perfected in practice. Although some stakeholder opinions supported greater use of simulation, this was overshadowed by caution about the actual extent and the assurance needed that this would be supplementary and supportive of learning rather than a wholesale substitute for direct contact with women and their families. As such, simulation at present is only permitted in skills midwifery students may not experience within the clinical area such as vaginal breech, episiotomy and perineal suturing.

To facilitate easy movement of the midwifery workforce across the UK's close geographical partners in Europe, the EU directive regarding the specific number of occasions a skill is performed remains (Table 12.1). However, with increasing maternal complexity and caesarean section leading to falling vaginal deliveries concerns regarding students being able to logistically obtain 40 births personally facilitated remain high. As a result, work within both the areas stated above remains ongoing.

Inconsistencies in terminology, approaches to assessment and grading of practice have been a core concern to nursing and midwifery educationalists for several years (Fisher et al., 2017; 2019; Mårtensson et al., 2020). This was often exacerbated further since the removal of commissioned National Health System (NHS) placement for students resulting in placement providers that hosted multiple AEI students. As a result, to ensure standardisation and consistency to all midwifery students one generic clinical assessment document known as the MORA (Midwifery Ongoing Record of Achievement) was developed and approved for England and Northern Ireland, aligned with Standards for Student Supervision and Assessment (SSSA) and the new

TABLE 12.1 EU Directive 2005/36/EC

Advising of pregnant women, involving at least 100 pre-natal examinations

Supervision and care of at least 40 pregnant women.

Conduct by the student of at least 40 deliveries; where this number cannot be reached owing to the lack of available women in labour, it may be reduced to a minimum of 30, provided that the student assists with 20 further deliveries

Active participation with breech deliveries. Where this is not possible because of lack of breech deliveries, practice may be in a simulated situation

Performance of episiotomy and initiation into suturing. Initiation shall include theoretical instruction and clinical practice. The practice of suturing includes suturing of the wound following an episiotomy and a simple perineal laceration. This may be in a simulated situation if absolutely necessary

Supervision and care of 40 women at risk in pregnancy, or labour or post-natal period

Supervision and care (including examination) of at least 100 post-natal women and healthy newborn infants

Observation and care of the newborn requiring special care, including those born pre-term, post-term, underweight or ill.

Care of women with pathological conditions in the fields of gynaecology and obstetrics

Initiation into care in the field of medicine and surgery. Initiation shall include theoretical instruction and clinical practice.

---

midwifery standards and proficiencies as set out within the NMC six domains (Figure 12.1).

Background to Clinical Assessment Within the UK

For nurses and midwives who assess the clinical practice of pre-registration students in the UK, the NMC states that they are accountable for confirming that students have met, or not met, the NMC standards. Professional accountability involves accepting responsibility for professional decisions. Stated more simply, practitioners are 'entrusted with, answerable for, take the credit and blame for and can be judged within legal and moral boundaries' (Castledine, 1991).

NMC Standards to Support Learning and Assessment in Practice (SLAiP) (2008-2019)

However, it was not until the publication of the NMC standards to SLAiP (NMC, 2008) that professional accountability for student learning and assessment in clinical practice in the UK started to receive due attention. Within

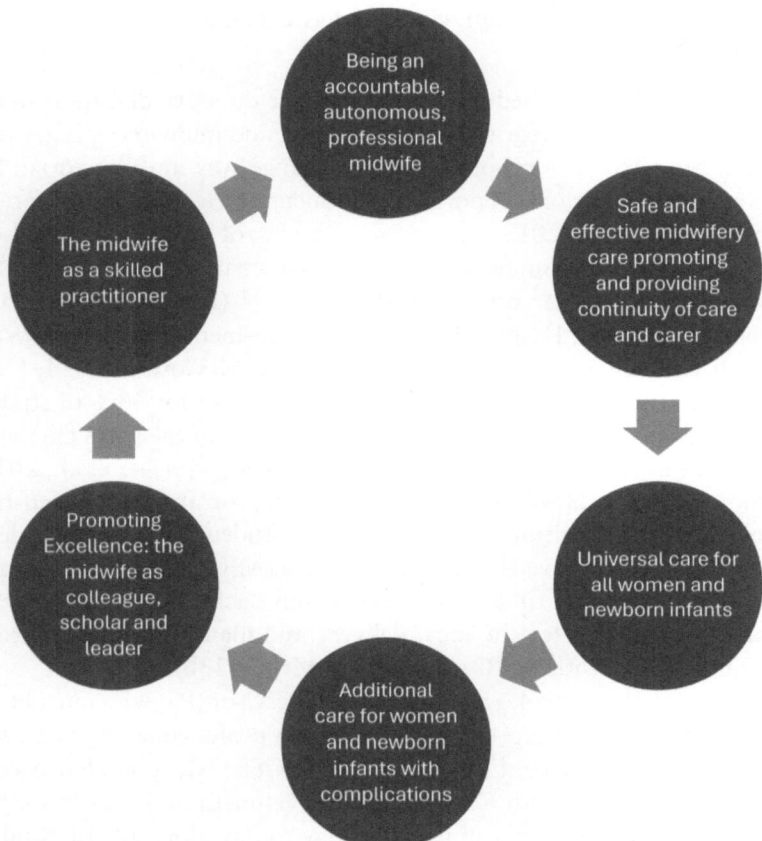

FIGURE 12.1 The NMC six domains (NMC, 2023c)

these NMC registrants that support pre-registration midwifery students and make summative assessments were expected to work at least 40% of their time with a mentor and be signed off as proficient by a sign-off mentor (an experienced mentor that had undergone further education) at the end of their programme. The only caveat to note here was that a mentor or sign-off mentor could only sign off students that would be qualifying on the same part of the NMC register as themselves.

Within the SLAiP standards, the NMC also set out clear expectations of the requirements for mentor preparation programmes which included academic level (HE Intermediate); Length of time (minimum of 10 days of which 5 days were protected learning time); learning both in academic and practice settings; relevant work-based learning (mentoring a student under supervision of a qualified mentor with the opportunity to reflect on the experience); and normally completed within three months.

NMC Standards for Student Supervision and Assessment (SSA) (2019 – Present)

In 2018, the NMC published their SSSA with the directive that these needed to be in place for all pre-registration UK nursing and midwifery programmes by September 2020. The rationale for this change was multi-factorial. Successive concerning national reports (Department of Health, 2013; National Health Service (NHS), 2013) had led to a review of health and social care regulation and training and recommendations for change (Willis, 2015). Failure to fail remained ever present in the literature (Bachman et al., 2019; Bradshaw et al., 2019; Duffy, 2003); close student-mentor relationships had led to concerns regarding subjectivity (Bennett & McGowan, 2014; Helminen et al., 2016); and finally the previous requirement for 40% of students time to be spent with a mentor who was a registrant on the same part of the programme was seen to be limiting placement capacity (Fisher et al., 2022).

Within SSSA, the NMC replaced the term mentor and introduced three new roles to the supervision and assessment of students. Their rationale for the change to give approved education institutes (AEIs) and practice learning partners more flexibility to develop creative approaches to education whilst still being accountable for the local delivery and management of approved programmes in line with NMC standards (NMC, 2023b).

The first of these new roles is the practice supervisor (PS) who must be registered health and social care professional with a professional regulator such as the NMC, GMC (General Medical Council, GPhc (General Pharmaceutical Council), HCPC (Health Care Professions Council) or Social Work England. These practitioners very much work day-to-day alongside the students in clinical practice providing ongoing feedback to the student with a focus on their knowledge, performance and professional behaviour.

Each student then has a nominated practice assessor (PA), who must be an NMC registered midwife, who is assigned for a practice placement or a series of practice placements. These meet with their assigned students at the beginning of the year, or part of the programme, to plan practice learning. Taking on more of a helicopter view of student progression they do not work directly with their assigned student or sign off any proficiencies. Instead, they schedule periodical observations with the student and rely on reviews from the practice supervisors to make their assessments and progression decisions, completing all reviews and summative holistic assessment.

Working alongside the PA, each student also has a nominated academic assessor (AA) for each year/part of the programme. Again, a registered midwife reviews the student's progress at designated points within the programme. Make decisions about student progression in partnership with the practice assessor and review and verify student achievement, completing the progression summary within the clinical assessment document.

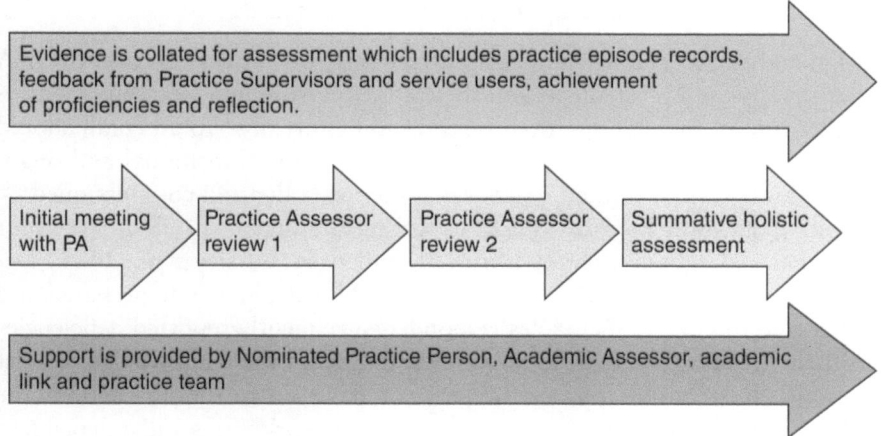

FIGURE 12.2   Roles and process of assessment following SSSA

The roles and process of assessment are outlined within Figure 12.2.

Whilst preparation of professionals for these roles is mandatory taking an outcome-focused approach, the NMC states this preparation can be done in several different ways and does not have to be limited to a formal preparatory course (NMC, 2018). The only stipulation mentioned being that AEI's with its practice learning partners, are responsible for making sure the right support, education and training is provided which upholds public protection and enables students to meet their programme outcomes and relevant NMC standards. Another important point to note is the same person cannot simultaneously be the PS, PA or AA for the same student.

REFLECTIVE ACTIVITY 1

The issue of subjectivity is not new within the assessment process. In your role as assessor:

- What steps do you take to minimise this?

The Helicopter view that the PA brings to clinical assessment of students can be viewed as a novel approach.

- What do you consider are the potential advantages and disadvantages of such an approach?

Current Review of the Implementation of SSSA Standards

Leigh and Roberts (2018) emphasised very early on in the swap over to SSSA that there would be challenges in the transition from long-standing mentoring traditions, highlighting that the time and effort this would entail should not be underestimated and that further preparatory, transitional and ongoing training was warranted. However, a service evaluation commissioned by Health Education England (HEE) exploring the impact of SSSA over four years has highlighted several unresolved challenges (Whaley et al., 2023). Despite the NMC stating, all PAs and PSs should feel adequately prepared and supported to take on their roles respondents frequently reported deficiencies in their preparation resulting in persistent gaps in their knowledge. Whilst the outcome-focused approach appears to have led to the innovations the NMC wanted, such as online guidance/training, workbooks and independent study (Pearce, 2019), the lack of consistency in content has also led to varied levels of preparation across geographical locations dependant on the robustness of their approach. As such, recommendations include a more standardised approach to the preparation of PAs and PSs supported by the creation of appropriate training resources.

The development of the AA role was to provide a more collaborative approach to practice assessment (NMC, 2023a). However, to date there is little evidence that this has been the case (Drayton & Edmonds, 2020; Whaley et al., 2023). A key challenge here is the managing of clear communication channels between AEIs and their practice learning partners. The development of electronic assessment documents has played a part in facilitating these channels, but the evaluation still highlighted that PAs' and PSs' knowledge of the documentation remains poor. Therefore, alongside further training and support for the role, exploration of how these communication links could be improved is key to ensuring they feel supported by their affiliated AEIs.

Unfortunately, a lack of protected time for practitioners to undertake their PA and PS roles remains a frequent issue for SSSA as well as it did for (formerly titled) mentors as they balance the demands of hands-on direct service user care, increased workload pressures, as well as their supervisory role all often exacerbated further by frequent staff shortages (Newton et al., 2017; Panda et al., 2021). As a result, assessors often report the amount of work associated with their role as overwhelming, especially regarding the completion of student assessment documentation; with the potential, in turn, to negatively impact the learner experience with limited exposure to positive role modelling, insufficient feedback and missed learning opportunities (Hughes et al., 2019). As a result, PAs and PSs are often using their own time to fulfil their roles despite previous recommendations that practice educators have their clinical workload decreased and are afforded protected time to provide effective assessment and supervision for students (Newton et al., 2017). This is significant as all NHS Trusts have access to education and training tariffs (DHSC, 2024) with the aim to ensure providers are reimbursed consistently for the training placements they provide, ensuring placements are high quality and meet the appropriate supervisory teaching and support as defined by the NMC.

Due in part to these concerns in December 2024, the NMC suggested the following actions:

- Clearer guidance and consistent standards to support consistency regarding SSSA,
- Better organisation and co-ordination of placements with enhanced support for those undertaking the SSSA roles, and
- Strengthening supervision and assessment with a focus on increasing numbers of PAs and PSs with clearer expectations of training and support available to them.

As such, the landscape around SSSA is likely to change with the NMC due to report to Council at the end of January 2025.

REFLECTIVE ACTIVITY 2

Take a few moments to write down some thoughts on the three questions below:

1 Consider how you prepare and maintain current knowledge and expertise that is relevant for the proficiencies of your professional programme outcomes.
2 In your assessor role, consider how you communicate and collaborate in assessment decision-making with your local education provider.
   - Reflect on how this could be enhanced.
3 Identify the local support mechanisms available to you to help you develop and maintain emotional resilience and personal support strategies within your role as assessor.

Preceptorship

Whilst at the point of registration, newly qualified midwives (NQM) must have the knowledge and skills and behaviours required to join the professional register due to the autonomy of midwifery practice, midwives are usually considered as newly qualified up to a year post-qualification or not more than two years (NHS, 2023; Scott & Poat, 2025). However, extensive evidence shows us that NQM feel unprepared and struggle with the sudden increase of responsibility likening it to a roller coaster of emotions both high and low with the potential to influence their journey to becoming a confident and competent practitioner (Kitson-Reynolds et al., 2014; Nolan et al., 2022; Norris, 2019; Wain, 2017; Watson & Brown, 2021; Weir & Lake, 2022).

Therefore, akin to most countries within the UK, it is recognised that a supported structured period of preceptorship has benefits for employers, preceptees and service users. Not only can it influence recruitment, but it can increase confidence and promote a sense of belonging with greater professional and team identity leading preceptees to feel valued by their employer and ultimately improve retention. Vital factors when successive maternity investigations have highlighted understaffing and culture as key components contributing to a lack of safe care (Knight et al., 2022; Ockenden, 2022; Renfrew et al., 2014)

Not surprisingly then, concerns regarding recruitment and retention of all healthcare practitioners, including midwives, are also of concern to the UK government from both financial and political standpoints and as a result are often a political weapon used within election campaigns (Labour Party, 2024; Office for National Statistics, 2024; Savage et al., 2023). As a result, it is also a common feature within NMC publications (Figure 12.3) and the Royal colleges including the Royal College of Midwives (RCM) (NMC, 2023d; RCM, 2022).

However, many of the issues discussed relating to PAs and PSs are also commonplace with preceptorship and concerns regarding a lack of continuity of preceptor, staff shortages, increased workload, lack of supernumerary time and structured rotations, a lack of support from colleagues all leading to NQM struggling with their own expectations but also those of others (Foster & Aswin, 2014; Scott & Poat, 2025). As a result, NHS trusts have invested heavily within preceptorship in the recruitment of preceptorship

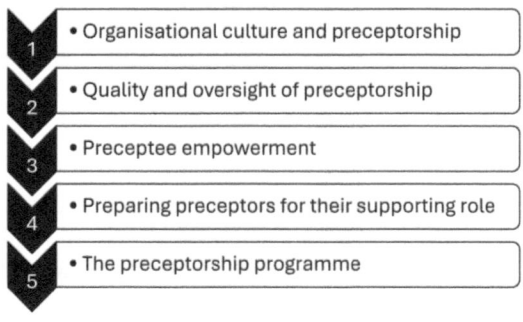

- 1 • Organisational culture and preceptorship
- 2 • Quality and oversight of preceptorship
- 3 • Preceptee empowerment
- 4 • Preparing preceptors for their supporting role
- 5 • The preceptorship programme

FIGURE 12.3 NMC principles of preceptorship (2023)

leads within their education teams and the development of robust preceptorship programmes. In the NHS quest for standardised guidance on key elements and expectations of a good preceptorship following the success of the Capital Midwife preceptorship framework (2019), in 2023 it published the national preceptorship framework for midwifery, which states roles and responsibilities minimum standards and quality standards to follow (NHS, 2023).

The NMC in writing their SSSA standards was clear that any practitioner that had undergone the requisite training could take on the role of supporting and assessing students, recommending that this be integrated into pre-registration curriculum (NMC, 2023b). However, this issue remains a hotly debated issue regarding preceptorship with many believing they should be protected from this role as they consolidate their own learning (Kitson-Reynolds et al., 2014; Norris, 2019; Wain, 2017). As such, this remains very much a local decision.

REFLECTIVE ACTIVITY 3

Reflect on when you were newly qualified.

- What were the barriers and facilitators to you feeling both confident and competent?

Peer support has been found to improve the transition through the sharing of experiences.

- Is this available where you work? If not could such an approach be easily implemented?

References

Bachman L, Groenvik CKU, Hauge KW, Julnes S. (2019). Failing to fail nursing students among mentors: a confirmatory factor analysis of the failing to fail scale. Nursing Open. 6(3):966–973. https://doi.org/10.1002/nop2.276

Bennett M, McGowan B. (2014). Assessment matters – mentors need support in their role. British Journal of Nursing. 23(9):454–458. https://doi.org/10.12968/bjon.2014.23.9.454

Bradshaw C, Pettigrew J, Fitzpatrick M. (2019). Safety first: factors affecting preceptor midwives experiences of competency assessment failure among midwifery students. Midwifery. 74:29–35. https://doi.org/10.1016/j.midw.2019.03.012

Capital Midwife. (2019). Preceptorship programme framework. Available at Communications and Engagement Workshop.

Castledine G. (1991). The advanced nurse practitioner. Part 1. Nursing Standard. 5(43):34–36. https://doi.org/10.7748/ns.5.43.34.s43

Department of Health. (2013). Report of the Mid Staffordshire NHS Foundation Trust Public Inquiry (Francis Report). The Stationery Office. https://webarchive.nationalarchives.gov.uk/20150407084231/http://www.midstaffspublicinquiry.com/report

DHSC. (2024). Guidance. Healthcare Education and Training Tariff 2024 to 2025. Available at https://www.gov.uk/government/publications/healthcare-education-and-training-tariff-2024-to-2025

Drayton L, Edmonds M. Understanding the role of the academic assessor. Nursing Standard. 35(9):41–45. https://doi.org/10.7748/ns.2020.e11463

Duffy K. (2003). Failing Students: a Qualitative Study of Factors That Influence the Decisions Regarding Assessment of Students' Competence in Practice. Glasgow Caledonian University, Caledonian Nursing and Midwifery Research Centre. http://citeseerx.ist.psu.edu/viewdoc/download?doi=10.1.1.515.2467&rep=rep1&type=pdf

Fisher M, Bower H, Chenery-Morris S, Galloway F, Jackson J, Way S, Fisher M. (2019). National survey: developing a common approach to grading of practice in pre-registration midwifery. Nurse Education in Practice. 34:150–160. https://doi.org/10.1016/j.nepr.2018.11.014

Fisher M, Tomson A, Chenery-Morris S. (2022). Supervision and assessment in midwifery practice during a global pandemic: a cohort study. Nurse Education in Practice. 60:103318. https://doi.org/10.1016/j.nepr.2022.103318

Fisher M, Way S, Chenery-Morris S, Jackson J, Bower H. (2017). Core principles to reduce current variations that exist in grading of midwifery practice in the United Kingdom. Nurse Education in Practice. 23:54–60. http://dx.doi.org/10.1016/j.nepr.2017.02.006

Foster J, Ashwin C. (2014). Newly qualified midwives' experiences of preceptorship: a qualitative study. MIDIRS Midwifery Digest. 24(2):151–157. https://www.researchgate.net/profile/JoanneFoster/publication/309012908

Helminen K, Coco K, Johnson M, Turunen H, Tossavainen K. (2016). Summative assessment of clinical practice of student nurses: a review of the literature. International Journal of Nursing Studies. 53:308–319. https://doi.org/10.1016/j.ijnurstu.2015.09.014

Hughes LJ, Mitchell ML, Johnston ANB. (2019). Just how bad does it have to be? Industry and academic assessors' experiences of failing to fail – a descriptive study. Nurse Education Today. 76:206–215. https://doi.org/10.1016/j.nedt.2019.02.011

Kitson-Reynolds E, Cluett E, Le-May A. (2014). Fairy tale midwifery – fact or fiction: the lived experiences of newly qualified midwives. British Journal of Midwifery. 22(9):660–668. https://doi.org/10.12968/bjom.2014.22.9.660

Knight M, Bunch K, Patel R, Shakespeare J, Kotnis R, Kenyon S, Kurinczuk JJ. (2022). Saving Lives, Improving Mothers' Care Core Report – Lessons Learned to Inform Maternity Care from the UK and Ireland Confidential Enquiries into Maternal Deaths and Morbidity 2018–20. Available at https://www.npeu.ox.ac.uk/assets/downloads/mbrrace-uk/reports/maternal-report-2022/MBRRACE-UK_Maternal_CORE_Report_2022_v10.pdf

Labour Party. (2024). Change: Labour Party Manifesto 2024. Available at https://labour.org.uk/wp-content/uploads/2024/06/Labour-Party-manifesto-2024.pdf

Leigh J, Roberts D. (2018). Critical exploration of the new NMC standards of proficiency for registered nurses. British Journal Nursing. 27(18):1068–1072. https://doi.org/10.12968/bjon.2018.27.18.1068

Mårtensson G, Lind V, Edin K, Hedberg A, Löfmark A. (2020). Development and validation of a clinical assessment tool for postgraduate nursing education: a consensus-group study. Nurse Education in Practice. 44:102741. https://doi.org/10.1016/j.nepr.2020.102741

Newton J, Taylor RM, Crighton L. (2017). A mixed-methods study exploring sign-off mentorship practices in relation to the nursing and midwifery council standards. Journal Clinical Nursing. 26:19–20:3056–3066. https://pubmed.ncbi.nlm.nih.gov/27865010/

NHS. (2023). National Preceptorship Framework for Midwifery. Available at NHS England » National preceptorship framework for midwifery.

NHS England. (2013). Review into the Quality of Care and Treatment Provided by 14 Hospital Trusts in England: Rapid Responsive Review Report for Risk Summit (Keogh Report). Colchester Hospital University NHS Foundation Trust. https://www.nhs.uk/NHSEngland/bruce-keogh-review/Documents/outcomes/Colchester%20Hospital%20University%20NHS%20Foundation%20Trust%20RRR%20report.pdf

NMC. (2001). The Nursing and Midwifery Order (SI 2002/253). The Stationary Office. https://www.nmc.org.uk/globalassets/sitedocuments/legislation/the-nursing-and-midwifery-order-2001-consolidated-text.pdf

NMC. (2008). The Code: Standards of Conduct, Performance and Ethics for Nurses and Midwives. Nursing and Midwifery Council, London, UK.

NMC. (2018a). The Code: Professional Standards of Practice and Behaviour for Nurses, Midwives and Nursing Associates. Available at The Code: Professional standards of practice and behaviour for nurses, midwives and nursing associates – The Nursing and Midwifery Council (accessed 15 December 2024).

NMC. (2023a). Standards Framework for Nursing and Midwifery Education. Available at Standards framework for nursing and midwifery education.

NMC. (2023b). Standards for Student Supervision and Assessment. Available at Standards for student supervision and assessment – The Nursing and Midwifery Council.

NMC. (2023c). Standards for Pre-Registration Midwifery Programmes. Available at Standards for pre-registration midwifery programmes – The Nursing and Midwifery Council.

NMC. (2023d). Principles of Preceptorship 2023. Available at https://www.nmc.org.uk/standards/guidance/preceptorship/

NMC. (2024) The Code Professional Standards of Practice and Behaviour for Nurses, Midwives and Nursing Associates. Nursing and Midwifery Council. London UK. https://www.nmc.org.uk/globalassets/sitedocuments/nmc-publications/nmc-code.pdf

Nolan S, Baird K, McInnes RJ. (2022). What strategies facilitate & support the successful transition of newly qualified midwives into practice: an integrative literature review. Nurse Education Today. 118:105497. https://doi.org/10.1016/j.nedt.2022.105497

Norris S. (2019). In the wilderness: An action-research study to explore the transition from student to newly qualified midwife. Evidence Based Midwifery. 17:4:128–134. Available at https://rcm.org.uk/wp-content/uploads/2024/06/ebm-dec19.pdf

Ockenden D. (2022). Ockenden Report – Final: Findings, Conclusions and Essential Actions from the Independent Review of Maternity Services at The Shrewsbury and Telford Hospital NHS Trust. Available at Final Report of the Ockenden Review – GOV.UK

Office for National Statistics. (2024). Healthcare Expenditure. UK Health Accounts. Available at https://www.ons.gov.uk/peoplepopulationandcommunity/healthandsocialcare/healthcaresystem/bulletins/ukhealthaccounts/2022and2023

Palmer W, Reed S, Hemmings N, Julian S, Bodea M, Oaten R, Plotkin L. (2024). Practice Learning in Nursing and Midwifery Education: An Independent Rapid Review. Nuffield Trust & Florence Nightingale Foundation. Research report.pdf.

Panda S, Dash M, John J, et al. (2021). Challenges faced by student nurses and midwives in clinical learning environment – a systematic review and meta-synthesis. Nurse Education Today. 2021(101):104875. https://doi.org/10.1016/j.nedt.2021.104875

Pearce L. (2019). New approach to nurse education affects every registrant – but are you ready? Nursing Standard. 34:9:24–26. https://doi.org/10.7748/ns.34.9.24.s12

Renfrew, MJ, McFadden, A, Bastos, BH, et al. (2014). Midwifery and quality care: findings from a new evidence-informed framework for maternal and newborn care. The Lancet. 384(9948):1129–1145. https://doi.org/10.1016/S0140-6736(14)60789-3

Royal College of Midwives (RCM). (2022). Position Statement: Preceptorship for Newly Qualified Midwives. Available at https://www.rcm.org.uk/media/6529/rcm-position-statement-preceptorship-for-newly-qualified-midwives-2022_2.pdf

Savage M, Tapper J, Helm T. (2023). Tories fear blue wall will crumble at local elections over NHS crisis | Politics | The Guardian.

Scott R, Poat R. (2025). An exploration into the experiences of newly qualified midwives during their transition to practice in the UK: a systematic review. Midwifery. https://doi.org/10.1016/j.midw.2025.104307

Wain A. (2017). Examining the lived experiences of newly qualified midwives during their preceptorship. British Journal of Midwifery. 25(7):451–457. https://doi.org/10.12968/bjom.2017.25.7.451

Watson H, Brown D. (2021). Experiences of newly qualified midwives working in clinical practice during their transition period. British Journal of Midwifery. 29(9):524–530. https://doi.org/10.12968/bjom.2021.29.9.524

Whaley V, Hay J, Knight KH. (2023). Preparing nurse educators for NMC standards for student supervision and assessment: the impact 4 yrs on. British Journal of Nursing. 32(3):130–135. https://doi.org/10.12968/bjon.2023.32.3.130

Wier J, Lake K. (2022). Making the transition: a focus group study which explores third year student and newly qualified midwives' perceptions and experiences of becoming a registrant midwife. Midwifery. 111(1):103377. https://doi.org/10.1016/j.midw.2022.103377

Willis D. (2015). Raising the Bar. Shape of Caring: A Review of the Future Education and Training of Registered Nurses and Care Assistants. Health Education England. https://www.hee.nhs.uk/sites/default/files/documents/2348-Shape-of-caring-review-FINAL.pdf (accessed 14 January 2025)

13

MIDWIFERY MENTORSHIP IN IRELAND

Deirdre Daly, Vivienne Brady, and Louise Gallagher

GLOSSARY OF TERMS

Preceptor

A preceptor is a registered nurse or registered midwife who has undertaken preparation for the role and who supports undergraduate nursing or midwifery students in their learning in the practice setting and assumes the role of supervisor and assessor of the students' achievement of clinical learning outcomes and competence.

Practice placement

A clinical site, approved by NMBI, to provide appropriate learning experiences for undergraduate or postgraduate nursing or midwifery students.

Clinical placement co-ordinator (CPC)

A CPC is an experienced registered nurse or registered midwife who supports the facilitation of learning, and assessment of competence, among nursing/midwifery undergraduate students in the practice setting.

DOI: 10.4324/9781003533733-14

Mentorship or clinical supervision

Mentorship or clinical supervision is an important component of competence development in advanced practice. This is facilitation of learning through the formal reviewing of clinical experiences with a professional colleague(s) who shares useful and insightful feedback. Mentorship or clinical supervision involves reflection and is an opportunity for the professionals involved to explore alternative perspectives with a commitment to enhancing clinical outcomes. It is central to the development and maintenance of high standards of professional performance and competence.

Source: https://www.nmbi.ie/Standards-Guidance/Glossary

Becoming a Midwife in Ireland

There are two routes to registration as a midwife in Ireland: an 18-month education programme for registered general nurses (RGNs) (NMBI, 2017), and a 4-year BSc in Midwifery for direct entry candidates (NMBI, 2022a), both of which must comply with the EU Directive 2013/55/EU and the amending Directive 2005/36/EC on the recognition of professional qualifications and regulation of midwives. The 18-month post-RGN education programme must have a minimum of 3,000 hours, with 26 weeks of theoretical content and 52 weeks of practical content (NMBI, 2017). Post-RGN midwifery students are paid employees of a maternity hospital. The four-year BSc in Midwifery programme must have 4,600 hours, with 58 weeks of theoretical content and 81 weeks of clinical practice content (45 weeks of supernumerary clinical placement and 36 weeks of paid internship clinical placement which occurs at the latter end of the fourth year of the programme) (NMBI, 2022a). These programmes are delivered by six Higher Education Institutions (HEIs) each affiliated with one or more of the country's 19 maternity hospitals (Associated Healthcare Providers (AHPs)).

Legislation and Regulation

Preceptorship is the preferred term used by the professional regulatory authority, the Nursing and Midwifery Board of Ireland (NMBI) (NMBI, 2017; 2022a), to support pre-registration midwifery students, midwives undertaking a return to midwifery practice programme (NMBI, 2020c) and midwives who are seeking employment in Ireland but whose midwife registration education programme did not comply with the EU Directives (NMBI, 2015a). The role of the preceptor is one of gatekeeper to the midwifery profession (NMBI, 2020b) and involves assessing and supporting students' achievement of pre-identified clinical learning outcomes and competence in designated areas. Mentorship or clinical supervision is the term preferred by the NMBI for qualified midwives who are undertaking Master of Science level of education to become an AMP and midwives who are undertaking the prescribing course in order to become registered midwife prescribers (NMBI, 2015b).

Midwifery legislation in Ireland was first enacted for the Island of Ireland in 1918 with the aim of increasing standards of professional education and moving away from the traditional handywoman role (Smith, 2024). The Act regulated training standards for midwives for the first time in Ireland and led to the establishment of the Central Midwives Board (CMB) (Smith, 2024). The CMB developed 'Rules for Midwives' who were noted to have developed their skills by 'working alongside other midwives' (O'Connell, 2019, p. 22). The first regulatory board – An Bord Altranais (Irish Nursing Board) was established in June 1951 (O'Connell, 2019).

Subsequent decades of the free state in Ireland have seen several Midwives Acts; however, most notably in 1985, the Nurses Act defined midwifery as a branch of nursing (Government of Ireland, 1985). This Act undermined the title and profession of Midwifery, as a midwife became a person whose name was on the '*Midwives' Division of the Nursing Register*' (Government of Ireland, 1985, Part I:2). In 1998, arising from a series of disputes between health service employers and nurses' and midwives' trade unions, and in recognition that there had been extensive changes in the requirements placed on nurses and midwives, both in training and in the delivery of service, the Commission on Nursing *A Blueprint for the Future* was published and made numerous recommendations for nursing and midwifery employment conditions and education (Government of Ireland, 1998). Following considerable midwifery representations, the Commission recommended a '*midwives amendment*' to the 1985 Nurses Act to strengthen midwifery in Ireland by establishing a Statutory Midwives Committee and recognising midwifery as a distinct profession, separate from nursing (Government of Ireland, 1998, pp. 110–111). It took until 2011 to enact the legislation, the Nurses and Midwives Act (Government of Ireland, 2011; 2023). This Act stated '*For the avoidance of doubt, it is hereby declared and recognised that midwifery is a separate profession to nursing*' (Government of Ireland, 2023, p. 10(2)). This acknowledgement was critical for midwives who, for the first time in Ireland, had commenced a direct entry four-year pre-registration midwifery education programme in 2006.

Whilst the terms 'preceptorship' and 'mentorship' of midwives are not referred to specifically in Irish legislation pertaining to Midwifery, the Nurses and Midwives Act (2011) states that '*a registered nurse and a registered midwife shall maintain professional competence on an ongoing basis*' (Government of Ireland, 2023, p. 67:77(1)). The Act charged the NMBI (formerly An Bord Altranais (The Nursing Board)) with detailing how registered nurses and registered midwives are expected to maintain their professional competence. The legislation also places a duty on the midwife's employer to facilitate the maintenance of professional competence by providing opportunities for learning.

Maintenance of Professional Competence

The first draft of the proposed professional competence scheme was not published by the NMBI until 2023, some 12 years after the legislation was first published. In the intervening years, preceptorship was not legislated for midwives, but the terms 'preceptorship' and 'supervision' featured in several professional standards and educational requirement documents. The Scope of Nursing and Midwifery Practice Framework (NMBI, 2015c) tasks the individual midwife with determining their own level of competence, alongside acknowledgement that midwives have a role in supervising and educating students and other healthcare workers as part of the multidisciplinary team. Preceptorship, mentorship and clinical supervision are identified as activities that contribute to midwives' continuing professional development. This supervisory role is also referred to in the Midwife Registration Programme Standards and Requirements where the role of a preceptor is acknowledged as key to the development of the midwifery profession (NMBI, 2017; 2022a). Support for the preceptor in their role in supporting students is also acknowledged, and the AHPs are charged with ensuring that preceptors have undertaken the required preparatory education and, together with the HEIs, monitor and report on the number of preceptors, midwives and nurses to facilitate student support, assessment and supervision. Every five years, all HEI and their AHPs must self-audit the clinical learning environment to demonstrate their level of compliance with the NMBI's Midwife Registration Programme standards and requirements, theoretical and clinical, by submitting a National Quality Clinical Learning Environment Audit Tool to the NMBI (NMBI, 2022a; 2020b). As part of these quality assurance processes, the NMBI will also conduct at least one site visit to the HEI and the AHP once every five years to review their continuing suitability as clinical learning environments for midwifery students (NMBI, 2022a).

The Introduction of Formal Preceptorship Education

Until 2000, all midwifery students in Ireland were required to be RGNs. Students completed a two-year midwife registration education programme were paid employees and supervised in practice by midwives who did not always have formal preceptorship education or preparation for the role. Midwives who were educated in Ireland did not complete a preceptorship education programme but midwives who were educated elsewhere, particularly in the United Kingdom (UK), may have. Research with these midwifery students revealed that they perceived themselves to be part of the workforce, believed they were given little clinical teaching and guidance (Begley, 1999) and that they were *'thrown in the deep end'* with little support (Begley, 2001, pp. 26–27). Completion of the programme led to registration as a midwife and the award of a Postgraduate Diploma in Midwifery, Higher Diploma in Midwifery from 2007 onwards.

A three-year Direct Entry to Midwifery (Pilot) programme commenced in 2000. Extensive consultation with midwives, midwife managers and midwife educators took place during the planning phase and this led to the inclusion of an 18-week supernumerary preceptorship period. This supernumerary preceptorship period was unique to midwifery and did not exist in any discipline of nursing. Preceptors were experienced midwives, appointed to the role, and were supernumerary to the rostered clinical midwifery team. They did not carry a midwifery practice caseload during the 18-week supernumerary preceptorship period except for the *sole* purpose of teaching/modelling midwifery practice for students. A 40-hour *'Teaching, Learning and Assessing in Midwifery Practice'* education programme (Table 13.1) was developed, implemented and evaluated (Carroll, Daly, Higgins, & Begley, 2005).

The curriculum for the three-year Direct Entry to Midwifery (Pilot) registration programme formed the basis of the curriculum of the national four-year BSc in Midwifery programme which started in 2006, and the content of the preceptorship programme formed the basis of the subsequent preceptorship preparation programme. Unfortunately, the period of supernumerary preceptorship was no longer funded by the Government; rather, all practising midwives were required to undertake a prescribed preceptorship course and preceptor midwifery students alongside and in addition to their midwifery practice caseload.

TABLE 13.1 Content of 40-hour Teaching, Learning and Assessing in Midwifery Practice Education Programme

Content
• An introduction to Direct Entry to Midwifery requirements and standards, the education programme and learning outcomes for the first year of the programme
• Reflection on experiences teaching post-RGN student midwives, and what works and does not work
• Theories of learning (andragogy and pedagogy); how adults learn
• Teaching communication in midwifery and maternity care, and teaching clinical skills

• Extensive role play covering scenarios including when a student:
  • was achieving the required level of practice,
  • was not achieving the required,
  • required a plan of action to be addressed in the next placement, and
  • disagreed with the preceptor's assessment

• Role clarification – the preceptor, the student, the midwife lecturer; sources of help and support and when to seek help or confidential advice

Currently, all midwives must complete a national mandatory NMBI approved preceptorship programme, usually within three months of commencing employment with the AHP. This programme is self-directed and online and comprises three modules; Module 1: *Introducing Preceptorship*, Module 2: *Supporting a Student on a Placement*, Module 3: *Supporting a Student Who is Not Achieving Competency*, and a Preceptorship in Practice Assessment. Each AHP can also include extra context-specific in-person content. Completing the preceptorship programme is part of all midwives' mandatory education, which must be undertaken every two years. All midwives are given time by their AHP to attend the programme which is available at no cost to the midwife.

How Preceptorship Works in Practice for Midwifery Students

Successful preceptorship has a significant influence on student learning and development (Livingstone, 2024). The preceptor orientates and socialises the student to the clinical practice environment, acts as role model and demonstrates best practice (NMBI, 2020b).

Each preceptor must be a member of the relevant division of the Register of Nurses and Midwives maintained by the NMBI, and they must have suitable clinical experience and must have completed the NMBI approved preceptorship course in preparation for the role. Education and preparation regarding assessment of student learning, competence and the required documentation is essential to the success and sustainability of preceptorship (Bradshaw, Noonan, Barry, & Atkinson, 2013). As stated earlier, undertaking a preceptorship course, and a refresher course every two years, is mandatory and monitored by the AHP and HEI jointly during five-yearly self-audits of the clinical learning environment.

The AHP and linked HEI are responsible for ensuring there are sufficient preceptors or named midwives available and able to support students to meet the requirements set out by the NMBI (NMBI, 2020b). The Clinical Midwife Manager in each practice area is accountable for preceptor allocation for the duration of the clinical placement, having assessed the registered practitioner's suitability and preparation for the role[1]. When the preceptor is absent, the student will learn alongside a named midwife or nurse, depending on the placement area.

At the start of every clinical placement[2], each midwifery student is allocated a named preceptor, who is a registered midwife (or a registered nurse/ midwife in a placement in gynaecological, operating theatre or neonatal intensive care departments) to provide support, guidance, supervision (at varying levels from direct in first year to distant in the fourth and final year) and assessment of competence. The preceptor should be available to assess the student for a minimum of *two thirds* of the duration of their clinical learning placement (NMBI, 2020a). In the absence of being able to allocate a preceptor (i.e., because of shift patterns, absences from practice, etc.), a named midwife or nurse must be allocated to support and supervise the student. The national student midwife competence assessment tool, based on the philosophy, values and five practice standards for midwifery (NMBI, 2022b), was developed by the NMBI with significant input from the six HEIs, AHPs and midwifery students (NMBI, 2015a). These standards and values are: 1. Respect for the dignity of the person; 2. Professional responsibility and accountability; 3. Quality of practice; 4. Trust and confidentiality; and 5. Collaboration with others (NMBI, 2022b). Each HEI and their AHP must use this national competence assessment tool (NMBI, 2015a) but can implement it according to local preference and organisation of clinical placements.

Learning outcomes and strategies to achieve learning experiences are discussed and agreed by the preceptor and student on commencement of the learning placement. These are recorded in a competence assessment tool (NMBI, 2015a) and are revisited continuously throughout the placement and in response to the student's learning needs and to progress made. Formal meetings to discuss learning progress and assessment take place at initial, midpoint and end of the clinical learning placement.

Midwifery student learning in clinical practice is facilitated by paired allocation of a preceptor (or named midwife) who is responsible for the care of a caseload of women and infants. This means that student access to women and their babies, and their personal data, is supervised by the preceptor (or named midwife). The level of student supervision and proximity of the midwife to student whilst on placement depends on the learner's stage of midwifery education, and in accordance with their individual level of competence set against predetermined safety and performance criteria set out by the NMBI in the competence assessment tool (NMBI, 2015a). Each AHP also has a Midwifery Practice Development Unit, and midwives employed as CPCs whose role is to support the delivery of the educational programme at a ratio of one CPC to every 15 midwifery students registered on the programme (NMBI, 2022a, p. 52). The CPC's role is to guide and support midwifery students in the clinical areas by ensuring that the clinical placements meet the requirements of the education programme regarding the planned experience and specified outcomes. This could involve providing students with support with clinical skills, setting clear learning objectives, communicating with the preceptor, or, in some HEIs and AHPs, linking in with/involving lecturer if concerns are emerging about a student's practice or conduct.

Each registered midwife is bound by a professional code of conduct to ensure that factors enabling quality clinical learning environments for midwifery students are established and maintained (NMBI, 2021). The preceptor provides continuous supervision, assessment and support over a longer period of time or number of shifts whilst named midwives may assess aspects of student competence in a particular activity, task or skill (such as a birth or antenatal/postnatal examination). Positive relationships and continuity in communication and support of the preceptor are essential elements of assessment and learning (Bradshaw, Murphy Tighe, & Doody, 2018; Thunes, & Sekse, 2015), and impact on safety and quality of care and on staff retention (Livingstone, 2024). At all times, respectful confidentiality regarding a student's progress is expected (NMBI, 2020b). Scenario 1 offers an example of how the preceptorship process works in practice.

SCENARIO 1 THE PRECEPTORSHIP PROCESS IN PRACTICE

Scenario: First Meeting Midwife Tom and First-Year Midwifery and Student, Anne

Tom is a registered midwife of one year working in the labour ward of a teaching hospital. He has completed the NMBI-approved mandatory learning in student preceptorship. He is preceptor to first-year midwifery student, Anne. On their initial meeting and Anne's orientation to the ward, Tom and Anne have a private discussion to ensure that Anne is familiar with the process of competence assessment and the relevant documents. Together, they agree learning objectives specific to Anne's labour ward placement as a first-year student, and discuss opportunities, resources for learning and a plan to achieve the stated learning objectives. Tom and Anne discuss the level of supervision that Anne needs (direct), as prescribed by the Midwife Registration Programme Standards and Requirements (NMBI, 2022a) and the assessment criteria and skills outlined in her Competence Assessment Document. They remind each other of the importance of honest, clear and documented feedback at all times throughout the placement between student and preceptor.

At the initial meeting, dates for the intermediate and final interviews are agreed and recorded.

Tom knows that if Anne has challenges in meeting her learning objectives or needs additional support, in consultation with Anne, he can call on a member of the hospital's Midwifery Practice Development Unit. In addition, a link lecturer (from the linked HEI) may also become involved to work with Tom and Anne to develop a plan to support Anne to achieve her clinical learning.

This scenario demonstrates:

i A concrete example of the preceptorship process
ii The student–preceptor relationship and confidentiality
iii The resources available to both the preceptor and the student.

It is acknowledged that the preceptor needs support to conduct the role when students are unsuccessful in their learning, or when learning is challenging (Cusack et al., 2020). In some HEIs, a named university academic midwife or link lecturer may be identified for all clinical placements to provide student and preceptor support (NMBI, 2020b). When in place, the link lecturer's role is to support the assessment process and to meet with the student and preceptor to discuss learning progress and outcomes at intersections where required. Support is also offered by the CPC responsible for co-ordinating students' placements in the practice area. Learning outcomes are available in each practice area to guide student learning, and these are reviewed jointly on an annual basis by the AHP and their linked HEI.

Advanced Midwife Practitioners

AMP roles were recommended by the Commission on Nursing in 1998 (Government of Ireland, 1998). The Commission recommended the development of a three-step clinical career pathway by the creation of clinical nurse or midwife specialist (CNS, CMS) posts and advanced nurse or midwife practitioner (ANP, AMP) posts which matched with specific posts within the health service. Essentially, these roles were recommended in order to develop a clinical career pathway and offer new promotional, and remunerated, opportunities to midwives who wish to remain in clinical practice rather than pursuing a career in management or education.

Whilst there are arguments about advanced practice in midwifery in that all midwives work towards fulfilling the ICM's definition of a midwife (ICM, 2024), achieving the full scope of activities can be enabled or limited, and regulated differently throughout the world. In practice, advanced practice in midwifery roles have been implemented internationally under various names to acknowledge, remunerate and promote expanded midwifery scope (Toll, Sharp, Reynolds, & Bradfield, 2024). These advanced roles can include research, leadership, advanced assessment and decision making (Begley et al., 2013; Begley, Murphy, Higgins, & Cooney, 2014).

In Ireland, midwives with AMP status are characterised by having extensive relevant experience, are expected to conduct research into clinical midwifery issues and have protected research time to achieve this, be prepared to Master's degree level and have an extended scope of practice (Government of Ireland, 1998). The framework for their approval/accreditation was established by the National Council for the Professional Development of Nursing and Midwifery (NCNM, 2008a; 2008b) which defined the required experience and appropriate post-registration education. Currently, AMPs in Ireland typically lead new service developments such as establishing new midwifery-led services in the AHPs and in the community. Examples include establishing midwifery-led clinics and services in diabetes (pre-existing and gestational), emergency care, postnatal complications, perinatal mental health urodynamics, antenatal clinics for women with complex needs and extended postnatal care services in the community. A key feature of their role is that they are the *lead* healthcare professional for the women and babies in their area of practice and are accountable and responsible for senior clinical decision-making. Their role is different from the midwife's role in that they *lead* and *develop* new services, as well as delivery midwifery care, and they must be registered medication prescribers.

The AMP role is registerable with the NMBI. Mentorship or clinical supervision is an essential component of competence development in advanced practice (NMBI, 2018). Currently, AMP candidates are usually supervised by a medical practitioner but this will change in the future as the numbers increase and AMPs have the capacity to take on supervision of candidate AMPs (cAMPs). Though the number of supervised hours in clinical practice are not specified, they must provide evidence of validated competencies relevant to the context of their practice. In 2023, there were 30 AMPs registered in Ireland (NMBI, 2023 pp. 62–63), an increase from just one AMP in 2014, and the numbers are expected to increase in the coming years as the Government of Ireland aims to have at least 3% of all registrants (midwives and nurses) practising at an advanced level (Government of Ireland, 2022).

The Future

Like many other countries throughout the world, Ireland is experiencing a shortage of midwives. To increase the number of midwives being educated in Ireland, additional pathways to registration are being considered. Any increase in the number of students in clinical practice will be challenging for AHPs and accessing midwifery placements whilst, at the same time, continuing to fulfil the EU's and NMBI's requirements. It will require alternative, innovative and creative meaningful 'practice' exposure and will necessitate an increase in the use of gaining exposure in simulation suites. This has the potential to place additional demands on preceptors who, as practising midwives with caseloads, will need to adapt how they support students with reduced clinical practise and *in vivo* experience to develop their skills and achieve competence.

Conclusion

Preceptorship is very satisfying and rewarding role for midwives. For newly qualified midwives, the process of becoming a preceptor continues and a whole new suite of learning has to be achieved as they embark on their new role. Without doubt, their experiences of being preceptored and supported to learn in practice will shape how they preceptor students and future midwives. Regular refreshers courses are also required to maintain competence and relevance to future students' needs.

Notes

1 In some Associated Healthcare Providers and, ideally, factors that may influence a midwife's suitability to be a preceptor are that the midwife has (i) a minimum of 6 months post-registration midwifery experience; (ii) completed a preceptorship programme and (iii) capacity to preceptor a midwifery student with the clinical caseload.
2 Students are allocated to placements of varying duration, depending on the type of placement. Some placements are of one to two weeks' duration, in areas such as gynaecology and operating departments, whilst midwifery-specific placement can be four to eight weeks' duration.

References

Begley, C. M. (1999). Student midwives' views of 'learning to be a midwife' in Ireland. Midwifery, 15(4), 264–273. doi:10.1054/midw.1999.0184.

Begley, C. M. (2001). 'Giving midwifery care: Student midwives' views of their working role. Midwifery, 17(1), 24–34. doi:10.1054/midw.2000.0232.

Begley, C. M., Elliott, N., Lalor, J., Coyne, I., Higgins, A., & Comiskey, C. (2013). Differences between clinical specialist and advanced practitioner clinical practice, leadership, and research roles, responsibilities, and perceived outcomes (the SCAPE study). J Adv Nurs, 69(6), 1323–1337. doi:10.1111/j.1365-2648.2012. 06124.x.

Begley, C., Murphy, K., Higgins, A., & Cooney, A. (2014). Policy-makers' views on impact of specialist and advanced practitioner roles in Ireland: the SCAPE study. J Nurs Manag, 22(4), 410–422. https://doi.org/10.1111/jonm.12018.

Bradshaw, C., Murphy Tighe, S., & Doody, O. (2018). Midwifery students' experiences of their clinical internship: A qualitative descriptive study. Nurse Educ Today, 68, 213–217. doi:10.1016/j.nedt.2018.06.019.

Bradshaw, C., Noonan, M., Barry, M., & Atkinson, S. (2013). Working and learning: Post-registration student midwives' experience of the competency assessment process. Midwifery, 29(5), 519–525. doi:10.1016/j.midw.2012.04.010.

Carroll, M., Daly, C. D., Higgins, A., & Begley, C. M. (2005). Supernumerary preceptorship – The key to learning midwifery skills in a direct-entry programme in the Republic of Ireland. Evidence-Based Midwifery, 3, 39+ https://go-gale-com. elib.tcd.ie/ps/retrieve.do?tabID=T002&resultListType=RESULT_LIST&search ResultsType=SingleTab&retrievalId=e7b7c5d9-e172-4e0d-9239-8f8b66ca799 a&hitCount=9&searchType=AdvancedSearchForm&currentPosition=6&docI-d=GALE%7CA167030934&docType=Article&sort=Relevance&contentSegmen t=ZONE-MOD1&prodId=AONE&pageNum=1&contentSet=GALE%7CA1670 30934&searchId=R1&userGroupName=tcd&inPS=true

Cusack, L., Thornton, K., Drioli-Phillips, P. G., Cockburn, T., Jones, L., Whitehead, M., Prior, E., & Alderman, J. (2020). Are nurses recognised, prepared and supported to teach nursing students: Mixed methods study. Nurse Educ Today, 90, 104434. doi:10.1016/j.nedt.2020.104434.

Directive 2013/55/EU of the European Parliament and of the Council of 20 November 2013 amending Directive 2005/36/EC on the recognition of professional qualifications. Available at: https://eur-lex.europa.eu/legal-content/EN/TXT/PDF/?uri= CELEX:32013L0055

Government of Ireland. (1985). The Nurses Act. Dublin. https://www.irishstatutebook. ie/eli/1985/act/18/enacted/en/html

Government of Ireland. (1998). Report of The Commission on Nursing. A Blueprint for the Future. Dublin. https://www.lenus.ie/bitstream/handle/10147/627027/ Report-of-The-Commision-on-Nursing.pdf

Government of Ireland. (2011). Nurses and Midwives Act 2011. Dublin. https://www.nmbi.ie/What-We-Do/Legislation

Government of Ireland. (2022). Graduate and Advanced Practice. Government of Ireland. Dublin. https://www.gov.ie/en/publication/96ce55-a-policy-on-the-development-of-graduate-to-advanced-nursing-and-midw/

Government of Ireland. (2023). The Nurses and Midwives Act 2011 (Updates to 2023). Dublin. https://revisedacts.lawreform.ie/eli/2011/act/41/revised/en/pdf?annotations=false

ICM. (2024). International Definition and Scope of Practice of the Midwife. https://internationalmidwives.org/resources/international-definition-of-the-midwife/

Livingstone, K. (2024). How lack of support and recognition for RN preceptors is affecting nursing students' learning on placement. Nurse Educ Today, 138, 106192. doi:10.1016/j.nedt.2024.106192.

NCNM. (2008a). Accreditation of Advanced Nurse Practitioners and Advanced Midwife Practitioners. https://www.lenus.ie/bitstream/handle/10147/254053/nc003.pdf?sequence=1&isAllowed=y

NCNM. (2008b). Framework for the Establishment of Clinical Nurse/Midwife Specialist Posts. https://www.lenus.ie/bitstream/handle/10147/44769/6340.pdf?sequence=1&isAllowed=y

NMBI. (2020a). National Quality Clinical Learning Environment Audit Tool (2020). Nursing and Midwifery Board of Ireland, Dublin. https://www.nmbi.ie/NMBI/media/NMBI/NMBI-NQCLE-Audit-Tool-(2020).pdf?ext=.pdf

NMBI. (2020b). National Quality Clinical Learning Environment Professional Guidance Document (2020). Nursing and Midwifery Board of Ireland, Dublin. https://www.nmbi.ie/NMBI/media/NMBI/NQCLE-Professional-Guidance-Document-(2020).pdf?ext=.pdf

NMBI. (2015a). Competence Assessment Tool for Midwives. Nursing and Midwifery Board of Ireland, Dublin. https://www.nmbi.ie/nmbi/media/NMBI/Publications/competence-assessment-tool-for-midwives.pdf?ext=.pdf

NMBI. (2015b). Prescriptive Authority for Nurses and Midwives: Standards and Requirements. Nursing and Midwifery Board of Ireland, Dublin. https://www.nmbi.ie/NMBI/media/NMBI/NMBI-Practice-Standards-Guidelines-02-03-2020_2.pdf?ext=.pdf

NMBI. (2015c). Scope of Nursing and Midwifery Practice Framework. Nursing and Midwifery Board of Ireland, Dublin. https://www.nmbi.ie/nmbi/media/NMBI/Publications/Scope-of-Nursing-Midwifery-Practice-Framework.pdf?ext=.pdf

NMBI. (2017). Midwife Registration Education Post-RGN Programme Standards and Requirements. Nursing and Midwifery Board of Ireland, Dublin. https://www.nmbi.ie/NMBI/media/NMBI/Publications/NMBI-Midwife-Reg-Education-(P1)-18-month.pdf?ext=.pdf

NMBI. (2018). Advanced Practice (Midwifery) Standards and Requirements. Nursing and Midwifery Board of Ireland, Dublin. https://www.nmbi.ie/NMBI/media/NMBI/Advanced-Practice-(Midwifery)-Standards-and-Requirements-2018-final_4.pdf?ext=.pdf

NMBI. (2020c). Return to Midwifery Practice Courses: Standards and Requirements. Nursing and Midwifery Board of Ireland, Dublin. https://www.nmbi.ie/NMBI/media/NMBI/Publications/Return-to-Midwifery-Practice-Standards-and-Requirements.pdf?ext=.pdf

NMBI. (2021). Code of Professional Conduct and Ethics for Registered Nurses and Registered Midwives. Nursing and Midwifery Board of Ireland, Dublin. https://www.nmbi.ie/NMBI/media/NMBI/Code-of-Professional-Conduct-and-Ethics.pdf

NMBI. (2022a). Midwife Registration Programme Standards and Requirements. Nursing and Midwifery Board of Ireland, Dublin. https://www.nmbi.ie/nmbi/media/NMBI/Publications/midwife-registration-programmes-standards-requirements.pdf?ext=.pdf

NMBI. (2022b). Practice Standards for Midwives. Nursing and Midwifery Board of Ireland, Dublin. https://www.nmbi.ie/NMBI/media/NMBI/NMBI-Practice-Standards-for-Midwives.pdf?ext=.pdf

NMBI. (2023). State of the Register. Nursing and Midwives Board Ireland. https://www.nmbi.ie/Registration/NMBI-state-of-the-Register

O'Connell, R. (2019). Midwifery 1918–2018: Coming full circle. WIN: World of Irish nursing and midwifery. J Ir Nurs Midwives Org, 26(10), 21–23. https://cora.ucc.ie/server/api/core/bitstreams/2d55de41-851d-4277-9209-23e7981c76df/content

Smith, C. (2024). Regulating Midwifery in Early 20th-Century. Epidemic Belfast. https://epidemic-belfast.com/regulating-midwifery-in-early-20th-century-belfast/#:~:text=The%20regulation%20of%20midwifery%20in,city%20to%20control%20this%20occupation

Thunes, S., & Sekse, R. J. (2015). Midwifery students first encounter with the maternity ward. Nurse Educ Pract, 15(3), 243–248. doi:10.1016/j.nepr.2015.01.012.

Toll, K., Sharp, T., Reynolds, K., & Bradfield, Z. (2024). Advanced midwifery practice: A scoping review. Women Birth, 37(1), 106–117. doi:10.1016/j.wombi.2023.10.001.

14

MIDWIFERY MENTORSHIP IN JAPAN

Akemi Mochizuki and Yuri Kasamatsu

History and Current Midwifery Education in Japan

In Japanese history, the role of assisting with childbirth was often carried out by elderly women in the local community, and their experience and knowledge was passed down from generation to generation. Before the Meiji era of 1868–1912, it took a long period of training to become a fully qualified midwife (direct entry) (Hinokuma, 2003). At the time, home births were common, so having an apprentice midwife work as an assistant was a very useful form of training. Midwifery students could receive guidance, support, and education from their 'master', who had a wealth of clinical experience. However, following the outcome of the Second World War when Japan came under the influence of the United States, midwifery education changed. It became necessary to receive three years of education at a nursing school and one year of education at a midwifery school to become a midwife (non-direct entry) (Yoshida, 2014). Nowadays, it is not possible to obtain a midwife's licence without also having a nurse's licence.

Despite the Japanese requirement to be a nurse as well as a midwife, the Medical Care Act (Act No. 25 of 1948) clearly states that Japanese midwives have the right to open their own midwifery clinics, as a privately practicing midwife. Further, the Act on Public Health Nurses, Midwives, and Nurses (Act No. 203 of 1948) states midwives do not need instruction from a doctor for low-risk births. In effect, midwives may work autonmoulsy outside of the hospital environment and without instruction from a doctor, if the woman is considered low risk. As a result of the

DOI: 10.4324/9781003533733-15

promotion of the American obstetric care model after the war, the place of birth shifted from the home to hospital facilities, the number of practicing midwives decreased, and the number of hospital-based midwives who also work as nurses increased.

(Japanese Nursing Association, 2013)

According to a 2022 report by the Ministry of Health, Labour and Welfare, 38,063 people were working as midwives, of which 76.8% were working in hospital facilities, and only 5.8% were working as private practice midwives (Ministry of Health, Labour and Welfare, 2022). In hospital facilities, the birth rate has decreased by about 32% over the past 38 years (Ministry of Health, Labour and Welfare, 2023). The birth rate has declined from 1.76 in 1985, 1.33 in 2000, to 1.20 in 2023. The decline in birth rate has led to a decline in the number of maternity wards, and an increase in mixed wards such as gynaecology, internal medicine, and paediatrics (Japanese Nursing Association, 2013). For midwives working in hospital facilities, where they cannot concentrate solely on midwifery duties it can be difficult to maintain or develop their diagnostic and technical skills as midwives. Despite this situation, midwives are expected to maintain their competencies around recognition and response to maternal deterioration and provide best care practices for birthing women. Midwives are held to the same high standard as their medical colleagues, despite having limited opportunities to maintain their scope of practice. Should medical event occur, resulting in a poor outcome, the midwife will be held responsible. Many midwives working in hospitals in Japan are expected to become nurses first and then to enhance their skills in order to take on the additional roles and responsibilities required as a midwife. After a few years of employment, without maintaining clinical currency in the maternity environment, midwives may find their midwifery identity threatened and may find themselves in a professional dilemma (attempt to maintain midwifery skills or leave and work in nursing only). Additionally, the high level of emotional workload required in the healthcare setting such as interprofessional and therapeutic communication skills, medical and technical procedure skills, and legal and ethical issues often leads to nurses/midwives experiencing mental health challenges. These reasons may increase the risk of midwives leaving the profession, further reducing the midwifery workforce and midwifery care options available for childbearing women.

In order to secure nursing staff (the term 'nursing staff' used in this chapter includes midwives), the 'Guidelines for Training of New Nursing Staff' (Ministry of Health, Labour and Welfare, 2014) and the 'Training guide for new graduate midwives' (Japan Nursing Association, 2012) have been created. According to these guidelines, against a background of changes in public needs, such as the increasing sophistication of medical care and heightened awareness of medical safety, there is a divergence between the clinical practice skills required in clinical settings and the nursing practice skills acquired through basic nursing education at educational institutions, and this divergence is pointed out as a factor in the turnover of nursing staff. In order to bridge this gap, it is necessary to improve basic nursing education and to provide more training to improve the practical skills of new nursing staff. One way to improve the practical skills and knowledge of students and new staff is mentorship.

Student Midwife Education in the Clinical Setting

The usual system of supervision, in the clinical setting, for midwifery students is a mixture of the preceptorship and team support methods. For further information regarding the different terms used, see Table XX Definitions and terms used in nursing professional education support. In Japan, the person responsible for supervising students in the clinical setting is called a 'clinical field supervisor', and this term is used in the following text.

The usual supervision system for midwifery students in clinical settings is a mixture of preceptorship and team support methods (see Figure 14.1: General system for supervising midwifery students in practical training) In the preceptorship system, clinical field supervisors work with midwifery school faculty to support midwifery students during their practical training. In addition to providing instruction on midwifery care, teaching midwifery skills, and providing mental support, they are also expected to act as role models for midwives. The team support method is based on the idea that multiple clinical field supervisor provide support as a team, rather than a specific someone. Midwifery school faculty play a major role in maintaining the relationship between the clinical field supervisor and the student. In addition to providing guidance and mental support to students, they also coordinate with clinical field supervisors, report, and share information, and work to ensure that the practical training progresses smoothly.

There are currently more than 200 midwife training schools in Japan. The education courses for becoming a midwife vary, including graduate schools where you study for two years, one-year specialist courses, university specialist courses, and special training schools. There are dual qualification courses, studying midwifery and nursing (limited to 5–10 students) over four years at university. Regardless of the course undertaken clinical experience in the midwifery, clinical setting is required. The number of births required to become qualified as a midwife in Japan is stipulated as a minimum of 10 in the 'Regulations for the Designation of Schools and Training Institutes for Public Health Nurses, Midwives and Nurses' (Act of 1951). Considering that in other countries you need to have assisted with over 30 births, 10 in Japan is relatively low. However, due to the declining birth rate in Japan, the decrease in the number

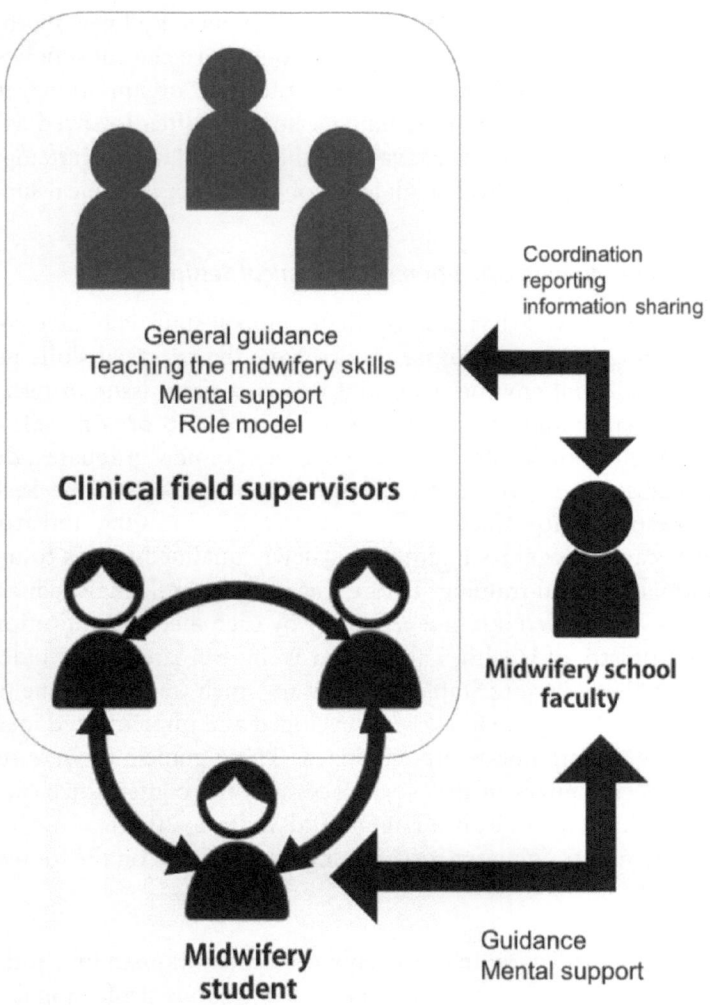

FIGURE 14.1 General system for supervising midwifery students in practical training

of normal births at hospitals, the difficulty of maintaining a 24-hour clinical environment (budget, equipment, human resources), and the shortage of clinical supervisors, it is becoming increasingly difficult for midwifery students to achieve even the required 10 births over the duration of their course.

The length of the practical training period differs depending on the training school, but many schools offer midwifery practical training for around three to six months. The clinical setting in which their practical training occurs varies and may entail one or more of the following: university hospitals, clinics or maternity hospitals. In order to provide education and guidance to midwifery students while ensuring the safety of pregnant women and new mothers, hospitals and facilities that accept students not only have clinical supervisors, but also provide practical training guidance as a team or organisational structure. Furthermore, teachers from the training school are often involved as supervisors. Conditional to the staffing available the training facility, attempts to appoint midwives with relatively high levels of experience as clinical supervisors.

New Graduate Midwife Education in the Clinical Setting

In Japan, it is believed that new graduate nursing staff who have completed a basic nursing education course do not have the practical skills needed to work in the clinical environment, and this is seen an issue in terms of ensuring the quality and safety of patients. In order to provide safe care for patients and promote professional development of new graduates, the Public Health Nurses, Midwives and Nurses Act and the Act on the Securing of Human Resources for Nursing Care were revised in 2009, and from April 2010, it became a legal requirement for newly qualified nurses to undertake post-graduate clinical training. Before the revision of this law, education for new nurses was carried out independently by each medical institution, but in 2010 the Ministry of Health, Labour and Welfare created the 'Guidelines for Training of New Nursing Staff'. A system in which training for new nursing staff, based on these guidelines, was developed and implemented in all places where new graduate nurses are employed. These guidelines were revised in 2014 to reflect changes in the workplaces and the content of basic nursing education (Ministry of Health, Labour and Welfare, 2014).

This system of training for new nursing staff is based on the following two principles.

1 Nursing is a profession that is deeply involved in human life, and requires continuous professional development. Continuous professional development and ongoing clinical skills training underpins best practice.
2 In order to support new nursing staff, it is important to foster an organisational culture in which all staff, take an interest in new nursing staff and work together to support them.

These guidelines for training new nursing staff aim to support new nursing staff and to encourage all staff to support the colleagues and professionally develop the profession as a whole.

Supporting Student Midwives in Japan

The clinical supervisor system is used to support students in the clinical context in Japan, primarily to assist students in the practice of labour and childbirth. For midwifery students, being able to assist in childbirth is an important part of their identity as midwives, as well as being a requirement for their course. For midwifery students, the practical training in assisting in childbirth is very stressful, with a lot of tension and anxiety (Kobayashi et al., 2024). The clinical field supervisor provides technical guidance and emotional support with the positive support of the supervisor facilitating a safe learning environment for student. During labour, the clinical supervisor midwife and the midwifery student work together to provide midwifery care from the first stage to the fourth stage of labour for each woman. After the birth, the clinical field supervisor follows up on the student's practice by checking their knowledge and skills against observed behaviours and actions, using their experience and performance evaluation sheets. It is common for the same clinical field supervisor to provide careful support for each case of labour assistance. However, for students who are on call 24 hours a day and waiting for a birth, this process could happen at any time, and it is not possible to have the same clinical field supervisor for different situations. Multiple clinical field supervisors (including teachers from the training school) may be involved. Having multiple supervisors means students will receive valuable insights, encouragement and support not only from a specific midwife, but from many midwives, and this can deepen their learning and increase their chances of finding the best role model for their personal learning (Taniguchi et al., 2015). While the multi-faceted guidance provided by multiple supervisors can broaden the scope of learning for students, the challenge is to make the necessary arrangements to ensure continuity of guidance.

Supporting New Midwives in Japan

In addition to clinical supervision for student midwives, support is provided for new graduates and new staff to organisations. When implementing training within a hospital, it is recommended:

1 A system to support new nursing staff is developed,
2 A training programme is planned,
3 Training is implemented for all staff, and, if required,
4 External organisations are sourced, to support training in facilities with few new nursing staff resources smaller hospitals.

The organisational systems that support new nursing staff include the preceptor system, the tutor system, the mentor system, and team support. To improve job satisfaction and employee retention rates, a system of intentional psychological support is provided. The definition/naming of support strategies in the midwifery clinical context, their primary objectives are shown in Table 14.1.

TABLE 14.1 Definitions and Terms Used in Nursing Professional Education Support (Adapted From 'Guidelines for Training of New Nursing Staff' (Ministry of Health, Labour and Welfare, 2014))

Name	Definition/Roles	Objective
Preceptorship	One nursing staff member (the preceptee) is paired with an experienced senior nursing staff member (the preceptor), who works with them for a fixed period of time. The preceptor's role is to help the preceptee learn independently.	This is effective to use in the early stages of employment for new nursing staff. The preceptor provides nursing care for the patient they are in charge of, while also providing assessment, nursing techniques, interpersonal relationships, the structure of medical and nursing services, self-management as a nursing professional, employment regulations, etc., while providing care, and acts as a model for a wide range of areas.
Tutorship	A tutor is a person who provides consultation and support to a nurse, covering a wide range of topics including work methods, study methods, worries, mental health, and lifestyle.	Having a designated mentor is seen as a reassuring support for new nurses. It is a good idea to assign a tutor throughout the nursing training period. However, it is not always possible to provide practical guidance on day-to-day work.
Mentorship	Mentors assist, support, guide, advise, and counsel new nursing staff. They provide a supportive role as well as being directly involved in offering guidance.	Mentors are suitable for supporting new nursing staff after the second half of their training, as they are involved in providing medium- to long-term career support, motivation, and support for professional development.
Team-based support	Rather than having a specific mentor, the nursing team will educate and support new staff members.	Each team member offers support and guidance in their area of expertise.

In clinical settings, these support systems can vary and are tailored to the facilities' resources and staffing capacity. The turnover of new nursing staff in 2023 is problematic, with a high turnover rate of 10.2% (Japanese Nursing Association, 2024). Factors leading to job loss include psychological stress, concerns about suitability to the profession, maintenance of technical/clinical skills, and interpersonal relationships. As mental health and wellbeing is becoming increasingly important to job retention, many facilities are introducing team-based support centred around preceptorship, which is said to be effective in reducing reality shock when entering the profession and improve psychological health.

Mentorship in the Education of New Midwives (Nursing Staff)

The number of births in Japan has decreased from 1.08 million in 2005 to 810,000 in 2021, and the number of facilities handling births has also decreased from 3,991 in 1996 (1,720 hospitals, 2,271 clinics) to 1,945 in 2021 (946 hospitals, 999 clinics) (Ministry of Health, Labour and Welfare, 2021). In line with the decline in the birth rate (noted above), in 2022, 23.7% of maternity wards were maternity wards only, 17.3% were mixed maternity and gynaecology wards, and mixed wards with multiple departments accounted for 60.5% (Japanese Nursing Association, 2024). Mixed ward environments can result in new midwives being responsible for providing non-midwifery care as well as care for women needing gynaecological care. The requirement to provide general nursing care as a new staff member, in conjunction with the minimal number of births undertaken during their student days, is having an impact not only on the physical health of new midwives, but also on their mental health. It is necessary therefore, to create an environment where midwives can concentrate on acquiring knowledge and skills related to midwifery without being caught up in multiple tasks and interruptions. Mentorship can support both future midwives (students and new staff).

As midwives are responsible for work that involves the safety and quality of care for women and their babies during childbirth, the mental burden can be overwhelming. It is essential therefore to provide support for new midwives. As stated earlier, each facility creates its own programme for training new midwives, the 'Training guide for new graduate midwives' (Japanese Nursing Association, 2012), and CLoCMiP (Clinical Ladder of Competence for Midwifery Practice) (Japanese Nursing Association, 2022) is used to develop and implement education for new midwives. This education is carried out by forming a team centred around preceptorship, with team members, including the preceptor, the 'education supervisor' who supports the preceptor, and the 'manager/supervisor' who supports the entire team.

Guidelines for Midwife Education

The 'Training guide for new graduate midwives' was created by the Japanese Nursing Association as a supplement to the specific training content for newly graduated midwives in the 'Guidelines for Training of New Nursing Staff' (Ministry of Health, Labour and Welfare, 2021). The 'Training guide for new graduate midwives' was developed with the aim of clarifying the ideal scope of practice for midwives, based on the current state of healthcare in Japan. It is made up of five sections:

  i 'Basic Approach to the Guide',
 ii 'Training for Newly Graduated Midwives',
iii 'Training for Supervisors of Newly Graduated Midwives',
 iv 'Training for Educators of Newly Graduated Midwives', and
  v 'Evaluation of Training Plans, Training Systems, etc.'

The guide recommends the creation of a career path that enables new midwives to plan how they will develop their careers while maintaining a balance between work, study, and life.

CLoCMiP (Clinical Ladder of Competence for Midwifery Practice)

CLoCMiP mandates the level of proficiency required in midwifery practice and describes the practical skills (core competencies) and proficiency levels that Japanese midwives will need to acquire as they progress through their career. The four practical, or core, skills are 'ethical sensitivity', 'maternity care skills', 'professional autonomy', and 'women's healthcare skills' (Japanese Midwives Association, 2021) (see Figure 14.2 Core competencies and proficiency levels that Japanese midwives should acquire). The proficiency levels are divided into five levels: beginner, Level I to Level IV. By linking these to career stages, it is possible to acquire the practical skills required of midwives in phases, in line with each person's growth. It is hoped that this will contribute to the development of midwifery in response to the increasingly diverse and complex needs of society.

In 2015, the CLoCMiP Level III certification system was launched. The midwives who have received certification can practice midwifery care autonomously, taking into account the individuality of the midwife, without limiting the location of midwifery practice, such as outpatients or wards.

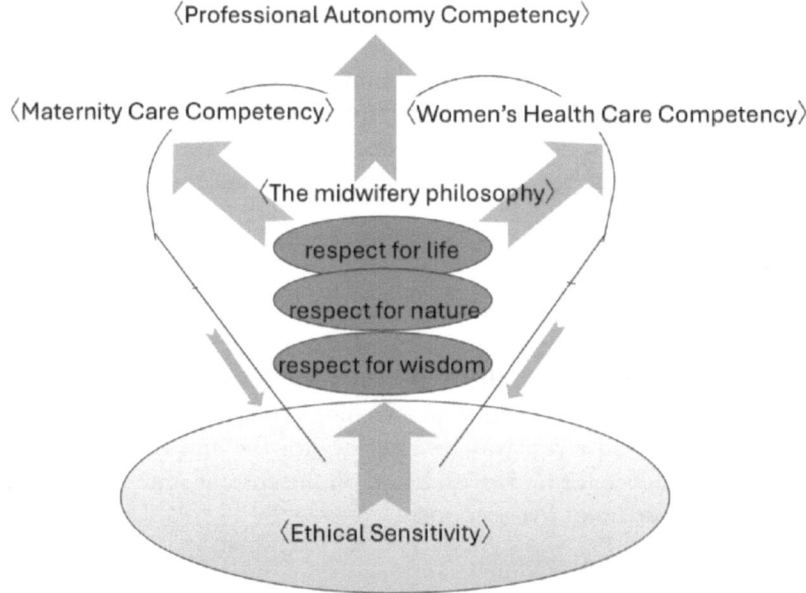

FIGURE 14.2 Core competencies and proficiency levels that Japanese midwives should acquire

Also they are able to identify and deal with transitions to high risk at an early stage and take a leadership role. In 2023, 8,951 people had received certification.

Models of Educational Support for New Midwives

In Japan, education for new midwives is carried out at each facility, with reference to 'Training guide for new graduate midwives' (Japanese Midwives Association, 2021) and CLoCMiP (Japanese Nursing Association, 2022). In this section, we will introduce two case studies. The first one, implemented at Higashiosaka-city Medical Centre, is based on successful preceptor–preceptee pairing. The second case study, introduced at Osaka General Medical Center, developed an education programme tailored to the individuality of the preceptee. Both these examples are underpinned by the Training guide for new graduate midwives' (Japanese Midwives Association, 2021) and CLoC-MiP (Japanese Nursing Association, 2022).

CASE STUDY 1 – HIGASHIOSAKA-CITY MEDICAL CENTRE

Higashi Osaka City is located in the east of Osaka City. With a population of around 480,000. Higashi Osaka City is the third most populous city in Osaka Prefecture and is famous as a 'city of rugby' and a 'city of manufacturing'. Higashi Osaka Medical Centre is a 520-bed medical facility that has participated in the Ministry of Health, Labour and Welfare's 'Project to Improve Clinical Practice Skills of New Midwives' in 2005, 2008, and 2009 and is committed to the education of new midwives. It has 19 maternity beds with approximately 350 births a year. There are 24 midwives working in two shifts, and on average, two to four new midwives are employed each year.

This hospital revised its new midwife training programme at the perinatal centre in 2024, with reference to CLoCMiP, and set clear achievement targets in four areas: midwifery and nursing practice skills, interpersonal skills, learning, teaching and research skills, and management skills. In order to become independent, new midwives usually need to have assisted in 12–14 births and will be able to perform normal births independently after one and a half years. From the second year to the fifth year, they will become fully fledged midwives, and from the sixth year onwards, they will be able to provide guidance to midwifery students.

A preceptor system was introduced, with importance placed on the compatibility of the pairing. Consideration of the personality and learning/teaching styles of the preceptee and preceptor, before deciding on the pairing of preceptor and preceptee. The preceptor's teaching style is emphasised in order to ensure the psychological safety of the new midwives. The preceptorship period is one year, but there is also a follow-up system in place after that, and from the second year onwards, the follow-up person is changed so that everyone has a follow-up person who can guide junior staff up to Level III. The new midwives set their own goals for 'birth', 'obstetrics', and 'newborn care', and their preceptors draw up a one-year education plan. Every month, new staff set their goals with their preceptors, and at the end of the month they assess their progress towards achieving these goals, checking their own and others' evaluations on a checklist. The midwives in charge of training new midwives participate in preceptor training and leadership training held at the facility, and acquire the skills necessary for training. In addition, midwives are encouraged to obtain advanced midwife qualifications, and after obtaining these qualifications, they are awarded a certification badge by the Japan Midwives Association.

CASE STUDY 2 – OSAKA GENERAL MEDICAL CENTER

Osaka Prefectural General Hospital for Acute and General Medicine, with 865 beds, is a general hospital in Osaka Prefecture. This hospital is certified according to the ISO 9001 standard for quality management systems, established in 2019 by the International Organisation for Standardisation, a non-governmental organisation based in Geneva, Switzerland. It has a total of 46 beds, including 6 MFICU beds and 40 general beds in the perinatal and maternal health centre. Around 1,000 births occur each year and have 54 midwives on staff. Every year, 6'10 midwives are employed, and there are 22 midwives in their first to fourth year of employment. New midwives undertake births, with support from midwives in their fifth year or more. The preceptor midwives who are in charge of training new midwives are midwives who have been in the job for at least four years, and these preceptor midwives are supported by the midwives in charge of education.

The mentor for new midwives is a midwife with at least four years' experience, and the midwife in charge of education supports fourth-year or higher level midwives. The instruction of new midwives in birth assistance is handled by a senior midwife at Level III. It takes more than two years for a new midwife to become independent, as they need to experience ten deliveries during the day shift and handle multiple tasks such as caring for multiple women. For this reason, preceptorship is carried out continuously from the time of employment until the new midwife has obtained their Level 3 qualification and become an advanced midwife, and a support system as a team is in place.

They have created their own midwife education programme based on CLoCMiP, and the programme clearly states the required number of care and midwifery practice skills for each stage of pregnancy, labour, the postpartum period, newborns, and primary care, as well as the goals to be achieved from the novice to Level IV and the goal of becoming an advanced midwife. New midwives receive education with the aim of being able to provide midwifery care while receiving guidance, and are assessed based on a review report for each of the ten deliveries they have attended, a checklist of knowledge and skills, and a portfolio. If they achieve 80% or more, they are promoted to Level I. Level I is aimed at those with two to three years of experience, but the education for new midwives is tailored to the abilities of each individual, and steady growth is emphasised over speed. In the past, to increase the number of births attended by midwives, new midwives had to assist with a large number of births, which placed a heavy mental burden on them. Now, taking into account the low competitiveness of Generation Z, we have changed our education to match the speed of each individual, and there are no longer any new midwives complaining of mental health problems, and we have been able to provide effective education.

The education of supervisors is shared by the team through in-house preceptor training, participation in external training, and communication training for participants, and the methods of instruction are unified. In addition, Level III midwives are working on self-improvement by attending seminars that are essential for obtaining the qualification of advanced midwife, which is certified by the Japan Nursing Association.

Education for Instructors

CLoCMiP is a measure of proficiency in midwifery practice, and Level II is considered to be the level at which one can instruct midwifery students, while Level III is the level at which one can train junior staff. For this reason, many preceptors for new midwives have a career of four to five years or more.

As the development of instructors is important for the effective implementation of training for new nursing staff, the 'Guidelines for Training of New Nursing Staff' (Ministry of Health, Labour and Welfare, 2014).also stipulate the abilities required of instructors, the goals to be achieved through training, and the content of training programmes. The guidelines also clearly state the roles of preceptors (on-the-job supervisors) and the educators (those in charge of training) who support them, and it is recommended that those in charge of training at organisations not only train new staff, but also evaluate the training plans and systems for on-the-job supervisors and educators, and use the results of this evaluation after the training. If there is a shortage of educators or if training cannot be provided at the facility due to its small size, there are also options such as using external organisations such as the Japan Midwives Association or general hospitals that accept nurse training from the local area. The aforementioned Osaka General Medical Center is one such general hospital, and it also takes on midwife education for the surrounding area.

REFLECTIVE ACTIVITY 1 SUPPORTING NEW MIDWIVES IN YOUR UNIT

1 Look at the educational and competency and capability frameworks guiding midwifery practice in your midwifery unit.
2 Design a sustainable support strategy for new midwives and or new staff in your unit (underpinned by your professional frameworks).
3 How would new staff and ongoing staff (permanent staff) benefit from your strategy?
4 What barriers might imped the strategy?

Optional task: Take your strategy to your midwifery manager / midwifery team to discuss implementation

---

Conclusion

In Japan, the number of births that midwifery students can experience during their practical training is limited, so they sometimes graduate without having acquired sufficient practical skills. However, by being carefully supervised by several midwives and faculties during their practical training, and by being exposed to safe, high-quality midwifery care, they can deepen their knowledge and skills, including their professional identity and ethical sensibilities, which are the most fundamental aspects of being a midwife. The Midwifery Practice Proficiency Level (Midwife Competency) and the CLoCMiP have been introduced for the mentorship of New midwives, and through hospital-level mentorship systems that respond to the characteristics of each hospital. Continuous and thorough training in the practical skills required of midwives is required. However, each institution faces challenges such as the difficulty of improving the delivery assistance skills of New midwives due to the declining birth rate, the increase in the number of staff leaving due to mental health problems, and the difficulty of applying teaching methods due to the changing values of Generation Z. One strategy to address these issues is to focus on the development of trainers/mentors. By having the Japan Midwives

Association and major hospitals take on the role of training midwifery leaders in regional hospitals, midwifery mentorship will develop, expertise will improve and leadership will be promoted. It is hoped that this kind of collaboration between the education system will support the mental health of new midwives, support the development of future midwifery leaders, and lead to higher-quality midwifery practice.

References

Hinokuma, F. (2003) The future of midwifery education. Bulletin of the Junior College of Medical Technology, Annual reports of the College of Medical Technology, Kyoto University, 23, 1–11

Japanese Nursing Association. (2012) Training Guide for New Graduate Midwives. https://www.nurse.or.jp/nursing/home/publication/pdf/guideline/shinsotsuguide.pdf (viewed on 2024/09/21)

Japanese Nursing Association. (2013) A Guide to Introducing Unit Management in Obstetric Wards for More Comprehensive Mother and Child Care. https://www.nurse.or.jp/nursing/home/publication/pdf/guideline/sankakongo.pdf (viewed on 2024/09/21)

Japan Ministry of Health, Labour and Welfare. (2014) Guidelines for Training of New Nursing Staff [Revised]. https://www.mhlw.go.jp/file/06-Seisakujouhou-10800000-Iseikyoku/0000049466_1.pdf (viewed on 2024/09/21)

Japan Ministry of Health, Labour and Welfare. (2021) Guideline for the Establishment of Perinatal Care System. https://www.mhlw.go.jp/content/10800000/001118039.pdf (viewed on 2024/21/09/)

Japanese Midwives Association. (2021) Midwifery Core Competencies 2021. https://www.midwife.or.jp/midwife/competency.html (viewed on 2024/09/21)

Japanese Nursing Association. (2022) Midwifery Practice Competencies Proficiency Stage Utilisation Guide 2022. https://www.nurse.or.jp/nursing/home/publication/pdf/guideline/CLoCMiP_katsuyo.pdf?ver=2 (viewed on 2024/09/13)

Japanese Nursing Association. (2023) 2022 Hospital Nursing and Midwifery Fact-Finding Survey Report. https://www.nurse.or.jp/nursing/home/publication/pdf/research/99.pdf (viewed on 2024/09/02)

Japanese Nursing Association. (2024) Hospital Nursing Fact-Finding Survey 2023. https://www.nurse.or.jp/home/assets/20240329_nl04.pdf (see 2024/09/21)

Japanese Nursing Association. (2024) New Release https://www.nurse.or.jp/home/assets/20240329_nl04.pdf (viewed on 2024/9/21)

Kobayashi, M., Kubota, M., Kojima, S., Morita, C., Ikeda, K., Watanabe N. (2024) Students' learnings regarding the midwifery diagnosis process in the first stage of delivery during delivery assistance training – Focusing on the first to third cases of delivery assistance. Niigata Seiryo Gakkai-shi. 17 (1), 20–26. https://ndlsearch.ndl.go.jp/books/R000000025-I011010006136182

Ministry of Health, Labour and Welfare. (2009) Trainig for New Nursing Staff https://www.mhlw.go.jp/file/05-Shingikai-10801000-Iseikyoku-Soumuka/0000029067.pdf (viewed on 2024/10/28)

Ministry of Health, Labour and Welfare. (2014) Guidelines for Training of New Nursing Staff https://www.mhlw.go.jp/file/05-Shingikai-10801000-Iseikyoku-Soumuka/0000049472.pdf. (viewed on 2024/09/03)

Ministry of Health, Labour and Welfare. (2022) Summary of the 2022 Health Administration Report (Employment Medical Personnel). https://www.mhlw.go.jp/toukei/saikin/hw/eisei/22/dl/gaikyo.pdf (viewed on 2024/09/03)

Ministry of Health, Labour and Welfare. (2023) 2023 Population Dynamics Monthly Report (Summary) https://www.mhlw.go.jp/toukei/saikin/hw/jinkou/geppo/nengai23/dl/gaikyouR5.pdf (viewed on 2024/10/15)

Taniguchi, H., Gabeyama, K., Noguchi, Y., Nakamichi, Y. (2015) Identifying the current issues of midwifery clinical practice and education: From viewpoint of undergraduate midwifery students. Journal of Japan Academy of Midwifery, 29 (2), 283–292

Yoshida, K. (2014) Development of midwives into professionals: History of midwives: its historical development. Kumamoto University Socio-Cultural Studies Departmental Bulletin Paper, 12, 211–227.

15

MIDWIFERY MENTORSHIP IN MALTA

Nicole Borg Cunen and Georgette Spiteri

Introduction

Midwifery plays a crucial role in Malta's healthcare system, ensuring the well-being of mothers and their newborns. According to the International Confederation of Midwives (ICM, 2020), with support from the United Nations Population Fund, mentoring is defined as:

> a reciprocal learning relationship in which a mentor and mentee agree to a partnership where they work together toward achievement of mutually defined goals that will develop a mentee's skills, abilities, knowledge and/ or thinking.
>
> *(p. 24)*

Preceptorship, in contrast, is described as a foundational phase at the beginning of a midwife's career, designed to provide newly qualified practitioners, or preceptees, with a structured and designated period of support from an experienced professional. This guidance helps foster their growth, development, and confidence in practice (O'Malley et al., 2000).

A robust mentoring and preceptorship framework is essential for nurturing competent and confident midwives in the Maltese Islands. Coaching students and newly registered midwives through these systems plays a crucial role in shaping their professional development and the impact of this is profoundly felt within the maternity health services.

Malta recognises the importance of equipping future midwives with the skills necessary to excel in their roles. Since midwives are directly involved in the provision of care during pregnancy, childbirth, and the postnatal period,

DOI: 10.4324/9781003533733-16

their training is essential for ensuring positive outcomes for both mothers and their babies. This rigorous preparation ensures:

1 **High-Quality Maternal Care:** Midwives are at the forefront of maternal health services, and their competence directly impacts the quality-of-care women and infants receive. Malta like many other countries all over the world recognises that well-trained midwives reduce the risk of maternal and infant mortality, birth complications, and unnecessary medical interventions. Through comprehensive training programmes, Malta aims to ensure that midwives can identify and manage complications, provide emotional support and guidance to women and their families, and foster safe and natural birth practice, encouraging non-invasive interventions unless absolutely necessary.

2 **Building Confidence Through Education and Practice:** Helping to develop confident midwives is key to ensuring successful outcomes. Malta's midwifery education focuses on a combination of theoretical knowledge and hands-on clinical practice to ensure future midwives feel prepared for the challenges they may face in real-life situations. Through supervised placements and practical simulations, midwifery students gain real-world experience in diverse clinical settings such as hospitals and health centres. This helps them practice essential skills, which include but are not limited to antenatal care, intrapartum care, and postpartum care within home and hospital settings. This supervision helps students to develop their problem-solving abilities and decision-making skills, particularly in urgent or emergency situations.

3 **Promoting Person-Centred Care:** Midwives in Malta are trained to provide holistic, person-centred care that respects the needs, preferences, and cultural backgrounds of women and their families. This approach encourages greater trust between the midwife and the patient, which in turn can lead to more positive experiences and health outcomes. By building confidence in communication and empathy, Malta aims to develop midwives who can support informed decision-making and provide individualised care that addresses the emotional, social, and physical needs of both mother and baby.

Historical Context of Midwifery Education in Malta

Midwifery in Malta has a rich history, deeply rooted in the country's cultural and social fabric. Historically, midwives were respected figures in the community, often learning their trade through apprenticeship and hands-on experience (Savona-Ventura, 2009). It was in the early 19th century, exactly March 1802, that Dr Francesco Buttigieg, the appointed teacher of obstetrics at the Woman's Hospital in Valletta, Malta's capital, delivered lectures about midwifery practice (Savona-Ventura, 2009). This school, however, was later closed, causing a deterioration in the practice of midwifery in Malta (Savona-Ventura, 2009). It is interesting to note that in 1842, 49 women were registered on the population census as midwives (Savona-Ventura, 2009). It was in 1915 the school was integrated into Malta's University, whereby a course leading to a Diploma of Midwife was offered (Savona-Ventura, 2009). However, this course only ran for a few years. By 1946, the teaching of midwifery was taken up by the Medical and Health Department and was delivered up until 1960. For the following decade, individuals who wanted to pursue education in midwifery travelled to the United Kingdom (Vella Bondin, 1994).

Over the years, the formalisation of midwifery education has transformed the profession, aligning it with international standards and practices. In 1988, the Institute of Health Care was founded at the University of Malta. This was done to develop courses for the health professions. In 1990, a four-year direct entry diploma programme in Midwifery was set up, and in 2002, this programme was replaced by the direct entry B.Sc. (Hons.) Midwifery programme. Since then, three students have obtained a Bachelor's degree in Community Midwifery Studies, 189 students have obtained a Bachelor's degree in Midwifery, and 18 students have graduated at Master's level.

Currently, the University of Malta is the only institution on the island delivering midwifery education. There are several courses delivered by the Department of Midwifery, including the four-year full-time B.Sc. (Hons) programme. This programme aims to prepare students to achieve the competencies required to be a midwife, as stipulated by the ICM (2024). The programme complies with the European Union, Midwives Directives 80/154/EEC Article 4, Directive 2005/36/EC Article 42, amended by Directive 2013/55/EU, and with the Maltese Health Care Professions Act [cap. 464, p4, art IV, 23(5)]. Students pursuing a Bachelor's degree in Malta complete a total of 2,400 clinical placement hours during their training. During their clinical placement periods, students are required to compile a register of accomplishments and a record of achievements together with their mentors or clinical supervisors.

Following successful completion of their undergraduate studies, students may opt to pursue a full-time M.Sc. in Midwifery via a taught programme which spans over three semesters or else the M.Sc. in Midwifery (by research), which is a part-time programme. PhD programmes in midwifery are also offered.

Current State of Midwifery Practice in Malta

Today, midwives in Malta operate within a well-structured healthcare system that emphasises maternal and child health. All midwives are required to be registered with the Maltese Council for Nurses and Midwives (CNM). This council regulates the Nursing and Midwifery Professions in Malta. Its function is defined in the Health Care Professions Act (2003). The Council is responsible for the upholding of high professional and educational standards for both professions. The CNM published the Code of Ethics for Midwives and Nurses in 1997, with this document being replaced by the Code of Ethics and Standards of Professional Conduct for Nurses and Midwives in January 2020. Although this document stands independently, it closely aligns with the International Code of Ethics for Midwives issued by the International Confederation of Midwives (ICM, 2014). The Council for Nurses and Midwives is committed towards the attainment of excellence in the delivery of professional care by encouraging continuing professional development amongst its registrants. In relation to mentorship and preceptorship, the Code of Ethics (Council for Nurses and Midwives Malta, 2000) gives midwives the responsibility of supporting both students and staff more junior than themselves, stating the following:

> Nurses and midwives should be ever ready to share their knowledge, competence, experience and resources with others, particularly with junior staff. Nurses and midwifery administrators and educators are morally obliged to provide timely and accurate feedback to nurses, midwives, and their supervisors, student nurses and student midwives and their teachers/mentors.
>
> *(p. 17)*

Midwives in Malta provide comprehensive care, from prenatal to postnatal services, and play a pivotal role in ensuring positive health outcomes. Despite the progress, the profession faces challenges such as resource constraints, the need for further continuous professional development opportunities, and adapting to evolving healthcare demands and the changing demographics of Maltese society.

Mentorship in Undergraduate Midwifery Education

As previously described, midwifery education in Malta is structured to include both academic and practical components. Mentorship plays a crucial role in bridging the gap between theoretical knowledge and practical application in the undergraduate midwifery programme, providing students with the opportunity to gain hands-on experience in real-world settings and to receive real-time feedback from experienced midwives. This experiential learning helps students to apply what they have learnt in the classroom to specific clinical situations, and thus facilitates an understanding of how academic knowledge informs real-life midwifery practice. Midwifery mentors in Malta do not use a structured assessment framework, rather an individual approach enabling them to tailor their teaching approach to each student's unique learning style. Mentors offer personalised guidance to ensure their mentees not only master clinical competencies but also develop a professional demeanour, facilitating a more holistic learning experience. They often serve as role models, demonstrating professional behaviour, ethical practices, and a commitment to continuous learning.

The mentor–mentee relationship encourages open communication, where students feel comfortable seeking advice and discussing challenges. Over the time they spend together, a sense of trust is built, and a safe, non-judgmental space is created. This encourages students to be open about their thoughts, questions, and uncertainties and concerns without fear of criticism, thus fostering a culture of mutual respect and support. The development of this relationship is fostered through processes that promote transparent dialogue from the start, such as completing a SWOT (Strengths, Weaknesses, Opportunities, and Threats) analysis, which will be explained later in the section.

REFLECTIVE ACTIVITY 1

Review the following scenario and consider how you, as a midwifery mentor, would approach the situation:

The student midwife you are mentoring is struggling with confidence during clinical placements, feeling overwhelmed by the transition from theoretical learning to hands-on practice. You notice the student hesitates to ask questions, fearing they might be perceived as incompetent.

Consider:

- How would you build trust and create an environment for open communication?
- What techniques would you use to help the student gain confidence and integrate theoretical knowledge into practice?

It is important midwifery mentors are approachable and practise active listening, giving their full attention to the student's concerns, validating their experiences, and responding thoughtfully. Knowing their mentor is willing to listen helps students feel supported and encourages more open and meaningful discourse. While this may come naturally to some, most midwives benefit from training that coaches on how to create a learning environment where students feel comfortable sharing openly and engaging in meaningful discussions.

In preparation for mentorship, midwives are encouraged to complete a stand-alone study unit, titled 'Applied Clinical Education in Health Care Practice', which is offered annually by the University of Malta and held over a single semester of 14 weeks. The study unit is offered at MQF level 7 which, according to the National Qualifications Framework, is at Master's level (Malta Further and Higher Education Authority, n.d.). This study unit is interdisciplinary and designed to empower healthcare professionals to develop the clinical setting into a meaningful learning environment. Delivered through a blended approach with both in-person and online components, the assessment includes contributions to online discussions and a case-study-based written exam. Although this study unit is not mandatory, and there is no associated remuneration, those who complete it are given preference when applying to be a mentor.

Any midwife working within the local public health services in a clinical role and for a minimum of 30 hours a week can apply to become a mentor, casually employed by the University of Malta. Applications for midwifery mentors are opened annually, and the contract period is for a one-year term. In addition to completing the aforementioned study unit, selection criteria include years of midwifery experience, further educational qualifications, and prior mentoring experience. Mentors are compensated based on the number of students they mentor, and each is assigned a maximum of two students at a time to ensure that they can provide them with individualised attention. The mentorship system is overseen by the academic staff of the Department of Midwifery. One of the initial steps in the process involves pairing mentors with students. Whenever possible, students are paired with mentors practising in clinical areas suited to their current stage in the undergraduate programme. Students in their penultimate year, for example, are often paired with mentors who practise in the labour ward to build intrapartum skills and complete necessary competencies.

Currently, formal mentorship is limited to students' summer clinical placements when they are free from academic obligations. This allows students to follow their mentor's shift pattern, including night duties and weekends. They are expected to complete a total of 240 hours with their mentor over two months and jointly formulate a schedule to ensure this requirement is met. During the remainder of the academic year, in the first and second semesters, the students attend non-mentored clinical placements. During these periods, they practise according to a fixed schedule, often rotating between several clinical areas, spending a few weeks in each. The 'Charge Midwife' of the clinical area assigns each student to work with a midwife who is on duty on that particular day, with this often being a different individual at each shift. These non-mentored placements, therefore, lack the continuity that comes with mentored placements.

Students are encouraged to complete a SWOT analysis with their mentor at the start of the placement. This is used as an opportunity to stimulate discussion between the pair about the students' perceived needs and the objectives to be achieved during their time together. These objectives may include opportunities such as increasing familiarity with the ward environment, increasing competence in clinical skills, and gaining confidence in interpersonal communication. There may also be more specific targets, such as completing portions of the students' achievement records or preparing for a specific practical examination. The mentors do not currently carry out any formal evaluation of student skills, with these being assessed during structured practical examinations overseen by clinical and academic midwives.

Effective communication between academic staff and mentors is critical for the success of the mentorship programme. An annual meeting involving all academic staff and mentors is held to clarify expectations, address common challenges, and suggest improvements. Mentors are also provided with a handbook that outlines the roles and responsibilities of each party and offers guidance in areas such as providing constructive feedback and supporting students who encounter difficulties. This is complimented by a designated link lecturer from the university who oversees ongoing communication with mentors and their assigned students, addressing any issues that arise during placements. If necessary, meetings between the link lecturer, mentor, and student are organised to review progress and identify how the student can be supported to achieve their goals. In these tripartite meetings, the student's progress to date is discussed, any obstacles to learning are identified and resolved, and an action plan is formulated for the remainder of the placement.

All parties complete feedback forms at the end of the placement. In the mentors' version of the form, individuals are encouraged to comment on the student's performance, including information about their attitude with staff and clients, skilfulness, and willingness to learn. They are also asked to identify areas where the student needs further practice and any issues encountered. The students' feedback form includes several open-ended questions about their mentor, exploring aspects such as communication ease, availability, teaching abilities, and effectiveness in providing feedback.

Students and Midwives' Perception of Mentoring

The impact of well-structured mentoring programmes is profound. Mentors contribute to the professional development of students, enhancing their clinical skills and confidence. Mentoring also leads to better care, as the midwives of the future are better equipped to handle complex situations and provide high-quality services.

Feedback from students and mentors regarding the mentorship system is overwhelmingly positive. Students can compare their mentored placements to those which are unmentored, with the former being regarded as the preferable option. Students value having a dedicated person who they can refer to. This helps them feel like an integral part of the ward complement rather than an outsider to the team. Over time, the mentor gets to know their capabilities and is thus able to help them build on their skills. Testimonials from mentors and mentees highlight the positive effects of these programmes. Mentees often express gratitude for the guidance and support they receive. The excerpt below is taken from the narrative of a recent graduate reflecting on the experience of being mentored:

> ... I worked with several midwives during my course, some of which shaped the midwife I am today and the care I try to give to mothers and their families. I viewed these midwives as role models and aspired to follow in their footsteps once I graduated as a midwife. Having a mentor meant having someone keeping track of your progress, trusting you little by little with more responsibilities and tasks and working together on improving your clinical skills whilst providing the best possible care. Having the same person supervising your work enables a trusting relationship to be built between the mentor and the student, whereby the mentor knows what the student is capable of doing and works hand-in-hand with the student whilst giving care. Personally, I used to feel more at ease discussing difficulties and concerns with those who monitored my progress over a period of time rather than those whom I worked with on occasional instances.

Mentors, in turn, report a sense of accomplishment as they witness students grow in competence and confidence. It is fulfilling for them to know they have played a part in their mentee's development, and, through their efforts, they are helping to shape the future of local midwifery practice. In the following excerpt, a midwife reflects on the experience of being a mentor:

> The biggest accomplishment in being a mentor is understanding the students' character, identifying their aims and what they wish to improve, and working thoroughly with them to achieve this. It is extremely rewarding being the student's role model while seeing them achieve their full potential with a little guidance from your end.

To ensure effective mentorship experiences for both the mentee and the mentor, both are encouraged to engage in an independent personal reflexive activity about the mentoring placement experience. This activity helps them to become more self-aware and identify areas that were beneficial to the overall experience and others which provided some difficulty so that potential improvements can be made, and support provided. Exemplar questions that facilitate this reflexive exercise include:

How did your mentor support your learning and professional growth?
Were there any challenges or gaps in the support provided?
How did these affect the learning experience?

Based on your reflections, identify one or two ways you can enhance your role as a mentor in the future.

How might you address challenges or build on the strengths of your previous experiences?

What do you think would help support your experience as a mentor or mentee?

REFLECTIVE ACTIVITY 2

As either a mentee or mentor, please take time to answer the above questions about a recent mentee or mentor experience you had.

Post-Registration Preceptorship

Following formal qualification from their undergraduate education, most midwifery graduates enter the local public health service, although some may choose to work in private practice or overseas. For those who chose to work within the local public system, their first two years involve rotating through different midwifery-related clinical areas, spending three to six months in each. This applies to both local graduates and those from equivalent programmes abroad, ensuring they gain a hands-on, holistic understanding of the full continuum of care that women and their families receive during the perinatal period and the interconnectedness of each stage of care within Malta.

The transition from student to qualified midwife is a complex journey, both challenging and rewarding. Preceptorship, as defined previously, enables professionals to apply and integrate their knowledge into daily practice, build confidence, and begin their careers with a strong foundation (NHS England, 2022). Consequently, within the Maltese public health service, newly registered midwives undergo a preceptorship period that spans one year. A period of preceptorship helps these midwives transition from students to autonomous professionals. Preceptorship commences with a week-long programme which includes refresher sessions regarding essential skills such as breastfeeding support, caring for bereaved families, and performing neonatal resuscitation, all delivered by experts in the field. The midwives are also expected to complete a competency booklet during their first year of practice, where they document skills attained, with these being signed off by experienced midwives. This is a staff training and support requirement imposed by the employer. The competencies include but are not limited to, physical skills, such as those concerning intravenous infusion management, to communication and problem-solving skills.

Reflective practice is another key component of the preceptorship and is led by a 'Practice Development Midwife'. In an initial reflective session, held during the first month of practice, the 'Practice Development Midwife' observes each newly qualified midwife individually over a morning shift in the clinical environment. This is followed by a joint reflection on the care provided, highlighting what was done well and what elements could have been improved. To avoid over-structuring the reflective process, and limiting flexibility, no particular reflective model is used. The aim is to encourage the midwives to critically evaluate their actions and decisions, leading them to provide a better quality of care.

In subsequent sessions, one held between the third and sixth month of practice, and one between the 10th and 12th month, the newly qualified midwife is encouraged to talk through further experiences they've encountered during their practice and to reflect on these. These reflective sessions also serve as an opportunity for the 'Practice Development Midwife' to touch base with the newly qualified midwife and assess how she is adjusting to her role. The following excerpt reflects the thoughts of a recently registered midwife regarding the value of such sessions:

> ... a practice development midwife observed my care [at the labour ward], providing me with an opportunity to reflect and receive feedback, which further reinforced my confidence and helped me continue developing my practice.

At the end of their first year of practice, the group of newly qualified midwives is brought back together to bring the preceptorship period to a close. This involves the midwives each presenting a reflective case study to their peers and a panel of experienced midwives. They are encouraged to draw on events they have encountered in practice. In this setting, the newly qualified midwives also derive support from one another. One such midwife reflected on this in the excerpt below:

> During this transition, the most valuable support I received came from my peers, especially those who were also newly qualified. Their shared experiences made me feel less isolated in facing the challenges associated with the transition from student to qualified midwife.

Challenges and Solutions

Despite their benefits, the mentorship and preceptorship systems are not without their challenges. Mentors and preceptors must balance their clinical responsibilities with the time and energy required to guide students or newly qualified midwives effectively. Varying learning styles and complex clinical environments can further complicate the role. This section will explore the common challenges faced in midwifery mentorship and preceptorship and, where feasible, discuss strategies to overcome these obstacles to ensure both mentor and student achieve the desired outcomes.

- Some of the shortcomings of the current mentorship system relate to the unpredictability of the applicants. Currently, there are not enough applicants to allow for much selectivity. While obvious outliers, such as those who work in non-clinical roles or do not work the required number of hours, are passed over, the mentoring allocations are otherwise largely dependent on the midwives who choose to apply and their places of work. The implication is that some clinical areas may have few or no mentors. This means students are sometimes assigned to work in clinical areas that are not considered ideal for their current needs, such as wards where they have already had sufficient non-mentored practice. Furthermore, where there are not enough applicants, some student cohorts may be required to practise without a mentor, at least for a portion of their placement hours, particularly if they require experience in a clinical area which lacks mentors. On the other hand, applicants may include many midwives who work in the same clinical area and on the same shift, which can lead to overcrowding in the clinical area. To overcome these challenges, increasing the number of applicants would allow for a better distribution of students across clinical areas.
- Reluctance to take on a mentoring role may be influenced by several factors. Mentors sometimes lament the fact that, as a consequence of their role, they are assigned a heavier workload. For instance, if a mentor is working with a student at the Delivery Suite, they are more likely to be consistently assigned to care for women in advanced labour so the student has the opportunity to complete competencies related to labour and delivery. This can lead to burnout for the mentor.
- Conflict between mentors and non-mentors can also cause issues. Non-mentors are sometimes reluctant to have students shadow them, even, for instance, on occasions when the mentor is unwell, citing the fact they are not getting paid for the role. This is despite the fact that the supervision of students falls directly under the midwives' role according to the Code of Ethics and Standards of Professional Conduct for Nurses and Midwives (Council for Nurses and Midwives Malta, 2020). Where this tension exists, it leads to further burnout for the mentors and to students feeling unwelcome in the clinical setting. Affected mentors may decide not to re-apply for the role in subsequent years.
- Midwives may also be hesitant to sign up for the recommended study unit that would better prepare them for their mentorship role. The time and effort required to undergo the course, alongside their clinical duties, is sometimes regarded to be too heavy a commitment, particularly given the content is regarded to be challenging. In the past, undergoing this training

within two years of commencing the mentorship role was a prerequisite for selection as a mentor, but this requirement has recently been removed to ensure that enough midwives qualify for the role.

- Other difficulties around mentorship concern individual mentor–student pairs, where one or both of the parties highlight obstacles such as inappropriate attitudes, a lack of communication, an unwillingness to teach or learn, or attendance issues. Not all mentors or students have the same level of enthusiasm for and commitment to working together, and some incompatibilities are inevitable. In such cases, the link lecturer investigates the problem from the perspective of both parties and steps in to try to resolve the dispute amicably. On rare occasions, re-assignment of the student is regarded as the best solution.

In the below excerpt, a midwifery mentor reflects on her experiences of encountering such challenges:

> A very challenging aspect I found in mentoring students is understanding that not all students have the same character and willingness to learn. Although I would have tried my best, certain students don't have the same goals and determination as others. It is quite discouraging to see little to no progress from their end after weeks of mentoring.

- In the past, mentors were asked to assign a mark to the student, which counted towards their final grade in associated study units. This element of continuous assessment was regarded as advantageous, given that it allowed for ongoing insights into students' progress and reduced the pressure associated with final examinations. However, many midwifery mentors, having built a close relationship with their mentees and/or often lacking the ability to compare their performance with their peers, would give unrealistically inflated marks to students. On the other hand, more experienced mentors often give more impartial marks to their students. This inconsistent marking led to the discontinuation of the practice. Training mentors in fair and objective student evaluation may resolve this issue if the system were to be re-introduced.

- Ideally, students would be mentored throughout the year rather than solely during the summer period. However, students are bound to attend physical timetabled lectures during the first two semesters of the academic year. It would thus be challenging to organise a schedule that both fit with their mentors' shift pattern and respected the students' academic commitments while ensuring they worked the required hours. This issue could be resolved through the re-organisation of the academic calendar to include learning blocks in each semester, where lectures would be fit into the first half of the period, and the remainder would be reserved for clinical practice. This solution has, however, so far been met with resistance by the University as it would require changes to several systems, including the assessment period.

- While mentorship has many associated advantages, a potential drawback of the arrangement is that it limits the number of midwives that the students observe in practice. This narrows students' exposure to different practice styles and potentially limits their understanding of alternative approaches, making it harder for them to develop a well-rounded skill set. Students might also unconsciously mimic their mentors without exploring other ways of thinking or practising. If the mentors observed do not consistently adhere to best practices or up-to-date guidelines, students may adopt outdated or suboptimal practices. To minimise this effect, mentors are provided with an updated clinical skills book to which they can refer if in doubt about the latest practice guidelines. Finally, mentorship may reduce networking opportunities, limiting the opportunities for students to build connections with a greater number of midwives.

- In relation to post-registration preceptorship, the system could be improved through formalising the process of shadowing. Shadowing, in this context, involves the newly qualified midwife working with an experienced midwife for a period each time they rotate to work in a new clinical environment. This allows the newly qualified midwives time to re-orient themselves to the clinical area and gives them access to a reference person from whom they can easily seek support and guidance as they gain confidence. While shadowing is often done informally, formalising this would improve its consistency, helping to reduce the stress and anxiety that new graduates often face. Knowing there is a clear support plan in place can help new midwives feel more secure in their new roles. This was reflected upon by two newly qualified midwives:

> One aspect that could have eased this transition would have been having a designated support figure, who is also a midwife, to maintain ongoing communication and frequent discussions, offering a safe space to discuss difficulties and concerns .... With appropriate support systems and structures in place, I believe that the transition from student to midwife can be smoother. New recruits would feel empowered and inspired to provide high-quality care, knowing that they have a robust network of guidance and support.

> Beginning my journey as a midwife was a combination of excitement and uncertainty, and the support I received during this time was instrumental in building my confidence and capabilities .... [At] my initial placement in the Neonatal and Paediatric Intensive Care Unit ... I was assigned a senior midwife who guided me and allowed me to reflect on my practice and identify areas for improvement. These elements made my transition from student to qualified midwife smoother and more reassuring ....

- Furthermore, while the preceptorship programme currently in place is perceived to be helpful, newly registered midwives often feel that more intensive and ongoing support would help to further facilitate their journey as they gradually gain confidence in their abilities as autonomous practitioners. One such midwife reflects on this in the excerpt below:

> One aspect I found challenging was the lack of ongoing, consistent feedback. While the initial feedback was invaluable, as time went on, it became less frequent. This left me to sometimes interpret "no feedback" as "no news is good news". In hindsight, having more regular feedback sessions, even informal ones, would have helped me continue to grow and feel reassured about my progress .... [Moreover], while I felt well-prepared overall, having more opportunities for structured reflective practice, particularly after handling complex or emotionally charged cases, would have been beneficial. Debriefing sessions where we could openly discuss challenges and emotional responses would offer additional layers of support and learning.

Conclusion

Mentoring and preceptorship are indispensable components of midwifery practice, contributing to the professional growth of midwives and the quality of care they provide. Entering the field of midwifery can be daunting due to the high stakes and emotional demands of the role. Through mentoring and preceptorship, students and newly registered midwives gain reassurance and support, which helps them overcome self-doubt and build a sense of competence. These supportive initiatives provide a safe space to discuss experiences, reflect on performance, and receive constructive feedback. This process not only boosts students' and new practitioners' confidence but also fosters resilience, enabling them to handle the pressures and challenges of midwifery with greater ease. By observing and interacting with experienced professionals, students and new practitioners gain insights into the various aspects of a midwifery career, including leadership, teamwork, and professional advocacy. This exposure helps them understand the broader context of their role and prepares them for future responsibilities, whether in clinical practice, research, or education. By addressing current challenges and building on successful initiatives, Malta can continue to enhance its midwifery workforce, ultimately benefiting mothers and their newborns. This chapter underscores the importance of sustained efforts to support midwifery through robust mentoring and preceptorship programmes, paving the way for a brighter future in maternal and child healthcare.

Policymakers should consider developing national standards for mentoring and preceptorship, ensuring consistency and quality across all programmes.

Additionally, fostering a culture that values and supports ongoing professional development is crucial for the future of midwifery in Malta.

References

Council for Nurses and Midwives Malta. (2020). *Code of ethics and standards of professional conduct for nurses and midwives.* https://nursing.gov.mt/wp-content/uploads/2024/04/Code_of_Ethics_and_Standards_of_Professional_Conduct_for_Nurses_and_Midwives.pdf

Health Care Professions Act. (2003). *Cap. 464 – Health Care Professions Act.* https://legislation.mt/eli/cap/464/20230922/eng

International Confederation of Midwives. (2014). *International Code of Ethics for Midwives: Philosophy and Model of Practice. https://internationalmidwives.org/resources/international-code-of-ethics-for-midwives/*

International Confederation of Midwives. (2020). *Mentoring Guidelines for Midwives 2020.* https://internationalmidwives.org/resources/mentoring-guidelines-for-midwives/

International Confederation of Midwives. (2024). *Essential Competencies for Midwifery Practice.* https://internationalmidwives.org/resources/essential-competencies-for-midwifery-practice/

Malta Further and Higher Education Authority. (n.d.). *Malta Qualifications Framework.* https://mfhea.mt/wp-content/uploads/2021/01/The-Framework.pdf

NHS England. (2022). *National Preceptorship Framework for Nursing.* https://www.england.nhs.uk/long-read/national-preceptorship-framework-for-nursing/

O'Malley C., Cuncliffe E., & Breeze J. (2000). Preceptorship in practice. Nursing Standard, 14(28):45–9.

Savona-Ventura, C. (2009). *The history of midwifery education in the Maltese Islands.* Department of Obstetrics and Gynaecology, Faculty of Medicine and Surgery, University of Malta.

Vella Bondin, M. (1994). Midwifery through the years. Midwives Journal, Midwives Association of Malta, 3, 20–25.

16

MIDWIFERY MENTORSHIP IN MEXICO

Akane Sugimoto Storey, Hannah Borboleta, and Yaredh Marín Vázquez

Introduction

The chapter was written by two preceptor midwives in Mexico, and one anthropologist specialised in urban autonomous midwifery in Mexico. In the chapter, we combined narratives in first person – as midwives – and the ethnography fieldwork – as researcher – regarding the daily life of midwifery. In Mexico, fieldwork and studies about midwifery training and educational processes are scarce. For this reason, we use our experiences as central data for constructing this chapter. Throughout this chapter, we refer to *apprenticeship* as a student midwife's or midwifery apprentice's route of experiential or clinical learning. We refer to *preceptorship* as the role of the midwife instructor or lead midwife in an aspiring midwife's clinical learning process in accordance with an apprenticeship/preceptorship training model. More commonly, you will see us refer to mentorship. In Mexico, the word *mentorship* is popularly used synonymously with the apprenticeship/preceptorship training model. As the preferred term in Mexico, we refer extensively to mentorship regarding apprenticeship/preceptorship training. As you will read throughout this chapter, mentorship goes much beyond the role of clinical supervision. We also refer to midwifery centres (Stevens & Alonso, 2020) with the term used in Mexico, 'casas de partería' (midwifery houses), which encompass many more services than childbirth alone and are community-based and not well-integrated into the health system.

What is Midwifery Mentorship in Mexico?

Midwifery mentorship in Mexico involves an extensive teaching and training process in which experienced midwives guide and instruct student midwives in all aspects of the full-scope midwifery practice. As synonymous to

DOI: 10.4324/9781003533733-17

apprenticeship/preceptorship training, this includes hands-on teaching of midwifery skills and knowledge through around-the-clock integration of student midwives into the midwife's casa de partería or homebirth practice. During midwifery mentorship, the supervising midwife retains full clinical responsibility while gradually and progressively transferring the primary role of delivering midwifery care to the student midwife. This is achieved through an ongoing and reciprocal training process that strengthens the student midwife's knowledge, skills, confidence, sense of responsibility, and embodiment of midwifery values and philosophy. It is an extensive and involved process. With midwifery poorly integrated into Mexico's health system, this process extends beyond a transfer of clinical knowledge and skills, and as a community-based process, midwifery mentorship occurs outside of formal, accredited educational settings. Before exploring the intricacies of midwifery mentorship, we first present a historical context of midwifery, the contemporary maternal health system, and the types of midwives in existence across Mexico.

How Midwifery Operates in Mexico: A Historical Context of Midwifery

Mexican midwifery has a rich historical and cultural background. Records of midwifery practice date back to pre-Hispanic times, with testimony of midwifery practice recorded in the Florentine Codex (Sahagún, 1577). Essentially, midwifery knowledge has been curated, transferred, replicated, and nurtured through time by traditional midwives from the numerous indigenous groups who inhabit this land currently known as Mexico. Mexico's establishment as a nation-state altered many relational processes of social life. As such, the traditional midwives who, during pre-Hispanic times, enjoyed high levels of legitimacy and social recognition have lost authority and legitimacy over the course of centuries.

As in many countries, Mexico's national laws and regulations have encouraged allopathic medicine and the biomedical system to be deemed the legitimate type of knowledge and practice for treating the human body. Consequently, midwives have been curtailed in their practices. Through the 19th century up until the 1950s, there were initiatives for the 'professionalisation' and recognition of midwives (Cházaro & Estrada, 2005). We added quotations to the previous sentence because, as historian Ana María Carrillo (1999) highlights, professionalisation was not about improving midwifery, but rather, to make midwifery subordinate to physician practice and keep traditional midwives in check. By 1960, midwives were outright prohibited from attending childbirth (Carrillo, 1999; Freyermuth Enciso & Argüello Avendaño, 2017).

Midwifery practice has since occurred against the grain outside of Mexico's formal health system. Although midwifery is not currently prohibited – largely due to the recognition of traditional midwifery as a practice of

> ancestral origin, consisting of comprehensive systems of care for pregnancy, childbirth and postpartum(...) (in which] knowledge and know-how have been preserved. With these systems pertaining to cosmovisions (...) [that are largely considered] biocultural heritage.
>
> *(Sevilla Villalobos et al., 2023, p. 8)*

It is also not sufficiently supported and sustained through public policy or socially. These complexities regarding midwifery practice imply adversity for the midwifery training process. Why train as a midwife? Who decides to teach midwifery? How can one train as a midwife? How can midwifery practices be sustained? Discussing the teaching–learning processes of midwifery in Mexico requires us to consider the risk of disappearance of the people and spaces in which this knowledge is found.

The Contemporary Maternal Health System

With midwives poorly integrated, over-intervention, coercion, and obstetric violence are normalised components of Mexico's modern maternity care system. To meet global targets[1,2], Mexico has long implemented policies tying social benefits to women's performance of health-related behaviours, including appearance at health facilities for antenatal care and facility-based childbirth. While these types of policies are often associated with reductions in maternal mortality, sustained reductions in maternal mortality have not been observed in Mexico (2000 to present) (World Bank, 2024). Moreover, moving childbirth from community to hospital-based settings has had unintended consequences. Mexico maintains a consistently high caesarean section rate, at 48.8% in public hospitals (2018–2019) (Lamadrid-Figueroa et al., 2021) and 77.7% in private facilities (2008–2017) (Uribe-Leitz et al., 2019). Obstetric violence is a well-recognised phenomenon globally (Bowser & Hill, 2010) and in Mexico (Castro & Frías, 2020). Smith-Oka (2009, 2012) elucidates how indigenous women are especially coerced to undergo certain reproductive medical procedures, including sterilisation, and experience obstetric violence. It is important to add that indigenous values and perspectives are not integrated into the curriculum of biomedically focused health providers, with 96.9% of births in Mexico occurring in hospitals (WHO, 2024) with 80% attended by medical residents in training (Instituto Nacional de Salud Pública (INSP), 2020). These normalised occurrences within Mexico's modern maternal healthcare system occur within wider contexts that treat feminised and racialised bodies as disposable (Sánchez Hernández et al., 2023).

While it is well established that midwifery is critical to the capacity of health systems to meet the health needs of women, newborns, and childbearing families (Renfrew et al., 2014), a longstanding campaign to delegitimise midwives means that no midwifery scope of practice has been recognised by the federal government (Arellano et al., 2020); not even that of the International Confederation of Midwives (ICM) (2019b), which is recognised around the world as the international definition of the midwife[3]. Loopholes in legislation have resulted in local variations in the treatment and integration of midwives by the health sector (Arellano et al., 2020; Atkin et al., 2017). In response to the culture of institutionalised birth in Mexico, there are specific efforts by independent midwives to provide home births and offer midwifery-led care through midwifery centres (Stevens & Alonso, 2020). These are opened by midwives and establish relationships with state administrative and health institutions, but they are not systematically supported, which results in obstacles. Recently, in 2023, the first government-recognised midwifery school designed, established, and taught by midwives was opened[4]. However, the lack of social support and institutional barriers limit the operational capacity of these initiatives and ultimately lead to their extinction.

Types of Midwives and Maternal Health Providers

Contemporary Mexican midwifery is diverse, pluralistic, and reflective of many social, political, and historical transformations. There is a wide range of 'types' of midwifery practices and training processes and, in turn, a diverse composition of midwives providing care across Mexico. Marín (2019) suggests grouping into the following four categories of self-identification, which are not mutually exclusive:

1 Training: empirical, in the tradition, in a programme without official recognition, technical, and professional.
2 Ethnic or national differentiation: indigenous, mestiza[5], and foreign.
3 The geopolitical demarcation where they practice: urban or rural.
4 Their political stance: autonomous, postmodern, and feminist.

Additionally, there are those who have initially trained as obstetric or perinatal nurses and who later decide to train or practice as midwives because they find this an alternative to the violence they witness daily in biomedical practice.

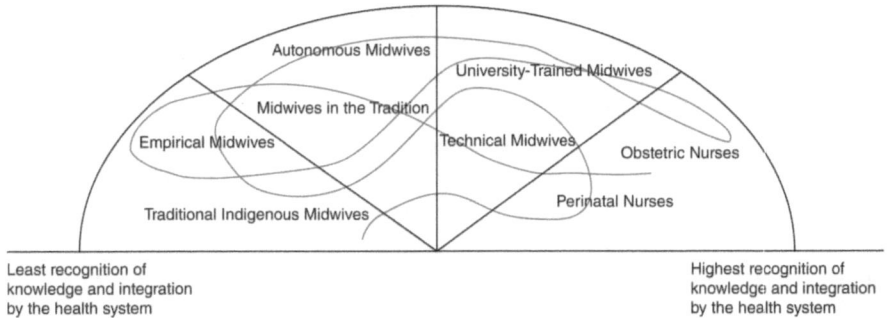

Least recognition of
knowledge and integration
by the health system

Highest recognition of
knowledge and integration
by the health system

FIGURE 16.1   Types of maternal health providers other than physicians

* the grey dotted line of Figure 16.1 represents the movement of providers among these quadrants

We highlight midwives, or rather, maternal health providers other than physicians, are recognised by the biomedical system to varying degrees, depending upon their type or affiliation and training route. We display this phenomenon through quadrants in Figure 16.1.

Midwifery practices most distanced from and less recognised and integrated by the biomedical hospital system are in the two left quadrants. We locate traditional indigenous and empirical midwives, whose learning processes and practices are strongly supported through cultural and community practices, in the lower left quadrant. We locate autonomous midwifery practices, midwives in the tradition and autonomous midwives, in the upper left quadrant. Midwives in the tradition are generally mestiza women who seek to practice a form of indigenous or traditional midwifery that includes a core practice on spiritual healing. Their practice attempts to model indigenous midwifery while also incorporating aspects of more formalised, westernised homebirth midwifery. Autonomous midwifery is also usually attended by mestiza women who train through extensive apprenticeship and mentoring through care models politically distanced from hospital-based settings: in homebirth and midwifery centre practices. Models more closely aligned to biomedicine and, therefore, poised to be integrated into the health system, are located in the two right quadrants. We locate technical and university-level midwifery in the upper right quadrant, as practices 'formally' recognised by the State, but poorly integrated. In the lower right quadrant, we locate obstetric and perinatal nursing practices. These final two are maternal health models that integrate some basic midwifery knowledge, but are almost exclusively aligned to biomedical knowledge. These nursing practices and training are generally recognised as 'professional' by State educational and health institutions. These two final models are also not well integrated. There is no public budget dedicated to these jobs at hospitals, and very few obstetric and perinatal nurses self-identify as midwives.

It is important to mention that people who practice midwifery move across these quadrants. They are not fixed or static categories. Rather, from this representation, one is able to look at the possibilities or impossibilities that each of the self-adscriptions acquires in relation to social perception (i.e., how service users see midwives) and the health and administrative policies of the State. Dixon (2020), Freyermuth (2018), and Laako (2017) confirm the conceptual framework of Figure 16.1.

Training Processes of Midwives

Each type of midwifery noted in Figure 16.1 has its unique pathway into practice. Traditional midwifery emerges from knowledge systems that resist, endure, and encompass specific cultural ways of looking at and experiencing the world. Traditional indigenous and empirical midwives (Murray de Lopez, 2015) inherit the gift of midwifery from **their families** or **communities**. They are trained by mothers, grandmothers, or women from their villages; some even become experts through their own experiences of giving birth. The community recognises their knowledge and legitimises it. There is substantial overlap between traditional indigenous and empirical midwifery. Our perceptions are that the distinction, if one could be named, is perhaps level of urbanisation and connection to indigenous cosmovision. Or, perhaps it is proximity to government-sponsored 'trainings' (El Kotni, 2019). The former is generally practised in more isolated rural and indigenous communities, and the latter is often practiced in semi-urban and urban communities. Many, though certainly not all traditional midwives identify as indigenous. Many, though certainly not all empirical midwives also identify as indigenous. Training for midwives in the tradition generally consists of shorter- to medium-term midwifery programmes or schools that are not formally accredited. Their training commonly includes shorter- to medium-term apprenticeship-based learning with one or more traditional or community-based midwives. Autonomous midwives learn through extensive homebirth and midwifery centre-based apprenticeship and mentoring, or other routes into autonomous practice (i.e., training outside of Mexico, etc.). A handful of accredited midwifery schools offer institutionalised training. Challenges with Mexico's accredited programmes are well-documented by Atkin et al. (2017). The midwifery mentorship we focus on in this chapter is primarily from the perspective of autonomous midwifery.

Midwifery Mentorship

Mexico's autonomous midwives primarily practice in urban areas. Feeling discontent regarding the dominant forms of gynaecological–obstetric care in their places of residence, autonomous midwives arrived to midwifery through seeking alternatives. Laako (2017) identifies the training trajectory of autonomous midwives:

1 training through midwifery programmes (i.e., those trained at CASA, in Guanajuato; Nueve Lunas, in Oaxaca[6]; Centro de Formación Profesional en Partería, in Jalisco; or Mujeres Aliadas A.C., in Michoácan).
2 training in the mentor-apprentice model (for example, those trained in casas de partería such as Luna Maya, Casa Aramara, or Morada Violeta) and
3 those registered in programmes in other countries (i.e., in the United States, Italy, Chile, or another country).

In most cases, autonomous midwives use a combination of these training pathways with aims of strengthening their practices, including mentorship, workshops, volunteer work (i.e., in casas de partería or with other midwives), and apprenticeship with traditional midwives. In general, autonomous midwives conceive this practice as their vocation. That is, they 'recognize midwifery as a passion or an inner calling' (Laako, 2017) and a way of life. They combine their formal training with extensive ongoing daily and empirical research. It is important to highlight that autonomous midwives are fully recognised as midwives by their communities and peers due to their continued commitment, skills, and ongoing training.

Hannah and Akane describe midwifery mentorship and explain that, in Mexico, the word mentorship is used synonymously with the apprenticeship/preceptorship training model. Hands-on, practice-based learning led by the mentor midwife or midwives, in most settings, is supplemented with theoretical and classroom-type learning, also led by the mentor midwife. As Mexico lacks a midwifery scope of practice, mentor midwives base their training and assessment process on internationally recognised standards and guidelines, including those of the ICM (2019a), World Health Organization (WHO) (2016, 2018b, 2022), and others (Escobar et al., 2022; International Federation of Gynecology and Obstetrics, 2023; Midwifery Education Accreditation Council, 2024; Morris et al., 2017; North American Registry of Midwives, 2024; Warren & MacDonald, 2021) to ensure their students learn full-scope midwifery practice.

When student midwives begin with their mentors, they are fully integrated into the practices' model of care. The student midwives are physically present during most to all care provision and introduced as part of the care provision team – sometimes rotating weeks for antenatal and postnatal visits at the casa de partería or client's home, depending upon the number of midwives and students in the practice or individual arrangements. As students become increasingly acquainted and acquire confidence and skills, they increasingly play active roles in the practices' midwifery care provision.

Students transition through phases of learning in which they first observe, then assist, and then attend the births of clientele families in the midwifery practices' care. Hannah and Akane each relate that they match requirements for the phases of learning with what is required of student midwives using the United States of America's direct-entry midwifery pathways (North American Registry of Midwives, 2024):

10 births in the observed phase,
20 births in the co-assistant phase, and
25 births in the primary midwife under supervision phase.

To acquire these numbers, students ultimately attend hundreds of antenatal and postnatal visits during the training period, also increasing their levels of involvement with care provision in these visits. The full training process through mentorship, when completed in full, takes approximately three to four years. This type of training pathway, though recognised as more than meeting international standards for practice (Faget & Capasso, 2017; International Confederation of Midwives, 2019a), as is autonomous midwifery practice, is unrecognised by the Mexican government.

The Challenges

Midwifery mentors working and practising outside of formal educational institutions do their best to train midwives based upon their practices, international guidelines, midwifery competencies, and our capabilities to generate learning resources. Mentorship entails ensuring students also acquire awareness about their positioning as midwives in community, clinical, and legal spaces. Students accompany in all midwifery-related interactions with families, including after hospital transports and in some interactions with the health sector. Mentorship entails the responsibility of teaching, and the challenge of being mindful about your practice so you can explain why you do what you do. It means being creative and finding numerous ways of explaining things because people learn in multiple ways, and there is no one correct way. It sometimes means taking on a mothering role because you teach students how to understand and deal with their emotions. This is especially relevant when families become upset after requiring hospital transport. It means teaching how to accept death and unexpected outcomes. It means teaching about loss, rejection, and reproach… as natural consequences that occur when families are belittled by hospital or medical personnel when transferred by their midwives for higher levels of care, for having even sought care with a midwife; or when the midwifery team itself is belittled during or after a hospital transport. As birth happens at all hours, being a mentor entails being available around the clock for providing midwifery care and teaching student midwives as events requiring midwifery care are often not schedulable. Our mentorship role includes preparing students on how to navigate our challenging relationship with the health system, with families, with the government, and with the wider community, all of whom, to some degree, adore midwives when all goes well and reproach them when an ideal birth does not occur.

It is important to mention that training autonomous midwives primarily occurs through one (or maybe two) midwives to another. There is no network of other educators. Rather, learning primarily occurs through transmission from one person to another. There is no financial support, and at the end of the journey, there is no certificate or recognition that legitimises the knowledge and skills gained to any external party, including the State. Autonomous midwives must, therefore, also become entrepreneurs and fund their own homebirth practice of midwifery centres that, again, exist outside of State regulation. This adds to the weight of responsibility and exhaustion.

Through dialogue with midwifery students – from both independent and school-based training – Yaredh has identified the feeling of frustration is constant. Some students consider the training processes are violent and deeply demanding. Students report feeling the demands arising from the pace of work are too much and the forms of communication between mentors and apprentices are unfriendly. On several occasions, this leads to abandoning the training process and even to the 'breaking' of the mentor/apprentice relationship. With care for the confidentiality of the narratives, Yaredh has discussed these findings with established parties, some of them mentors, who have agreed the processes can indeed be violent. The precariousness of midwifery practices, for example economic, material, didactic, and legal, generates precarious teaching–learning environments and these same conditions contribute to the generation of hostile dynamics.

There are other challenges in the training process. There is also a huge lack of training material, books, and articles. There are almost no midwifery books translated into Spanish, and where there are, they are hardly available in Mexico. Students who speak English have a much easier time finding material relevant to their training and philosophy of care. Two of the authors of this article, mentoring midwives themselves, know of the struggle of equipping students with training resources that make sense to them, are in Spanish and teach midwifery and not obstetrics. It finally comes down to each mentor's resources, as some midwives may purchase or get books and articles from others and then share them with their students. In a region such as ours, where inequity is unacceptably high (Inter-American Development Bank (IDB), 2024), we suggest that the vaster the mentor's social, cultural, and economic capital, using Bourdieu's (2002) framework of capital, the better-equipped students can become. Since there is more training material in English, one could think the solution is translating it but there are so few practising midwives in México and so little time available for them to translate and no resources to pay translators. Even regarding anatomy and physiology, very few texts and books reflect what we do as midwives and why we interpret many circumstances very differently than in a medical model of care.

Another challenge is that legal ambiguity has led to some individuals calling themselves midwives when they neither meet global standards for practice nor the criteria of traditional midwifery practice. Because no legislation recognises formal training or qualifications on non-institutionalised pathways, anyone in Mexico could mentor midwives. While lack of regulation provides more freedom, it also leads to undertrained midwives providing care and mentoring midwives. This can and has led to disastrous outcomes. Moreover, midwifery groups within and across categories do not always agree upon what the minimal standard of practice should be.

Being a midwifery student is not an easy pathway. This is true with all training routes. However, the autonomous pathway is especially challenging because it requires so much of students, with such little legitimacy as soon as a physician or a family member disagrees with what the midwife said or how she said it. It is challenging to teach students how to best navigate our extremely complex socio-political positioning, which often comes across as violence. Sadly, many students do not complete their training. Some students complete it and then soon leave practice. Though all of this, at the same time, midwifery students are resilient. However, things should be much easier for them and for midwives. One simply should not need to depend upon such high levels of resiliency to be a midwife.

Mentors of independent training and technical and professional programmes point out that the work of 'teaching' and accompanying the learning process requires more from them than the design of plans and programmes (in the case of independent training) and content for the development of 'clinical skills'. Mentoring involves emotional support for students, practical teaching of logistics to support the practice itself, and promoting the development of skills on how to respond and relate to midwifery service users, families, biomedical personnel, health institutions, bureaucrats, activists, and media, within wider contexts of political and gender-based violence. Coexistence is usually intense and for long periods of time. Tensions are accentuated by fatigue and the pressure of teaching and learning in precarious social frameworks.

The mistakes of students in contexts of tension can provoke visceral responses from mentors. We consider the lack of kindness of mentors should and is not justified, but it is inadequate to attribute individualised blame. We consider it pertinent to ask the following question: Why does a student's 'mistake' trigger harsh responses? In some cases, we consider that fatigue is an important factor, as is weariness due to long hours and the lack of interpersonal distance due to arduous coexistence. However, the status of midwifery in structural terms accentuates these tensions.

An error or mistake, in certain learning contexts when students have greater responsibility, is 'critical' because malpractice exposes the health of women, newborns, or the 'legitimacy of their mentor's practice' which in the Mexican context is grave. Yaredh observed in the field that mentor midwives feel their students do not measure the responsibility that being their guarantor in the learning process entails. The parties individually assume the cost of learning with their resources, prestige, and networks. The students also assume, with their own resources, the social, economic, and institutional cost of training as a midwife, a practice that carries the stigma of being obsolete and risky.

Before we move on to the final section of this chapter, we invite you to undertake the below activity. The following questions encourage you to reflect on midwifery mentorship in contexts like Mexico, considering how the legacies of colonisation and inequitable structures of power may have influenced midwifery in your country. We invite you to explore the tensions between traditional and institutionalised practices, legislative processes, and the exclusion of midwives from policymaking. Our aim is to generate dialogue about a future for midwifery that prioritises communities, cultural rights, and women through embracing diverse knowledge systems and fostering closer, more equitable collaboration between communities, midwives, healthcare systems, and actors in spheres of global health policy, as achieving equitable, safe, compassionate, culturally congruent practices depends on this collaboration.

REFLECTIVE ACTIVITY 1

1 How familiar are you with the history of midwifery in your country?
2 In what ways have colonisation and decolonisation impacted midwifery practices and beliefs about childbirth in your country?
3 How have historical power structures, including gender and race, influenced the development and regulation of midwifery practice?
4 How have colonial legacies shaped perceptions about midwives and their role in maternal and newborn health care?
5 In what ways do existing social power structures influence how midwifery is positioned within the broader healthcare system?
6 What are the primary risks associated with restrictive government legislation on midwifery, particularly when these restrictions limit midwives' autonomy in their professional practice?

7 What challenges arise when government policies on midwifery exclude midwives from the legislative process, especially in light of historical restrictions and a lack of trust?

8 How might midwives effectively advocate for legislative reform when governments have historically marginalised midwifery practices?

9 What are the potential benefits of midwives taking part in epistemological disobedience – challenging dominant knowledge frameworks – in order to create more inclusive models of midwifery? How can midwives in the Global North support this process?

10 How might collaborative relationships with other health professionals help midwives address and overcome legislative barriers?

11 What specific policies or reforms could help rebuild trust between midwives and government bodies to support more equitable and culturally respectful or congruent midwifery practices?

The Future

The practices we focus primarily upon in this chapter – urban and professional, autonomous, and feminist – a concept we do not expand upon here – exist within a framework of multiple contradictions, including the relationships between midwives and students that are not free of conflict and tensions. We agree with Laako (2017) when she says that autonomous midwives are at a crossroads between traditional and professional midwifery. With their legitimacy constantly being questioned, they are constantly challenged to 'demonstrate' their skills and knowledge due to the lack of a community that supports and recognises them. For Mexico, this encompasses and includes knowledge that is held and transferred by women who are caregivers to other women using knowledge systems tied to indigenous traditions. Among autonomous midwives, there is constant debating about their clinical relevance and levels of regulation and integration. They worry about establishing fair relationships with the women and families they serve, and question how to defend their practice without resulting in cultural appropriation or harm to 'traditional and indigenous midwifery'.

The authors identify that to ensure mentorship adequately prepares students for midwifery practice and midwifery itself survives, midwives must be at the forefront of defining what appropriate and culturally diverse midwifery training entails. Strengthening midwifery accreditation processes among midwifery stakeholders is crucial, especially considering the diverse types of training pathways.

Mentoring is crucial to midwifery training, but there are challenges such as those Yaredh has identified in her fieldwork. On more than one occasion, she has encountered urban women who, without any kind of serious training, introduce themselves as midwives. They usually refer to their title as having 'spent time with' traditional midwives, but unfortunately, it soon becomes visible these stays have been more of a first approach than a cultural, epistemological, and/or spiritual formation. Naming oneself in this way results in risky acts, uncomfortably weighs on the practice of autonomous midwifery, and reveals a 'utilitarian' treatment of traditional midwifery and traditional midwives. In several cases, they offer their so-called 'services' under the tutelage of a doctor, which weakens the understanding of midwifery as a legitimate practice and autonomous knowledge system.

The creation of education standards for autonomous midwifery pathways appears to be a reasonable next step for midwifery mentors to demonstrate alignment to global standards (International Confederation of Midwives, 2021) in the absence of government recognition. Recently, a group of Mexican midwives created a national certification process (Red de Parteras Certificadas, 2024). The process is coordinated by a technical committee composed of two traditional midwives, two technical midwives, two autonomous midwives, two obstetric nurses, and two perinatal nurses, aligned to global standards (ICM, 2019a). The certification process is an important step for midwives of multiple cosmovision's and worldviews to ensure they meet basic standards to, in turn, ensure quality midwifery care for the public. However, the Mexican government has yet to recognise or ratify Mexico's midwifery-led certification.

Midwives must also be at the forefront of designing public policy that recognises midwifery practices as legitimate knowledge. As we write this chapter, midwives, women, and users of midwifery services are campaigning for a critical review of 'PROY-NOM-020' (SEGOB, 2024). This is an initiative by the Mexican government to regulate and oversee midwifery practice and health facilities providing maternal and newborn care. The government argues this regulation will strengthen the health system and provide safety for service users and midwives. There is widespread concern about the risks this draft regulation poses to the practice of autonomous midwifery and the restrictions it will place on users for choosing out-of-hospital births attended by midwives. Initiatives to regulate midwifery in Mexico have a long history, dating back to colonial times and continuing to the present date. Most of these efforts fail to understand midwifery as a set of knowledge that articulates health, rights, and traditional and indigenous worldviews. Rather than benefiting health services users and midwives, the regulations have often triggered stigmatisation of midwifery. While, at first glance, the initiative's objective of incorporating 'professional' midwives into health services appears appropriate, the legislation overlooks Mexico's preexisting array of midwifery practices and establishes hierarchies among providers with midwives at the bottom and other midwives disappearing altogether. Midwives' voices and perspectives were not prioritised during the creation of the legislation, a process that included only a few midwives.

While, as midwives, we do not collectively object to the existence of a legislative framework that affects midwifery, we do advocate for the government to prioritise midwives' broad, pluralistic, collaborative, and participative engagement in the creation of public policy that recognises midwifery practices as legitimate knowledge. Certification processes for midwives designed by Mexican midwives should be recognised and strengthened. This can be done through supporting midwifery training designed and implemented by midwives, recognising Mexico's midwifery-led certification process, and designing public policies that guarantee decent living conditions for midwives.

For the future of midwifery, it is crucial to improve the working conditions of midwives today, strengthen current educational programmes, and prioritise midwifery training that is midwifery-led. Midwifery certification processes designed by Mexican midwives should be recognised and strengthened. Calling out to the global community, global definitions regarding midwifery must adapt to encompass the realities and contexts of communities in the Global South. This means recognising midwifery models as they exist and emerge in the Global South. Most importantly, midwives must be consulted regarding the public policies imposed on their practice and must be the main voice in making decisions about their work.

Notes

1 Millenium Development Goal 5, Target 1: Reduce by three-quarters, between 1990 and 2015, the maternal mortality ratio and achieve; Target 2: By 2015, universal access to reproductive health (United Nations, 2013).

2 Sustainable Development Goal (SDG) 3.1: By 2030, reduce the global maternal mortality ratio to less than 70 per 100,000 live births; SDG indicator 3.1.2: Proportion of births attended by skilled health personnel (United Nations, 2023).

3 The authors and others (Goodarzi, 2023) challenge global definitions from the International Confederation of Midwives (2019b), World Health Organization (2018a), and others (Stevens & Alonso, 2020) as needing to broaden in order to encompass the contexts and realities of countries in the global south, including Mexico.

4 Centro de Formación Profesional en Partería. https://www.escuelaprofesionalde-parteria.com/

5 Mestiza is the feminine version of the word mestizo, referring to a woman of mixed indigenous and European ancestry. The term mestizx is used throughout Latin America and originated during the colonial period when Spanish colonizers mixed with indigenous populations. It represents a blend of cultures, languages, and traditions from both heritages.

6 El Centro para los Adolescentes de San Miguel de Allende A.C. (CASA) (https://casa.org.mx/) was Mexico's first accredited midwifery school. CASA and Nueve Lunas (https://www.facebook.com/nuevelunasparteria/?locale=es_LA) no longer operate as midwifery schools.

References

Arellano, L. L., Ramírez, G. S., & Cárdenas, H. A. M. (2020). Professional midwives and their regulatory framework in Mexico. *Mexican Law Review*, 119–137. https://doi.org/10.22201/iij.24485306e.2020.2.14174

Atkin, L. C., Keith-Brown, K., Rees, M. W., & Sesia, P. (2017). *MacArthur Foundation's Initiative to Promote Midwifery in Mexico: Complete Baseline Report*. https://www.macfound.org/media/files/prh_baseline_report_revised_june2017_eng.pdf

Bourdieu, P. (2002). The forms of capital. In *Readings in Economic Sociology* (pp. 280–291). John Wiley & Sons, Ltd. https://doi.org/10.1002/9780470755679.ch15

Bowser, D., & Hill, K. (2010). *Exploring Evidence for Disrespect and Abuse in Facility-Based Childbirth: Report of a Landscape Analysis* (USAID-TRAction Project). Harvard School of Public Health, University Research Co., LLC. https://content.sph.harvard.edu/wwwhsph/sites/2413/2014/05/Exploring-Evidence-RMC_Bowser_rep_2010.pdf

Carrillo, A. M. (1999). Nacimiento y muerte de una profesión: Las parteras tituladas en México. *Dynamis*, *19*, 167–190.

Castro, R., & Frías, S. M. (2020). Obstetric violence in Mexico: Results from a 2016 national household survey. *Violence Against Women*, 26(6–7), 555–572. https://doi.org/10.1177/1077801219836732

Cházaro, L., & Estrada, R. (Eds.). (2005). *Colección debates. En el umbral de los cuerpos: Estudios de antropología e historia*. Colegio de Michoacán.

Dixon, L. Z. (2020). *Delivering Health: Midwifery and Development in Mexico*. Vanderbilt University Press.

El Kotni, M. (2019). Regulating traditional Mexican midwifery: Practices of control, strategies of resistance. *Medical Anthropology*, 38(2), 137–151. https://doi.org/10.1080/01459740.2018.1539974

Escobar, M. F., Nassar, A. H., Theron, G., Barnea, E. R., Nicholson, W., Ramasauskaite, D., Lloyd, I., Chandraharan, E., Miller, S., Burke, T., Ossanan, G., Andres Carvajal, J., Ramos, I., Hincapie, M. A., Loaiza, S., Nasner, D. & FIGO Safe Motherhood and Newborn Health Committee (2022). FIGO recommendations on the management of postpartum hemorrhage 2022. *International Journal of Gynecology & Obstetrics*, 157(S1), 3–50. https://doi.org/10.1002/ijgo.14116

Faget, M., & Capasso, A. (2017). *Midwifery in Mexico*. United Nations Population Fund, Management Sciences for Health, MacArthur Foundation, Comité Promotor Por Una Maternidad Segura. https://msh.org/wp-content/uploads/2017/06/midwifery_in_mexico_english.pdf

Freyermuth, G. (2018). *Los Caminos para parir en México en el siglo XXI: Experiencias de investigación, vinculación, formación y comunicación*. CIESAS, ACAS, A.C.

Freyermuth Enciso, G., & Argüello Avendaño, H. E. (Eds.). (2017). *Colección México. Salud y mortalidad aterna en México: Balances y perspectivas desde la antropología y la interdisciplinariedad* (Primera edición). Centro de Investigaciones y Estudios Superiores en Antropología Social.

Goodarzi, B. (2023). *Midwifery Misfits*. Amsterdam UMC Research Portal. https://pure.amsterdamumc.nl/en/activities/midwifery-misfits-2

Instituto Nacional de Salud Pública (INSP). (2020). *La partería profesional en México ¿hacia dónde va?* Instituto Nacional de Salud Pública. https://www.insp.mx/avisos/4315-seminario-parteria-insp.html

Inter-American Development Bank (IDB). (2024). *The Complexities of Inequality in Latin America and the Caribbean*. https://www.iadb.org/en/news/complexities-inequality-latin-america-and-caribbean

International Confederation of Midwives (ICM). (2019a). *Essential Competencies for Midwifery Practice: 2019 Update*. https://www.internationalmidwives.org/assets/files/general-files/2019/10/icm-competencies-en-print-october-2019_final_18-oct-5db05248843e8.pdf

International Confederation of Midwives (ICM). (2019b). *International Definition and Scope of Practice of the Midwife*. International Confederation of Midwives. https://internationalmidwives.org/resources/international-definition-of-the-midwife/

International Confederation of Midwives, J. (2021). *ICM Global Standards for Midwifery Education*. https://internationalmidwives.org/wp-content/uploads/global-standards-for-midwifery-education_2021_en.pdf

International Federation of Gynecology and Obstetrics. (2023). *FIGO Mifepristone & Misoprostol and Misoprostol Only Dosing Charts 2023*. https://www.figo.org/figo-mifepristone-misoprostol-and-misoprostol-only-dosing-charts-2023

Laako, H. (2017). *Mujeres situadas: Las parteras autónomas en México* (1a ed.). El Colegio de la Frontera Sur.

Lamadrid-Figueroa, H., Suárez-López, L., & González-Hernández, D. (2021). *La epidemia de cesáreas en México*. Instituto Nacional de Salud Pública. https://www.insp.mx/assets/documents/webinars/2021/CISP_Epidemia_Cesareas.pdf

Marín, Y. (2019). Nacer a contracorriente. Mujeres y familias urbanas usuarias de partería profesional en una metrópoli mexicana, 2015–2019. *Trabajo de Grado de Maestría, El Colegio de Michoacán*.

Midwifery Education Accreditation Council. (2024). Section I: Curriculum Checklist of Essential Competencies. In *Standards for Accreditation Handbook*. Midwifery Education Accreditation Council.

Morris, J. L., Winikoff, B., Dabash, R., Weeks, A., Faundes, A., Gemzell-Danielsson, K., Kapp, N., Castleman, L., Kim, C., Ho, P. C., & Visser, G. H. A. (2017). FIGO's updated recommendations for misoprostol used alone in gynecology and obstetrics. *International Journal of Gynecology & Obstetrics*, *138*(3), 363–366. https://doi.org/10.1002/ijgo.12181

Murray de Lopez, J. (2015). Conflict and reproductive health in urban Chiapas: Disappearing the partera empírica. *Anthropology Matters*, *16*(1). https://doi.org/10.22582/am.v16i1.339

North American Registry of Midwives. (2024). *Certified Professional Midwife Candidate Information Book (CIB)*. NARM. https://narm.org/pdffiles/CIB.pdf

Red de Parteras Certificadas. (2024). *Certificación*. Red de Parteras Certificadas. https://redparterascertificadas.org/certificaci%C3%B3n

Renfrew, M. J., McFadden, A., Bastos, M. H., Campbell, J., Channon, A. A., Cheung, N. F., Silva, D. R. A. D., Downe, S., Kennedy, H. P., Malata, A., McCormick, F., Wick, L., & Declercq, E. (2014). Midwifery and quality care: Findings from a new evidence-informed framework for maternal and newborn care. *The Lancet*, *384*(9948), 1129–1145. https://doi.org/10.1016/S0140-6736(14)60789-3

Sahagún, B. D. (1577). Historia General de las Cosas de la Nueva España. http://cdigital.dgb.uanl.mx/la/1080012524_C/1080012524_T1/1080012524_MA.PDF

Sánchez Hernández, A. L., Martínez Martínez, M. A., & Díaz Estrada, F. (Eds.). (2023). *Gender-Based Violence in Mexico: Narratives, the State, and Emancipation*. Routledge.

Secretaría de Gobernación (SEGOB). (2024). *Diario Oficial de la Federación. PROYECTO de Norma Oficial Mexicana PROY-NOM-020-SSA-2024, Para establecimientos de salud y para la práctica de la partería, en la atención integral materna y neonatal*. https://www.dof.gob.mx/nota_detalle_popup.php?codigo=5733911

Sevilla Villalobos, A., Galante, M. C., Alarcón, R., & Gallegos, A. R. (2023). Análisis del marco legal vinculado a la partería tradicional en México: Grupo de Trabajo Independiente sobre Partería Tradicional en México (1st ed.). Secretaría de Cultural Instituto Nacional de Antropología e Historia.

Smith-Oka, V. (2009). Unintended consequences: Exploring the tensions between development programs and indigenous women in Mexico in the context of reproductive health. *Social Science & Medicine*, *68*(11), 2069–2077. https://doi.org/10.1016/j.socscimed.2009.03.026

Smith-Oka, V. (2012). Bodies of risk: Constructing motherhood in a Mexican public hospital. *Social Science & Medicine, 75*(12), 2275–2282. https://doi.org/10.1016/j. socscimed.2012.08.029

Stevens, J. R., & Alonso, C. (2020). Commentary: Creating a definition for global midwifery centers. *Midwifery, 85,* 102684. https://doi.org/10.1016/j. midw.2020.102684

United Nations. (2013). *Millenium Development Goals and Beyond 2015: Goal 5 Fact Sheet—Improve Maternal Health.* United Nations. https://www.un.org/ millenniumgoals/pdf/Goal_5_fs.pdf

United Nations. (2023). *Global Indicator Framework for the Sustainable Development Goals and Targets of the 2030 Agenda for Sustainable Development, 2023 Refinement.* https://unstats.un.org/sdgs/indicators/indicators-list/

Uribe-Leitz, T., Barrero-Castillero, A., Cervantes-Trejo, A., Santos, J. M., de la Rosa-Rabago, A., Lipsitz, S. R., Basavilvazo-Rodriguez, M. A., Shah, N., & Molina, R. L. (2019). Trends of caesarean delivery from 2008 to 2017, Mexico. *Bulletin of the World Health Organization, 97*(7), 502–512. https://doi.org/10.2471/ BLT.18.224303

Warren, R., & MacDonald, T. (2021). *Clinical Practice Guideline 10. Management of the Uncomplicated Pregnancy Beyond 41+ Weeks Gestation.* Association of Ontario Midwives. https://www.ontariomidwives.ca/sites/default/files/2021-05/CPG-Management-uncomplicated-pregnancy-beyond-41-weeks-gestation-PUB.pdf

WHO. (2024). *Proportion of Births Delivered in a Health Facility.* WHO Data. https://platform.who.int/data/maternal-newborn-child-adolescent-ageing/ indicator-explorer-new/mca/proportion-of-births-delivered-in-a-health-facility

World Bank. (2024). *Maternal Mortality Ratio (Modeled Estimate, per 100,000 Live Births)—Mexico.* Data. https://data.worldbank.org/indicator/SH.STA.MMRT? locations=MX

World Health Organization. (2016). *WHO Recommendations on Antenatal Care for A Positive Pregnancy Experience.* https://www.who.int/publications-detail-redirect/9789241549912

World Health Organization. (2018a). *Definition of Skilled Health Personnel Providing Care During Childbirth: The 2018 Joint Statement by WHO, UNFPA, UNICEF, ICM, ICN, FIGO and IPA (WHO/RHR/18.14).* https://iris.who.int/bit-stream/handle/10665/272818/WHO-RHR-18.14-eng.pdf?sequence=1

World Health Organization. (2018b). *WHO Recommendations: Intrapartum Care for A Positive Childbirth Experience.* https://iris.who.int/bitstream/han dle/10665/260178/9789241550215-eng.pdf?sequence=1

World Health Organization. (2022). *WHO Recommendations on Maternal and Newborn Care for A Positive Postnatal Experience.* https://www.who.int/publications-detail-redirect/9789240045989

17

MIDWIFERY MENTORSHIP IN THE NETHERLANDS

*Tamar van Haaren-Ten Haken
and Marianne Nieuwenhuijze*

Introduction

For more than 150 years, midwifery students in the Netherlands have been formally educated as autonomous professionals who are officially recognised within the Dutch maternity care system (see Box 17.1). Their education meets legal requirements documented in national laws (since 1861) that also describe their field of expertise and scope of practice (Besluit Opleidingseisen en Deskundigheidsgebied Verloskundige 2008, n.d.). They are registered in the national registration for healthcare professionals and must apply for re-registration every five years.

Midwives offer full prenatal, natal and postnatal care in the community to women with a healthy profile. They function as 'gate-keepers' in Dutch maternity care, where almost 90% of all women start their prenatal care with a community midwife (Perined, 2022). Women with uncomplicated pregnancy are offered the choice to give birth at home or in the hospital with a known midwife from the midwifery practice where they received their prenatal care. Over the last four decades, midwives have also gained a position in the hospital where they are part of the maternity care team, including obstetrician, residents and (obstetric) nurses. In this setting, they add the perspective on the physiology of childbirth to the care of these women (Thompson et al., 2016). They care for women independently with the end-responsibility being that of an obstetrician.

After graduation, midwives are competent to start in the community as advanced beginners, equipped to offer the full scope of individual primary care to a pregnant woman. However, with the growing complexity of the maternity care system, newly graduated midwives rely on support

DOI: 10.4324/9781003533733-18

from senior colleague midwives for the organisational aspects around care (Kool et al., 2019; 2020). A recently established Master's programme offers opportunities to develop additional competences for this field as well as advanced research skills. Simultaneously, as a growing number of newly qualified midwives start working in hospital settings, students are also educated with basic competencies for the hospital setting, necessary to care for women with a higher chance of complications. For those midwives, additional education after graduation is also available, including a master programme.

BOX 17.1 SHORT OUTLINE OF THE DUTCH MATERNITY CARE SYSTEM

The Dutch maternity care system is based on a division between primary care provided in the community and secondary and tertiary care in hospitals (De Vries et al., 2013). Women's care is based on the assessment of the individual risk of each woman. Women with a low-risk pregnancy are cared for by community midwives in midwife-led, primary care, and have the option of birthing at home, in a birth centre or to have a midwife-led hospital birth. Women at intermediate or high risk are referred to obstetrician-led secondary or tertiary care where they are looked after by hospital-based midwives, nurses and obstetricians (Amelink-Verburg & Buitendijk, 2010).

The current funding system in the Netherlands entails that community midwives are compensated per care episode per client (pregnancy, labour and birth, postpartum) and hospitals are reimbursed based on 'diagnosis treatment combinations (DTCs)'. These DTCs are based on the type of services, treatments and procedures that will be carried out (Nederlandse Zorgautoriteit, 2023).

In this chapter, we will further explore the education and mentoring of student midwives in the past, the present and challenges for the future within the context of the unique maternity care system of the Netherlands.

Midwives' Education Over the Centuries

Midwives have been giving care to birthing women in the area that is now the Netherlands for many centuries. Official documentation refers to midwives ('vroedvrouw' or wies vrouw' ≈ wise/knowledgeable woman) from the Middle Ages, including court reports on witch trials (Rösslin, 1513; Vanysacker, 1988). Around the same time, education of midwives also became a topic that was considered and discussed. In the training of new midwives in the Netherlands, practising midwives have always played an important part, from early both in an official capacity and non-official capacity.

During the 18th century, midwives in Dutch towns (stadsvroedvrouwen) were gaining a stronger position (Marland, 1993). They had their own practice and were (partly) paid by the town council that also set up standards for quality and education. Midwives were expected to be able to read and write. During their training, they had to follow lessons given by physicians, conduct a number of births under the supervision of an experienced midwife and do an exam. In situations where the quality of care was regarded as being poor, midwives with a high reputation were brought in to further educate the established midwives. However, in rural areas, women were mainly looked after by women that were mentored by more experienced women without established education, regulation or overview on quality.

In the 19th century, the Dutch government started to regulate healthcare on a national level. In the Medical Practice Act of 1865, regulating healthcare professions, midwives were recognised as autonomous medical professionals immediately after doctors got recognised (Kroneman et al., 2016). Subsequently, midwifery schools with birthing facilities were established in different parts of the country, paid for by the government.

It is these early mechanisms of support and education of midwives – instead of marginalising them – that are the base for the unique Dutch system of independent midwives and home births (Marland, 1993). Over the years, the scope of practice of midwives expanded, for example adding prenatal care in the 1930s or suturing perineum lacerations in the 1970s, confirming these expansions in national regulations. The midwifery schools maintained under the supervision of the Ministry of Health and outside the formal education system, while recognised as a programme at the level of higher education. This lasted until the implementation of the European Bachelor-Master system for higher education became a reality in the Netherlands.

A New Era: Bachelor of Science in Midwifery

In 2002, the Bachelor-Master system for higher education was introduced in the Netherlands, in accordance with the Bologna Process of the European Union. This system aims to facilitate student and staff mobility and to make higher education more inclusive, accessible and competitive worldwide (European Commission: Directorate-General for Education Sport and Culture, 2018). In the Netherlands, higher education includes higher vocational education (hoger beroepsonderwijs, HBO) provided by universities of applied science and scientific/academic education (wetenschappelijk onderwijs, WO) provided by research universities. Higher vocational education programmes provide theoretical and practical education for occupations where a higher vocational qualification is required, as in midwifery, whereas research university educational programmes provide a research-oriented theoretical education.

Following the introduction of this new higher education system, the midwifery programmes became part of an existing university of applied science from 2008 as a higher vocational education programme (HBO) with a four-year Bachelor of Science degree. This marked the end of an era of independent, autonomous midwifery programmes.

In recent decades, the level of the programme has often been a topic of discussion. Compared to other medical courses, such as medicine, veterinary medicine, dentistry or pharmacy, the midwifery programme is the only medical programme with an HBO Bachelor's degree instead of a university (WO) Bachelor's degree where students are educated to become an independent, autonomous medical professional legally allowed to perform reserved medical procedures. For now, the midwifery programme remains an HBO Bachelor of Science. Nevertheless, developing academic skills at a high level is an important part of the programme to enable collaboration at an equivalent level with other academic professionals in maternity care, such as obstetricians, paediatricians and general practitioners.

In addition to the Bachelor's programme for midwifery, the Master of Science in Midwifery was launched in 2023. This is a joint degree Master of Science offered as one collective programme of all three midwifery programmes in the Netherlands. Developments in maternity care, with increasing complexity in professional practice and system, require that midwives take on tasks that necessitate a master's level of thinking and working. To maintain the strong, autonomous position of midwives within Dutch maternity care, further knowledge development and solid scientific underpinning are needed. This master level complements the current Bachelor of Science programme and contributes to an educational continuum from a Bachelor's degree to a master's degree to a PhD. Additionally, midwives also have access to a Physician Assistant Master programme, specialising in hospital-based maternity care.

Midwifery Curriculum

Midwifery education in the Netherlands is a direct-entry competency-based programme with no prerequisite of a nursing background. Students are educated solely to become a midwife; nursing is not part of the qualification. The Bachelor programme meets both EU directives and Dutch legal education requirements for midwives that specify the theoretical topics and the content and duration of the practical training needed, including a certain number of professional activities to be performed (e.g. births) (Besluit Opleidingseisen en Deskundigheidsgebied Verloskundige 2008, n.d.). The national midwifery education framework (Landelijke

Opleidingsprofiel Verloskunde, LPOV) is the fundament for the midwifery curriculum. This education framework is based on the national profile of the midwife drawn up by the professional organisation, Royal Dutch Organisation of Midwives (Koninklijke Nederlandse Organisatie van Verloskundigen, KNOV) and aligns with the 'Essential Competencies for Midwifery Practice' of the International Confederation of Midwives (ICM) (ICM, 2024).

The CanMEDS roles are used as the classification principle in the national education framework (Frank et al., 2015). The CanMEDS roles are widely used among healthcare professions and education programmes in the Dutch healthcare sector. A competent midwife integrates the competencies of all seven CanMEDS roles: Medical Expert, Communicator, Collaborator, Leader, Health Advocate, Scholar and Professional. The national education framework is based on four task areas in which the midwife fulfils the different roles (see Box 17.2).

BOX 17.2   MIDWIFERY TASK AREAS:

1 Reproductive care
   This has been further divided by the ICM into:

   a social, epidemical and cultural context of maternal and newborn care
   b pre-pregnancy care and family planning
   c care during pregnancy
   d care during labour and birth
   e care for women during the post-partum period
   f care of the newborn
   g facilitation of abortion-related care

2 Organisation of midwifery care
3 Scientific basis of the profession
4 Professionalisation of the profession

Theoretical learning at the university – 60% of the programme – and learning in the professional midwifery practice through internships (clinical practice) – 40% of the programme – take place alternately from the first year onwards. Internships take place both with community midwives as well as with hospital-based midwives. This strong integration of theory and practice in an authentic environment helps students to understand and apply acquired knowledge in a meaningful way. It also contributes to the development of their professional identity.

Assessment of Skills and Knowledge

All the midwifery programmes use a competency matrix translated into Entrustable Professional Activities (EPAs) or critical professional tasks, integrating the CanMEDS roles. EPAs are tasks of professional (e.g. midwifery) practice that can be fully entrusted to a student, once he/she has demonstrated the necessary competence to execute the activity within a clinical context (Ten Cate, 2005; Ten Cate & Taylor, 2021). An EPA reflects work that is essential and important for the profession, is specific and focused, is observable and measurable in outcome, requires application of knowledge, skills and attitudes acquired through training and involves application and integration of multiple domains of competence. EPAs can be conceived of a single task as well as groups of tasks. An example is the EPA 'assisting uncomplicated birth' (see Table 17.1). Five entrustment levels are described as the student is allowed to:

1 observe,
2 execute the EPA with direct, pro-active supervision,
3 carry out the EPA with minimal supervision,
4 execute the EPA unsupervised,
5 provide supervision to more junior learners.

To assess the level of entrustment, it is important for mentors to assess if the student knows what to do, if the student has adequate knowledge and skills and if the student is aware of possible complications and what to do in case of unusual findings or outcomes. EPAs or critical professional tasks serve as a framework for providing oral and written feedback to students and to assess if students have the necessary skills and knowledge to perform specific midwifery tasks independently. This ensures they have the knowledge and skills for unsupervised midwifery practice after graduation.

REFLECTIVE ACTIVITY 1

If you mentor a student, try to provide feedback based on the five entrustment levels of the EPA 'Assisting uncomplicated birth'.

If you are a midwifery student, can you estimate your current level of entrustment (how much supervision you need) and where you want to head in this or the next clinical placement?

- How valuable did you find it to use the EPA as a framework to provide feedback or to describe your own level of entrustment?

TABLE 17.1 EPA Assisting Uncomplicated Birth

EPA title: Assisting uncomplicated birth

Role (CanMEDS)	Action criteria
Medical Expert	• Assists birth while monitoring and promoting physiology appropriate to the woman's care and care needs • Creates and implements policies based on clinical reasoning, EBM (evidence-based midwifery) and SDM (shared decision-making) • Acts adequately in acute situations • Documents and evaluates the care provided
Communicator/Counsellor	• Considers the woman's social context • Coaches and supports with the woman's autonomy as starting point • Communicates timely and effectively with other professionals • Communicates clearly and transparently with the woman about progress, treatment options and comes to agreements
Health Advocate	• Recognises and acknowledges signs of problems and unsafe situations in the family in a timely manner and takes appropriate actions
Leader/Organiser	• Organises care efficiently and optimally, ensuring continuity of care for the woman • Distributes/delegates tasks among available professionals for the benefit of the care process
Collaborator	• Works respectfully and effectively together (within a multidisciplinary setting)
Scholar	• Is knowledgeable about new insights into natal care and critically analyses their applicability for practice and care population
Professional	• Is accountable as a professional for the choices made • Respects own limits of competence and authority

Mentoring Undergraduate Midwifery Students

There is a separation between lecturers working in a midwifery programme, teaching knowledge and skills in a simulated environment, and midwives working in a community practice or hospital with the role of a mentor in clinical practice. Midwives who mentor students in practice attend a specific course, consisting of four modules (one day each) and annual training days focusing on mentoring midwifery students. These courses are jointly organised by all Dutch midwifery programmes and free of charge. No *formal* qualification and registration are needed to be a mentor; however, students only do internships with midwives who have completed the course. In hospital, they are mentored by hospital-based midwives, not by obstetricians or nurses. The national midwifery profile describes the midwife's role to mentor as follows:

> The midwife contributes to professional development, among other things by providing education and mentoring to future colleagues, students, fellow professionals, and other healthcare providers in maternity care.

However, it is not mandated by regulation. Midwifery practices and hospitals receive a financial contribution for mentoring students.

Midwives are trained to guide students through stages of modelling, coaching, scaffolding and reflection. **Modelling** is the first stage and involves demonstrating a process or behaviour for students to learn from. In this phase, students observe what the midwife does. **Coaching** is a more interactive form of support where the midwife provides guidance, feedback and encouragement. It helps students to develop their skills over time. The concept of **scaffolding** involves providing support to help students to achieve their goals by gradually increasing the level of entrustment and reducing the level of supervision as the students become more competent, in concordance with the EPA's. Using **reflection**, students look back on their own experiences to understand and learn. In addition to individual reflection moments, regular supervision meetings are organised during the internships with a lecturer of the midwifery programme and peers. There, they reflect on their own experiences as well as on the experiences of their peers. During their internships, students also have a mentor from the programme in addition to the mentor in clinical practice. This mentor is a lecturer with a midwifery background. Halfway through and at the end of the internship, both mentors evaluate with the student the course of the internship and the competences achieved.

Throughout the whole midwifery programme, students are also assigned a study counsellor. They play a crucial role in supporting students throughout their study, helping them to plan their courses and develop effective study behaviours. They also provide personal and psychological support and help students with specific needs to connect with additional resources, for example in the case of dyslexia or financial issues. During their study, student midwives work on their portfolio as a personal development and evaluation tool. It helps students to reflect on their progress and to set learning goals for improvement.

Lecturers of the midwifery programme are responsible for the final assessment and the decision if a student can graduate as a midwife. However, this decision is always made with input from the practising, mentoring midwife of their final internship.

REFLECTIVE ACTIVITY 2

As a mentor to undergraduate midwifery students reflect on the following questions:

- Can you teach students to be autonomous professionals?
- Which competences do they need to develop to achieve greater autonomy and work to the full scope of midwifery practice as defined by the ICM?

Mentoring Young Professionals

Upon graduation, midwives work independently as advanced beginners. They are fully qualified to practice midwifery in line with the international definition and scope of practice from the ICM and are registered with the Dutch national registration for health professionals (Ministry of Health, n.d.). No mentoring or post-registration activities are formally required, and they can choose to work as a community or hospital-based midwife. Every five years, health professionals must re-register with the Dutch national registration. Criterion for this re-registration is active work experience or educational requirement. Midwives with a Bachelor's degree in midwifery from another European Union (EU) Member State can register and practice as a midwife in the Netherlands based on European agreements. They must master the Dutch language sufficiently. Midwives from countries outside the EU will be formally assessed considering their qualifications and experience. Based on this assessment, they are given advice for further education and internships before they can legally register as a midwife in the Netherlands. Mastering the Dutch language is also a requirement.

Newly qualified midwives are competent to start in the community as advanced beginners, equipped to offer the full scope of individual midwifery care to a pregnant woman. However, as young professionals they still need to develop their competences regarding transcending tasks related to the organisation and management of the midwifery practice and the larger maternity care system. Further supporting and mentoring of young professionals after graduation, helping them to socialise into midwifery, is the responsibility of experienced midwives in practice. Most newly qualified midwives start practising midwifery in a community practice or hospital with experienced midwives to rely on. There is no formal programme for this and the implementation of this varies per midwifery practice.

Recent studies on newly qualified midwives in the Netherlands showed they perceive the first years in midwifery practice as highly demanding and difficult due to the autonomous and solo nature of the work and the increasing complexity of care. Experienced midwives recognise the need to support the young professionals, but they face several barriers in practice such as a lack of time and capacity problems due to staff shortage (Kool et al., 2019; 2020). More attention is needed to improve the transition into practice of new professionals through mentoring and coaching by experienced midwives. The professional organisation of midwives (KNOV) has recently launched a programme to support the mentoring of newly qualified midwives. This programme involves the development of a toolkit that supports new midwives and their experienced colleagues in practice. For instance, by providing more in-depth information about what you need to arrange when starting as a self-employed midwife or how to implement a buddy system with an experienced colleague. At this moment, it is too early to evaluate the results of this programme and some components still need to be further developed.

REFLECTIVE ACTIVITY 3

Think about midwifery in your country of residence (practice) and answer the following questions:

- What is according to the law the scope of practice of midwives in your country?
- Do most midwives in your country actual perform their full scope of practice?
- If not, what is needed in midwives (and yourself) to change that?

Future Challenges in Mentoring Midwives: Sustainable Midwifery Care

Maternity care is changing, and this creates challenges for future education of midwives. Where midwifery practice used to be the unit of care and the home base for you as a midwife, care has now transformed into network care where midwives collaborate with many more professionals and organisations to shape the entirety of maternity care. This also raises questions about the professional identity of midwives in the Netherlands: What is their responsibility and what is not? The physiological approach remains central, but midwives are operating in a more complex environment. There is an increase in childbirth interventions and in the use of healthcare technology, requiring different care approaches. There is increasing attention for integrated maternity care, where different healthcare providers work interdisciplinary to provide continuous and appropriate care. In the context of improving outcomes of care, there is a growing awareness for the need of a stronger focus on social circumstances and women in vulnerable situations. A better collaboration between the social services and the healthcare domains in the light of socio-cultural challenges is needed. This requires that student midwives are prepared to take on their role in this, but also to recognise and acknowledge the boundaries of their own profession. The challenge is to mentor new midwives into gaining a sense of belonging as a midwife, as experienced midwives are facing a changing maternity care system with a renewed focus on their professional identity. Addressing these issues in the education programme helps students to actively think about their own, future role and identity. In addition, the occupational wellbeing of Dutch midwives is under pressure due to increasing job demands, shortage of staff and high workload.

Reflective Practitioner

In the context of increased medicalisation of childbirth, there is a need to enhance the reflectivity of student midwives. This involves critical thinking skills, the ability to assess evidence and recognition of evidence-and non-evidence-based care as well as communication and debating skills to effectively communicate considerations in clinical decision-making together with women and with other healthcare professionals. Currently, students are capable of reflection on action after an activity has been completed based on the reflection model of Korthagen (Korthagen, 2014). But a stronger focus on reflection in action is needed, by critically analysing and questioning choices and decisions while the actions are actually happening. Reflection in action can help students in being responsive and flexible in the moment (Zondag et al., 2022). A midwifery-specific reflective model like the model of holistic reflection of Bass et al. (2017) may be useful in this. Mentors can act in this as role models, as role models contribute to the development of students' skills, attitudes and behaviour (Nieuwenhuijze et al., 2020). Students identify professionals in maternity care who demonstrate attitudes and behaviours they appreciate. They learn from observing their role models, in particular interactions in challenging situations. Active observation can enrich student midwives with a broad range of professional behaviour, including that of a reflective practitioner. Focus on the development of students to a reflective practitioner also means awareness of the ethical, cultural, social and political context of pregnancy and childbirth in order to provide more personalised care.

Innovation Readiness

To strengthen midwives' power in their position and their work and to improve maternity care, it is important to pay attention to the innovation readiness of student midwives. Innovation readiness refers to the ability to adopt, implement and benefit from new innovative ideas, processes or technologies. New midwives need to be prepared to critically assess, generate, accept and put new, useful ideas into practice effectively in this fast-evolving world. They need not necessarily have to be innovators, but they must we ready and willing to innovate. This means that lecturers and mentors should foster a culture and mindset that encourages creativity, experimentation, leadership and acceptance of change.

Competent and Resilient

To educate resilient midwives who are competent to practice midwifery in their full scope, the midwifery programmes should not only focus on midwifery skills and competences, but also focus on a broader view of maternity care including students' own professional role and career pathways. The national midwifery education framework, and following this, the midwifery curriculum, needs a revision for this. The current midwifery curriculum is already overloaded, so choices must be made. A recently launched master in midwifery science programme offers opportunities for the future. After graduation, newly qualified midwives need a support system from colleague midwives, tailored to individual needs, for a better transition into practice. This will contribute to sustainable midwifery care.

Midwives and midwifery education have been around for many centuries in the Netherlands, with a strong autonomous position in the Dutch maternity care system. Still, to ensure that women continue to have access to midwifery care, it is essential to remain vigilant and dedicated. Midwives have to demonstrate their resilience and adaptability to the changing times, meeting the evolving needs of women while staying committed and alert to future challenges.

References

Amelink-Verburg, M. P., & Buitendijk, S. E. (2010). Pregnancy and labour in the Dutch maternity care system: What is normal? The role division between midwives and obstetricians. Journal of Midwifery & Women's Health, 55(3), 216–225. https://doi.org/10.1016/j.jmwh.2010.01.001

Bass, J., Fenwick, J., & Sidebotham, M. (2017). Development of a model of holistic reflection to facilitate transformative learning in student midwives. Women and Birth, 30(3), 227–235. https://doi.org/10.1016/j.wombi.2017.02.010

Besluit opleidingseisen en deskundigheidsgebied verloskundige 2008. [Decree on Midwife Training Requirements and Area of Expertise] (n.d.). Retrieved September 30, 2024, from https://wetten.overheid.nl/BWBR0024254/2023-01-01

De Vries, R., Nieuwenhuijze, M., & Buitendijk, S. E. (2013). What does it take to have a strong and independent profession of midwifery? Lessons from the Netherlands. Midwifery, 29(10), 1122–1128. https://doi.org/10.1016/j.midw.2013.07.007

European Commission: Directorate-General for Education Sport and Culture. (2018). The EU in Support of the Bologna Process. Publications Office. https://data.europa.eu/doi/10.2766/3596

Frank, J. R., Snell, L., & Sherbino, J. (2015). CanMEDS 2015 Physician Competency Framework. Royal College of Physicians and Surgeons of Canada.

ICM Essential Competencies for Midwifery Practice. (2024). The Hague: International Confederation of Midwives.

Kool, L., Feijen-de Jong, E. I., Schellevis, F. G., & Jaarsma, D. A. D. C. (2019). Perceived job demands and resources of newly qualified midwives working in primary care settings in the Netherlands. Midwifery, 69, 52–58. https://doi.org/10.1016/j.midw.2018.10.012

Kool, L. E., Schellevis, F. G., Jaarsma, D. A. D. C., & Feijen-De Jong, E. I. (2020). The initiation of Dutch newly qualified hospital-based midwives in practice, a qualitative study. Midwifery, 83, 102648. https://doi.org/10.1016/j.midw.2020.102648

Korthagen, F. A. J. (2014). Promoting core reflection in teacher education: Deepening professional growth. In L. Orland – Barak, & C. J. Craig (Eds.), International Teacher Education: Promising Pedagogies (pp. 79–89). Emerald.

Kroneman, M., Boerma, W., van den Berg, M., Groenewegen, P., de Jong, J., & van Ginneken, E. (2016). Netherlands: Health system review. Health Systems in Transition, 18(2), 1–240.

Marland, H. (1993). The Art of Midwifery: Early Modern Midwives in Europe. Routledge.

Ministry of Health, (n.d.). BIG-register. Retrieved September 30, 2024, from https://english.bigregister.nl/

Nederlandse Zorgautoriteit [Dutch Care Authority]. (2023). Beleidsregel prestaties en tarieven medisch specialistische zorg [Policy rule on performances and rates medical specialist care]. Retrieved September 30, 2024, from https://www.nza.nl/zorgsectoren/medisch-specialistische-zorg/registreren-en-declareren/welke-regels-gelden-voor-de-medisch-specialistische-zorg-in-2023

Nieuwenhuijze, M. J., Thompson, S. M., Gudmundsdottir, E. Y., & Gottfreðsdóttir, H. (2020). Midwifery students' perspectives on how role models contribute to becoming a midwife: A qualitative study. Women and Birth, 33(5), 433–439. https://doi.org/10.1016/j.wombi.2019.08.009

Perined. (2022). Utrecht. Retrieved September 30, 2024, from www.peristat.nl

Rösslin, E. (1513). Rosegarden for Pregnant Women and Midwives. Strassbourgh.

Ten Cate, O. (2005). Entrustability of professional activities and competency-based training. Medical Education, 39(12), 1176–1177. https://doi.org/10.1111/j.1365-2929.2005.02341.x

Ten Cate, O., & Taylor, D. (2021). The recommended description of an entrustable professional activity: AMEE guide no. 140. Medical Teacher, 43(10), 1106–1114. https://doi.org/10.1080/0142159X.2020.1838465

Thompson, S., Nieuwenhuijze, M. J., Kane Low, L., & de Vries, R. (2016). Exploring Dutch midwives attitudes to promoting physiological childbirth: A qualitative study. Midwifery, 42, 67–73. https://doi.org/10.1016/j.midw.2016.09.019

Vanysacker, D. (1988). Hekserij in Brugge: de magische leefwereld van een stadsbevolking 16de en 17de eeuw [Witchcraft in Bruges. The magical lifestyle of a city's population 16th and 17th centuries]. Genootschap voor Geschiedenis te Brugge, Ed.

Zondag, D. C., van Haaren-Ten Haken, T. M., Offerhaus, P. M., Maas, V. Y. F., & Nieuwenhuijze, M. J. (2022). Knowledge and skills used for clinical decision-making on childbirth interventions: A qualitative study among midwives in the Netherlands. European Journal of Midwifery, 6, 56. https://doi.org/10.18332/ejm/151653

18

MIDWIFERY MENTORING IN AOTEAROA NEW ZEALAND

Cara Baddington

The Aotearoa New Zealand Midwifery Context

Midwives in Aotearoa New Zealand practice in a unique social, historical, and cultural context. Key aspects of this include midwifery as an autonomous and self-regulating profession, midwives as the main providers of care in the childbearing year, and the significance of Te Tiriti o Waitangi as a constitutional document.

Te Tiriti o Waitangi

Te Tiriti o Waitangi is recognised as a foundational constitutional document, grounding the country in principles of partnership and biculturalism. It is also a document with a complex and contentious history (Tūpara & Tahere, 2020). Originally intended as a mutually beneficial agreement between Māori and the Crown, it has been an instrument of colonisation, often used to justify the marginalisation of Māori with significant resultant inequities. In contemporary healthcare in Aotearoa New Zealand, Te Tiriti o Waitangi mandates the Crown's duty to meet its commitments, ensuring services uphold Māori rights, perspectives, and hauora (wellbeing).

An Autonomous and Self-Regulating Profession

Midwives in Aotearoa New Zealand practice autonomously (i.e. independently of medical supervision) and work collaboratively with other health professionals. In 1971, this autonomy was then removed and later restored with the passing of the Nurses Amendment Act in 2003 (Humphrey &

DOI: 10.4324/9781003533733-19

Kumar-Hazard, 2023). Midwifery was then fully recognised as a separate profession from nursing with its own regulatory authority in 2003 (Health Practitioners' Competence Assurance Act, 2003, n.d.). *The Health Practitioners' Competence Assurance Act* established a regulatory authority for the midwifery profession with the overarching goal of protecting public health safety and ensuring practitioners are competent and fit to practise. Te Tatau o te Whare Kahu Midwifery Council (the Midwifery Council) sets pre-registration education requirements for midwives, manages registration of midwives, and oversees the ongoing competence assurance of midwives through their recertification programme (Midwifery Council of New Zealand, 2024a). When applying for an Annual Practicing Certificate, registered midwives must make a declaration they meet the recertification requirements and maintain a portfolio of evidence thereof. These requirements include continuing professional education, professional activities, and participation in a quality assurance programme on a regular basis (three-yearly for most midwives).

Pregnancy, birth, and postnatal care is publicly funded and universally available in Aotearoa New Zealand. It is largely a midwifery-led service (Midwifery Council of New Zealand, 2024a). Midwives choose to work in a range of settings. Lead Maternity Carer (LMC) midwives provide continuity of care to women throughout their pregnancy, birth, and postnatal experience up to six weeks postpartum. They usually work in small group practices and are responsible for coordinating and providing 24/7 primary care and, where appropriate, collaborate with other health professionals such as obstetricians, general practitioners, and others. LMC midwives are fully publicly funded and mostly self-employed, contracting directly to Health New Zealand Te Whatu Ora, a government entity. Core midwives are employed to work within primary, secondary, and tertiary care facilities, providing care to women who attend care in those settings. Midwives working in these settings, whilst working within the midwifery scope of practice and philosophy, are caring for women with sometimes complex needs and conditions. When LMC midwives attend intrapartum care in a facility, they collaborate with their core midwifery, obstetric, and other colleagues as needed.

Midwifery care in Aotearoa New Zealand is centred around partnership with the woman and their whānau (family). This partnership recognises the power dynamic that can exist in healthcare relationships and seeks to share responsibilities and support autonomy in the birthing experience (Pairman & Gray, 2023). Aotearoa New Zealand has a Code of Health and Disability Services Consumers' Rights enshrined in law that protects health consumers. The Code provides a broad set of rights, including the right to be fully informed, the right to informed choice and giving informed consent (or decline), and the right to support (Humphrey & Kumar-Hazard, 2023).

Midwifery mentoring in Aotearoa New Zealand

Mentoring within the midwifery profession is a well-established practice and, in its broadest sense, can be found in various forms between midwives, between midwives and students, and between students as well. There is, at times, confusion about the related but distinct practices of mentoring, preceptorship, and clinical supervision in Aotearoa New Zealand, as all have the shared goal of providing support. Lennox et al. (2008) set out the characteristics of the three concepts to facilitate a shared understanding of these professional support processes.

Preceptorship is generally a structured, time-limited relationship focused on the clinical learning and socialisation of newly qualified or student midwives, with a stronger emphasis on knowledge transfer and skill acquisition within the healthcare environment (Lennox et al., 2008). In Aotearoa New Zealand, preceptorship involves a senior midwife who guides a less experienced practitioner through the initial phases of clinical practice. This could be an undergraduate midwifery student, or post-registration, a new graduate midwife or a midwife new to the particular context. This approach is distinct from mentoring because it is more prescriptive and is typically assigned rather than chosen by the preceptee, with goals aligned to the institution's requirements rather than the learner's personal needs (Lennox et al., 2008).

Clinical supervision represents another support process that is sometimes confused with mentoring but is distinct in purpose and application (Gray, 2006). Clinical supervision can be sought by the practitioner for reflective practice and self-assessment; however, it can also be confused with supervision that is imposed by the regulatory authority (Lennox et al., 2008). Clinical supervision emphasises a supportive, non-assessing relationship that focuses on the practitioner's reflection, professional growth and self-directed learning. This is distinctive from the regulated supervision required by some health authorities. For example, the Midwifery Council requires midwives returning to practice after a significant period to 'practice under supervision'. This means meeting regularly with a Council-approved supervisor who reports to the Midwifery Council, rather than an 'over the shoulder' type supervision (Midwifery Council of New Zealand, 2022). Thus, the term 'supervision' in clinical contexts has been historically complicated by its association with institutional control, assessment, and regulatory oversight.

Mentoring, distinct from both preceptorship and clinical supervision, is rooted in a peer-based, non-hierarchical relationship where the mentor's role is more flexible and often self-directed by the mentee's goals. Mentoring takes place in the post-registration context. Mentorship encourages professional reflection, guidance, and support without formal assessment or predetermined institutional objectives. Mentoring fosters long-term professional and personal development, facilitating growth through trust and mutual respect. Mentoring relationships are chosen rather than assigned, enabling mentees to seek out mentors who align with their professional aspirations and values. The Midwifery Council sets out in the Standards of Competence for Kahu Pōkai I Midwives that midwives support students, new midwives, and colleagues to provide clinically and culturally safe care (Midwifery Council of New Zealand, 2024c).

Another professional supportive relationship is the recently established role of **Clinical Coach** within hospital facilities across Aotearoa New Zealand. The Clinical Coach role was established in 2021 with the goal that senior core midwives in these roles would provide additional support to midwives needing it (e.g. for midwives new to the area or new graduate midwives). Where there are core midwives requiring supervision mandated by the Midwifery Council (for example, midwives returning to practice or overseas trained midwives new to practice in Aotearoa New Zealand), clinical coaches are also able to provide that supervision. In addition, the Ngā Maia Trust has begun offering a pilot programme of tuakana teina clinical coaching for Māori midwives beyond their first two years of practice to support improved recruitment and retention.

The New Zealand College of Midwives I Te Kāreti o ngā Kaiwhakawhānau ki Aotearoa (the College) published a mentoring consensus statement in 2000, outlining the definition, structure, and key attributes of an effective midwifery mentor, modelling this relationship on the construct of the midwife/woman partnership (New Zealand College of Midwives, 2000). The statement describes mentoring as a negotiated partnership between two registered midwives, with a focus on enabling and developing professional confidence. The duration and structure of the mentoring relationship are collaboratively defined by both partners, allowing for a personalised approach that adapts to the mentee's specific needs. The mentor's role is not to provide answers but rather to encourage exploration, reflection, and critical thinking, fostering the mentee's independence and affirming their accountability for their own practice.

Prior to 2007, mentoring in Aotearoa New Zealand was largely informal (Daellenbach et al., 2024). With the introduction of a structured conceptual model for midwifery mentoring (Gray, 2006), formal mentoring programmes were established to support the retention and sustainability of midwives across various practice settings. Examples of these are the Midwifery First Year of Practice (MFYP) programme and the Rural Midwifery Recruitment and Retention programme discussed below.

The consensus statement outlines that mentors are registered, practising midwives who have demonstrated practice which reflects the midwifery model (New Zealand College of Midwives, 2000). The New Zealand

College of Midwives provides a 'Practicalities of Mentoring in Aotearoa' course. Participation in this education is a requirement for midwives mentoring in the MFYP programme. The course introduces professional support mechanisms and mentoring in Aotearoa New Zealand, alongside practical strategies for midwife mentors (New Zealand College of Midwives, 2024). This course is delivered as self-directed e-learning and reflective activities online and has previously been delivered by the College as an in-person workshop. The online course is free to undertake by any registered midwife, and midwives gain two professional development hours towards their recertification requirements and are eligible to provide mentoring within one of the College's mentoring programmes (e.g. MFYP). The education of mentors has been an evolving process as the profession has embraced the concept of mentoring as one tool of professional support. The lived experiences of both mentee and mentor have informed the education development to ensure it meets the needs of the midwifery profession in Aotearoa New Zealand.

Research from Aotearoa highlights the efficacy of midwifery mentoring, particularly for new graduate midwives. Mentorship not only strengthens professional confidence but also contributes to successful integration into the workforce by offering a support system grounded in shared experiences and professional values (Daellenbach et al., 2024). Recent research into the key attributes of the midwifery mentoring relationship in Aotearoa New Zealand identified four key elements (Daellenbach et al., 2024): creating an empowered, confidential, safe space where power is balanced and vulnerability is shared; building a support infrastructure in which mentee's development is the focus and professional networks are built; supporting professional cohesion, through which different ways of practising midwifery are recognised; and sustaining midwifery practice, through which there is reciprocity of benefit for both mentee and mentor, reinvigorating mentors' passion for midwifery and supporting sustainable practices to support wellbeing and balance.

Formal mentoring in Aotearoa New Zealand has thus become a crucial component of sustainable midwifery practice, aligned with the profession's core values and supportive of midwives' long-term development.

Māori Midwife Mentoring – Research

Pihema et al. (2023) sought to gain in-depth insight into the experiences of Māori midwife mentors as part of the broader research into mentor experiences reported in Daellenbach et al. (2024). They found that the mentoring relationship for Māori mentor midwives was grounded in the practice of decolonisation within a Pākehā system in a way that is different from the traditional idea of a negotiated partnership between two individuals. The research articulated four themes in this multi-faceted vision and identified the unique aspects of mentoring seen through a Te Ao Māori perspective:

- *Decolonising.* The importance of decolonising both educational and clinical spaces, with mentors supporting mentees in reclaiming a Māori approach to midwifery. It involves supporting the mentee's navigation of the Pākehā health system, in a culturally safe way for them, allowing mentees to uphold their mana, and filling gaps in their education relating to mātauranga Māori.
- *Te Kai a te Rangatira* (**The Food of the Chiefs**). Mentors create a culturally safe, collective space for mentors, mentees, and whānau (family), establishing trust through shared vulnerability and whakawhanaungatanga (building relationships). Shared kai (food) facilitates connection, equal power, and mutual respect, and builds te reo Māori and tikanga Māori into the mentoring relationship.
- *Te Ao Māori.* Key principles tika and pono (to be correct/just, to be true/honest) guide conduct and support mentees in balancing their responsibilities to whānau, both personal and professional. Integrating whānau in the mentoring process enhances sustainability for both mentors and mentees.
- *Filling the kete.* Mentoring as a decolonisation practice supports the collective strength and longevity of Māori midwives by sharing the taonga (treasures) of knowledge across generations. The mentors view their roles as both giving and receiving gifts, nourishing their commitment and enthusiasm for Māori midwifery through the presence and growth of young Māori midwives.

REFLECTIVE ACTIVITY 1

Midwifery in Aotearoa New Zealand is rooted in the concept of partnership between midwives and whānau (families). Similarly, a successful mentoring partnership is based on values of trust, reciprocity, and shared power and responsibility. Consider a mentoring relationship you have experienced or observed.

- How were those values demonstrated in that relationship?
- What challenges were encountered in maintaining a balanced and equitable partnership in that mentoring relationship?
- How might these insights inform your own practice of mentoring?

Aotearoa New Zealand has many examples of mentoring in practice, in both undergraduate and post-registration contexts.

Examples of Supportive Professional Relationships in Undergraduate Midwifery Programmes

In Aotearoa New Zealand, the most common pathway to become a registered midwife is to obtain a Bachelor of Midwifery and then seek entry to the register of midwives. Midwifery undergraduate study is a demanding course of study requiring a high level of commitment. Given the intensity of the programme and the exposure to the full spectrum of childbearing experiences, ākonga (students) are provided with significant pastoral care and support by staff within the midwifery schools. Students have a named kaiako (teacher) from the institution with whom they debrief with and seek guidance and support from regarding their practice experiences. This form of support takes place one-on-one or in group settings with other ākonga. The kaiako facilitates debriefing of practice experiences, teaches communication and practice skills, stimulates reflective learning and critical analysis, and enables ākonga to integrate theory and practice (Kensington et al., 2017).

Another fundamental aspect of support in undergraduate midwifery education is the preceptorship of students in midwifery practice settings. Student midwives of any level can be precepted by registered midwives who have at least one year of midwifery practice experience (Midwifery Council of New Zealand, 2024b). LMC midwives and maternity facilities that have students placed with them receive a payment from the midwifery schools for this preceptorship. Preceptor midwives undertake competency assessments of the students, as set and directed by the midwifery schools. There is no nationwide standard assessment; however, the competency assessments are based on the Standards of Competence for Kahu Pōkai I Midwives, as set by the Midwifery Council of New Zealand. While preceptor midwives are not required by the Midwifery Council to undertake education for their preceptor role, most midwives do take up the option of free online education or face-to-face workshops offered by midwifery schools as part of their professional development. Bilous (2018) found that the presence of a midwifery student offered midwife preceptors both practical support and the refreshment of a commitment to the midwifery profession. Midwives benefited from the students' fresh knowledge and perspectives, which enriched their own practice and encouraged reflection. This relationship fostered professional satisfaction, as midwives felt they were positively influencing and sustaining the midwifery workforce.

Te Ara ō Hine – Tapu Ora Programme

Informal mentoring has always taken place in Māori and Pasifika midwifery communities, for example, the 'Aunties Initiative' which paired Pasifika students ('nieces') with Pasifika midwife mentors ('aunties') and was early inspiration for more culturally grounded support which focused on wraparound care for the students (Hill, 2023). Since 2021, the Te Ara ō Hine-Tapu Ora programme has provided Māori and Pasifika midwifery students access to additional funded pastoral, cultural, academic, and financial support (Health New Zealand Te Whatu Ora, 2024). The programme grew out of a clearly identified need for culturally grounded mentoring and support to improve recruitment and retention of Māori and Pasifika midwifery students, to work towards a midwifery workforce that represents the communities midwives serve in (Tūpara & Tahere, 2020).

TE ARA Ō HINE LIAISON PROFILE – KAYLA

Ko Ngati Kahu ki Whangaroa te iwi.
No Kawakawa/Aorangi au, engari kei te noho au ki Otautahi.
He Kahu Pōkai ahau.
He Te Ara ō Hine liaison ki Otago Polytechnic ahau.
Ka Kayla Burnes tōku ingoa.

Te Ara ō Hine is essential to tautoko tauira Māori within the midwifery degree. Having Māori kahu pōkai for whānau Māori in Aotearoa is pivotal for outcomes and experiences in the maternity system. Walking alongside tauira Māori within the midwifery programme is an absolute honour as they navigate the system to receiving their tohu. Celebrating successes, building relationships with their whānau and creating solutions to challenges and difficulties with tauira is very special. We are all tuakana and all teina in the spaces we sit, I am grateful for the continuous tautoko that I receive, and this is something Māori midwives have done forever. Continuing to create a safe space for tauira Māori to be unapologetically Māori is the priority. 'Mā mua ka kite a muri, mā muri ka ora a mua'. Those who lead give sight to those who follow, those who follow give life to those that lead. (Kayla)

A focus of the programme is the role of the liaison who provides wraparound support, and connections to internal student services and external community-based ones, in a way that is accessible and culturally nuanced (Marsters, 2022). The liaison roles are embedded in the Schools of Midwifery and maintain close national networks with other liaison midwives.

KAIARĀHI TEINA PROFILE

Talofa lava, o lou'u igoa Kizzi. As a final-year midwifery student, I was a Kaiārahi Teina to our Pasifika students for the last two years. What I loved about my role is that I was able to individually cater to the needs of each student and being able to support them through the degree and some life changes that may arise. Seeing each student come into their own in midwifery has been a blessing and has helped shape me into a Pasifika Teina in my own right. The benefit of having Te Ara ō Hine-Tapu Ora and Kaiārahi Teina roles is having support systems that reflect our Pasifika ways. (Kizzi)

The programme also includes peer mentoring between students with the Kaiārahi Teina role, which is taken up by Māori and Pasifika students to support and guide their peers. As with midwife-student mentoring relationships, peer mentoring has always existed between Māori and Pasifika students rooted in the concepts of tuakana-teina and whanaungatanga. Tuakana-teina is a Te Ao Māori concept where a more experienced person (tuakana) supports the learning of a less experienced person (teina), and acknowledges that the role of teacher and learner can be reversed and reciprocated within that relationship (Royal-Tangaere, 1997). Whanaungatanga is a foundational Te Ao Māori principle of belonging, connection, and kinship (Le Grice et al., 2017). Relationships are formed through shared experiences and bring a sense of belonging and unity. Kinship development comes through duties and responsibilities that reinforce each member's role in the kin group. The role of Kaiārahi Teina within the Schools of Midwifery means that those Tuakana are now recognised for what they do and provided with funding to support them in these roles. They themselves are supported by the Te Ara ō Hine-Tapu Ora liaisons and are connected to peer mentors in other Schools of Midwifery, forming a collective of support around Māori and Pasifika students.

Examples of Mentoring Type Relationships in Post-Registration Midwifery

Midwifery First Year of Practice Programme

The (MFYP programme is a cornerstone of midwifery mentoring in Aotearoa New Zealand. This fully funded programme has been available since 2007, and engagement and completion of the programme is a mandatory requirement for all new graduate midwives (Midwifery Council of New Zealand, 2024b). The one-year programme includes mentoring support, professional education, consolidation of clinical practice, and participation in a quality assurance programme called the Midwifery Standards Review (Pairman et al., 2016). New midwives are immersed in practice and move from being competent practitioners, on registration, to becoming confident practitioners.

A significant feature of the programme is that the new graduate midwives (or mentees) choose their own mentor. Choosing the right mentor is critical to the success of the mentoring relationship (Dixon et al., 2015; Pairman et al., 2016). New graduate midwives are advised to choose mentors who do not work in their immediate work context to avoid an unequal power dynamic. There is no requirement that midwives choose a mentor in the same broader context as them (i.e. employed/core or LMC). Finding a mentor can be challenging when new graduates moving into a new location to begin practice (Chapman, 2018). It may also be challenging in locations where there are small numbers of midwives. Where possible, Māori mentee midwives choose Māori mentor midwives (Pihema et al., 2023). The College provides an online directory to assist graduating students in finding a suitable mentor.

MFYP mentors are required to meet criteria to ensure they bring both experience and dedication to the role (New Zealand College of Midwives, n.d.). This includes completion of the short Practicalities of Mentoring in Aotearoa' mentoring course described above within the past three years, if they have not been actively mentoring in that time. Mentors must hold a midwifery Annual Practising Certificate, be at least five years in practice, have met their recertification requirements, and be in good standing. Mentors are expected to be current members of the New Zealand College of Midwives and have strong collegial relationships within midwifery and the broader healthcare sector. Additionally, mentors are expected to demonstrate commitment to equity and cultural safety in their practice and to be able to meet the time commitments of the mentor role.

MFPY MENTEE PROFILE

I am a new graduate midwife nearing the end of my first year of practice. My mentor has helped me reflect on my practice and given me incredible support. Fortnightly mentoring sessions have been absolutely key in growing my confidence this year, providing a chance to debrief practice situations, get advice on clinical or professional issues, and receive encouragement. The mentoring partnership also provides challenge and accountability and is a powerful way to kickstart a new career. (Andrea)

Mentoring within the MFYP programme involves a structured yet supportive framework, where new graduate midwives and their mentor create a mentoring agreement, and the mentee is supported to develop a professional development plan for the year. Throughout the programme, the mentor and mentee must complete between 40 and 56 hours of mentoring across several face-to-face sessions (Pairman et al., 2016). These mentoring sessions facilitate reflective discussions, helping mentees to critically examine their own midwifery practice, identify their learning needs, and receive ongoing support throughout their transition year (Lennox & Foureur, 2012). The mentor's role extends beyond simple guidance; they encourage and challenge the graduate midwife to view their practice within a broader context, thereby developing confidence and critical thinking. Mentors serve as a sounding board, offering feedback and advice while fostering a reciprocal relationship that benefits both the mentee and mentor (Chapman, 2018). In addition to mentoring, the MFYP programme includes funded hands-on clinical support (Pairman et al., 2016). It is also noted that new graduate midwives receive significant support from the broader midwifery community in their local areas, including core midwives and other LMC midwives outside the boundaries of the MFYP programme relationships (Pairman et al., 2016).

Another essential component of the MFYP programme is the requirement for new graduates to participate in a quality assurance programme (the Midwifery Standards Review) at the end of their first year (Pairman et al., 2016). This provides midwives with the opportunity to reflect on their first year of practice and their progress towards the 'confident midwife' profile, and to set goals and plan their ongoing professional development.

The benefits of the MFYP programme are significant. New graduates recognise that mentoring facilitates reflection on their practice, bolsters confidence in practice, and has been linked to higher retention rates in the midwifery workforce (Chapman, 2018; Dixon et al., 2015; Kensington, 2006; Pairman et al., 2016). Since its inception, the MFYP programme has evolved to meet the changing needs of the profession and continues to do so.

Rural Midwifery Recruitment and Retention Programme

Aotearoa New Zealand encompasses many rural and remote communities that are characterised by sparse populations, challenging weather conditions, and infrastructure constraints, and are often geographically isolated from secondary health services. Time and distance for transfer to base hospitals can be significant, and availability of road or air ambulances can be challenging. LMC midwives practice from within these communities, providing primary care locally as well as linking to secondary care services. Rural healthcare in Aotearoa New Zealand faces significant pressures in attracting and retaining health professionals, including midwives.

The Rural Midwifery Recruitment and Retention (RMRR) initiative was established in 2009 to address these issues and support rural midwives (Crowther, 2016). This initiative offers 12 months of funded mentorship to rurally practising midwives, helping them manage the distinct personal and professional demands that come with rural practice. The rural mentors provide vital peer support, offering guidance and connection to help midwives sustain their commitment to rural communities despite the challenges (Crowther, 2016; Daellenbach et al., 2020).

> **RURAL MENTOR PROFILE**
>
> *I provided rural mentorship in the MFYP to new graduates who I had supervised as student midwives. What was unique is that they lived in the rural community in which I worked and knew they wished to work in the rural region. This meant they were committed and eager to integrate their learning into being a rural LMC direct from their studies and start taking on their own case load. It was vital for me to provide this mentorship for succession planning and to mitigate the growing population in the region – it was increasingly evident that my caseload was on course to keep growing and I had little local support and ability to take time off. Growing new graduates into rural practice from within the community is essential because often those new to the area without family and friends struggle to achieve a work-life balance whilst being 'stuck' in the rural region. If your life is local in the rural area, then a midwife is less likely to feel hemmed in by the 24/7 on calls. Also, the level of mentorship in rural regions entails considerable time and commitment because of the isolation that new graduates can feel when 'out and about' when other peers are at a distance. In addition, providing a buffer to base hospitals and local GP practices is essential because communication issues can intensify feelings of isolation and unsafety. Lots of face-to-face meet-ups over a cuppa are pivotal to the mentorship process in rural areas because of the sense of lone working that can overwhelm the new graduate, who can quickly become fearful especially in challenging situations when they are so visible in small communities. (Susan)*

Mentors within the RMRR programme play a critical role in helping rural midwives navigate the complex interface between urban and rural healthcare systems. Rural midwives often manage different expectations and perspectives across practice settings, which can lead to misunderstandings and professional tensions (Daellenbach et al., 2020; Daellenbach et al., 2024). By providing strategies for constructive, non-confrontational engagement, rural mentors support midwives in managing these logistical and relational complexities. In addition to offering guidance on the urban-rural interface, mentors help rural midwives strengthen their connections with other healthcare professionals and community services, addressing the risk of professional isolation inherent in rural practice.

The Future of Midwifery Mentoring in Aotearoa New Zealand

Midwifery mentoring in Aotearoa New Zealand is not a static process, and the evolution of mentoring as a professional support mechanism is continually evolving. Mentoring within midwifery has demonstrated considerable benefits for both mentors and mentees, enhancing professional confidence, cohesion, and resilience across the profession. With the potential for further development such as of kaupapa Māori mentoring models, there is an opportunity to enrich existing strong mentoring practices. Challenges also exist for the stability of mentoring programmes with the possibility for fluctuations in funding due to external economic pressures. Ensuring consistent support for these programmes is essential for the long-term sustainability of Aotearoa New Zealand's midwifery workforce. By building on existing successes and embracing innovation, midwifery mentoring can continue to foster a supportive, sustainable, and culturally responsive professional community.

Te Reo Māori Glossary

Ākonga	student/learner
Aotearoa	New Zealand
Hauora	wellbeing
Kahu pōkai	midwife
Kai	food
Kaiako	teacher/lecturer
Kaiārahi teina	peer mentor
Kete	basket
Mana	dignity, spiritual power in people, places, objects
Māori	indigenous person/people of Aotearoa New Zealand
Mātauranga Māori	Māori knowledge/wisdom, ways of knowing
Pākehā	non-Māori person/people
Pono	to be true/honest
Taonga	treasure(s)
Tautoko	support
Te Ao Māori	the Māori world, the Māori worldview
Te Reo Māori	the Māori language (indigenous language of Aotearoa New Zealand)
Te Tiriti o Waitangi	the Treaty of Waitangi (Māori version)
Teina	younger relative
Tika	to be correct/just
Tikanga Māori	Māori customary protocol
Tohu	qualification
Tuakana	older relative
Whakawhanaungatanga	process of building relationships, connection
Whānau	family group
Whanaungatanga	Relationship, sense of connection

References

Bilous, E. (2018). *Gaining from giving: The benefits for midwives of working with student midwives.* [Master's thesis, Otago Polytechnic]. Otago Polytechnic Research Repository. https://online.op.ac.nz/industry-and-research/research/otago-polytechnic-research-repository-opres/midwifery-theses/gaining-from-giving-the-benefits-for-midwives-of-working-with-student-midwives

Chapman, A. (2018). Developing confidence in competence: My experience of the Midwifery First Year of Practice programme. *New Zealand College of Midwives Journal, 54,* 58.

Crowther, S. (2016). Providing rural and remote rural midwifery care: An "expensive hobby". *New Zealand College of Midwives Journal, 52,* 26–34. https://doi.org/10.12784/nzcomjnl52.2016.4.26-34

Daellenbach, R., Davies, L., Kensington, M., Crowther, S., Gilkison, A., Deery, R., & Rankin, J. (2020). Rural midwifery practice in Aotearoa/New Zealand: Strengths, vulnerabilities, opportunities and challenges. *New Zealand College of Midwives Journal, 56*(56), 17–25. https://doi.org/10.12784/nzcomjnl56.2020.3.17-25

Daellenbach, S., Dixon, L., Kensington, M., Griffiths, C., Pihema, N., Huia, J., Te, Otukolo, D., & Gray, E. (2024). Midwifery mentorship in Aotearoa New Zealand: The mentors' perspective. *New Zealand College of Midwives Journal, 2024*(60). https://doi.org/10.12784/nzcomjnl.246002

Dixon, L., Calvert, S., Tumilty, E., Kensington, M., Gray, E., Lennox, S., Campbell, N., & Pairman, S. (2015). Supporting New Zealand graduate midwives to stay in the profession: An evaluation of the Midwifery First Year of Practice programme. *Midwifery, 31*(6), 633–639. https://doi.org/10.1016/j.midw.2015.02.010

Gray, E. (2006). Midwives as mentors. *New Zealand College of Midwives Journal, 34,* 24–27.

Health New Zealand Te Whatu Ora. (2024, June 24). *Midwifery.* https://www.tewhatuora.govt.nz/for-health-professionals/health-workforce-development/midwifery

Health Practitioners' Competence Assurance Act. (2003). Health Practitioners' Competence Assurance Act 2003. https://www.legislation.govt.nz/act/public/2003/0048/latest/DLM203312.html

Hill, R. (2023). "We created a wraparound awhi of them" - Aunties mentor Pacific midwives. *Radio New Zealand.* https://www.rnz.co.nz/news/national/493446/we-created-a-wraparound-awhi-of-them-aunties-mentor-pacific-midwives

Humphrey, C., & Kumar-Hazard, B. (2023). Legal frameworks for practice in Australia and New Zealand. In S. Pairman, S. K. Tracy, H. G. Dahlen, & L. Dixon (Eds.), *Midwifery: Preparation for Practice 2* (5th ed., pp. 290–323). Elsevier.

Kensington, M. (2006). The faces of mentoring in New Zealand: Realities for the new graduate midwife. *New Zealand College of Midwives Journal, 35,* 22–27. https://oxfordbrookes.idm.oclc.org/login?url=http://search.ebscohost.com/login.aspx?direct=true&db=cin20&AN=106124045&site=ehost-live

Kensington, M., Davies, L., Daellenbach, R., Dreary, R., & Richards, J. (2017). Using small tutorial groups within a blended Bachelor of Midwifery programme: Bridging the theory-practice divide. *New Zealand College of Midwives Journal, 53*(53), 38–44. https://doi.org/10.12784/nzcomjnl53.2017.5.38-44

Le Grice, J., Braun, V., & Wetherell, M. (2017). "What I reckon is, is that like the love you give to your kids they'll give to someone else and so on and so on": Whanaungatanga and mātauranga Māori in practice. *New Zealand Journal of Psychology, 46*(3), 88–97.

Lennox, S., & Foureur, M. (2012). Developmental mentoring: New graduates' confidence grows when their needs shape the relationship. *New Zealand College of Midwives Journal, 46,* 26–31. https://www.midwife.org.nz/wp-content/uploads/2019/01/JNL-46-June-2012.pdf

Lennox, S., Skinner, J., & Foureur, M. (2008). Mentorship, preceptorship and clinical supervision : Three key processes for supporting midwives. *New Zealand College of Midwives Journal, 39,* 7–12.

Marsters, N. (2022). Pasifika: Tapu Ora: Kua mua, ka muri. *Midwife Aotearoa New Zealand, 106,* 36–37. https://issuu.com/collegeofmidwives/docs/midwife_magazine_issue_106_digital/36

Midwifery Council of New Zealand. (2022). *Returning to practice after more than three years.* https://midwiferycouncil.health.nz/common/Uploaded%20files/Registration/20230126%20Returning%20to%20practice%20after%20more%20than%20three%20years.pdf

Midwifery Council of New Zealand. (2024a). *Midwifery in Aotearoa New Zealand.* www.midwiferycouncil.health.nz

Midwifery Council of New Zealand. (2024b). *Standards for Approval of Pre-Registration Midwifery Education Programmes and Accreditation of Tertiary Education Organisations* (3rd ed.). https://midwiferycouncil.health.nz/Public/Public/07.-I-want-to-be-a-midwife/1.-Midwifery-education-in-New-Zealand.aspx

Midwifery Council of New Zealand. (2024c). *Standards of Competence for kahu pōkai | midwives.* https://www.midwiferycouncil.health.nz/common/Uploaded files/Standards of Competence Final Nov 24.pdf

New Zealand College of Midwives. (n.d.). *Midwifery First Year of Practice programme (MFYP).* https://www.midwife.org.nz/midwives/mentoring/midwifery-first-year-of-practice-mfyp/

New Zealand College of Midwives. (2000). *Consensus statement : Mentoring.* New Zealand College of Midwives.

New Zealand College of Midwives. (2024). *Practicalities of mentoring in Aotearoa.* https://www.midwife.org.nz/midwives/education/elearning/practicalities-of-mentoring-in-aotearoa/

Pairman, S., Dixon, L., Tumilty, E., Gray, E., Campbell, N., Calvert, S., Lennox, S., & Kensington, M. (2016). The Midwifery First Year of Practice programme: Supporting New Zealand midwifery graduates in their transition to practice. *New Zealand College of Midwives Journal, 52*(52), 12–19. https://doi.org/10.12784/nzcomjnl52.2016.2.12-19

Pairman, S., & Gray, M. (2023). Professional frameworks for practice in Australia and New Zealand. In S. Pairman, S. K. Tracy, H. G. Dahlen, & L. Dixon (Eds.), *Midwifery: Preparation for Practice* (5th ed., pp. 257–289). Elsevier.

Pihema, N., Daellenbach, S., Te Huia, J., Dixon, L., Kensington, M., Griffiths, C., Gray, E., & Otukolo, D. (2023). A vision of decolonisation: Midwifery mentoring from the perspective of Māori mentors. *New Zealand College of Midwives Journal, 59,* 39–46.

Royal-Tangaere, A. (1997). Māori human development learning theory. In D. McCarthy & T. Whaīti (Eds.), *Mai i rangiātea: Māori Wellbeing and Development* (pp. 46–59). Auckland University Press.

Tūpara, H., & Tahere, M. (2020). *Rapua Te Aronga-a-Hine: the Māori midwifery workforce in Aotearoa, A literature review - February 2020* (Issue February). https://terauora.com/rapua-te-aronga-a-hine-the-maori-midwifery-workforce/

19

MIDWIFERY MENTORSHIP IN PAKISTAN

Musarrat Rani

Background

Pakistan is one country within South Asia. Pakistan is the fifth most populated country and has a population of around 242.9 million, of which 49.2% are female. There are two official languages spoken, Urdu and English, with the majority of the population being Muslim. Literacy rates for females are around 45.3% and 71.5% for men. In 2024, the birth rate was approximately 25.6 births per 1,000 people or 3.189 births per woman, which is a 1.51% decline from 2023. Some predict there will be around 19,791 live births on average per day (824.61 per hour) in 2025; hence the role of midwifery and midwives is key not only to mother and baby health but also to mentoring the next generation of midwives.

Pakistan Nursing and Midwifery Council

The National Assembly of Pakistan amended the Pakistan Nursing Council Act, 1973 and again on Thursday, January 19, 2023. We refer to the amendment act as the Pakistan Nursing and Midwifery Council (Amendment) Act, 2023 (Act No. V of 2023), which further solidified the legal framework for midwives by amending the Pakistan Nursing Council Act of 1973 to include midwifery. The Pakistan Nursing and Midwifery Council (PNMC), in its first meeting held on August 8, 2023, adopted all regulations and decisions established by the Pakistan Nursing Council under the PNC Act 1973. The Council recognises the following qualifications till date:

- Four-year BSM: BSM (Baccalaureate Studies of Midwifery) Degree Programme
- Two-year Post-RN-BSM
- Nurse-Midwife/Post Basic Specialisation: one-year diploma course in Midwifery

DOI: 10.4324/9781003533733-20

- Lady Health Visitor (LHV): 27-month Diploma Programme
- Community Midwife (CMW): Two-year Diploma Programme
- Associate Midwifery Degree: Associate degree for LHV and CMWs after LHV and CMW diploma course.
- Pupil Midwives – 15-Month Year Direct Entry Midwifery Programme – closed

Historical Evolution of Midwifery and Mentorship in Pakistan

At the time of Pakistan's independence in 1947, midwifery services were largely informal and traditional, provided by *dais* (traditional birth attendants) in rural and urban communities. These women, often without formal training, relied on mentorship passed down through generations. However, *dais* practices were limited by a lack of medical knowledge and facilities. This is acknowledged by the government as part of its broader healthcare strategy, deciding there was a need for professional midwives, to this end the Pakistan Nursing Council (PNC) was established in 1948 and began formalising midwifery curricula.[1]

Sir Ganga Ram Hospital, Lahore Nursing School opened its door in December 1948, and it has the distinction of being the first new school of nursing established in Pakistan after the country's independence (CON & Allied SGRH. FJMU.2024). It was not until 1950 that the first formal midwifery schools were established with basic training programmes under the supervision of nurses. Like other countries, the nurse-midwife pathway was a one-year diploma programme following a three-year nursing diploma. During this time mentorship was unstructured, often involving on-the-job guidance from senior nurses or doctors rather than specialised midwives.

Lady Health Visitor Diploma Programme

In 1951 LHVs, came into existence. LHVs aligned their practice with medicine although were originally registered with the Pakistan Nursing Council and had to complete one year of midwifery training programme (Upvall et al., 2002). Their role was a specific cadre of health care providers and was the initial point of contact with the healthcare system for underprivileged women in rural areas. Services provided to urban and rural communities, included promote health, basic nursing care, and maternal child health services addressing prenatal and postnatal care. (Hezekiah, 1993). A part of the LHV role is teaching, and training traditional birth attendants, and training of community workers. In 2024, the LHV programme continues in private and public nursing and midwifery institutions, although the training has elongated to a two-year diploma programme, which now consists of one year in public health nursing and one year in midwifery.

Mentorship in this era remained informal, with senior practitioners providing guidance to trainees in hospitals and rural health centres. However, the lack of a dedicated mentorship framework limited the effectiveness of knowledge transfer and skill development.

It was not until the early 2000s, Pakistan introduced major policy reforms aimed at strengthening midwifery education and practice. Midwifery was recognised as a distinct profession with a direct entry pathway, which was 15 months, although the pathway for registered nurses to become midwives remained at one year.

In the early 2000s, Pakistan introduced major policy reforms aimed at strengthening midwifery education and practice. Midwifery was recognised as a distinct profession with 15 months for pupil midwives (direct entry programme) and 12 months for nurse midwives (post-licensure) midwifery diploma programmes running at that time.

Community Midwifery Diploma Programme

The Ministry of Health established the National Maternal Newborn and Child Health Programme (NMNCHP) in 2006, with funding support from external organisations such as USAID's Pakistan Initiative for Mothers and Newborns (PAIMAN) and Technical Assistance for Capacity Building in Midwifery Information and Logistics (TACMIL). The MNCHP introduced a new cadre called "Community Midwives" (CMW), to address the high maternal mortality rates in rural areas. This programme aimed to train midwives over a period of 18 months to learn antenatal, intrapartum, postnatal, and newborn care, so they could provide home-based care and improve access to maternal health services. Candidates were trained by at least four tutors and two clinical instructors in designated midwifery schools, after which they received six months of practical training at practice sites in communities or health facilities with at least one instructor (WMO/LHV). Once the entire course was complete, CMWs received certificates from PNC were eligible to practice as a CMW and were given a catchment area of around 5,000 people (USAID, 2012). It was anticipated around 12,000 CMWs would be trained nationwide to increase coverage of MNCH services by skilled providers. These were rural women from the same community as their clients. By December 2011, 4,700 CMWs were trained and deployed.

Mentorship during this period gained prominence as part of community midwifery training. Midwives acted as mentors, helping new midwives adapt to rural healthcare challenges. However, these efforts were often ad hoc and dependent on donor funding, lacking sustainability and institutional backing.

Nevertheless, the CMWs recommended internships in the community with a mentor, after their graduation, and inclusion of management of birthing centres through coverage of entrepreneurial skills in the curriculum. (Ali et al., 2015). A pioneering study in Pakistan by Siyani, Jan, Lennonx and Mohammad (2017b) titled Development of Mentorship Module and its Feasibility for Community Midwives in Sindh, Pakistan: a pilot study, measuring the impact of mentorship training on CMWs found significant improvements in their knowledge about mentorship ($P \leq 0.001$), willingness to mentor ($P \leq 0.001$), and perceptions of the cost-benefit of mentoring ($P \leq 0.001$). Most participants reported beginning to work as mentors during follow-up. The study concluded that mentorship training effectively improves midwives' knowledge, perceptions, and willingness to mentor. It also demonstrated the feasibility of designing a successful mentorship module for CMWs. This module can be shared with other healthcare providers and students, potentially encouraging midwifery schools to integrate mentorship concepts into their curriculums from the start.

Further, the overall effectiveness of this programme cannot be assessed because of the absence of data on CMW deployment and the lack of surveys to measure maternal mortality following 2006–2007 (Mubeen et al., 2019) study on CMWs noted that although the outcomes for CMWs are better than for some other cadres in Pakistan; they are still inadequate compared to midwives trained to international standards. The outcomes presented in this study are in line with the challenges of CMW survival reported in earlier studies. This strongly indicates the need for improvement in CMW's pre-service and in-service education to meet the global standards for midwifery education (International Confederation of Midwives, 2021). Despite this the CMW service continues in private and public nursing and midwifery institutions today.

Post Registered Nurse Bachelor of Midwifery Programme

Prior to 2012, there were three pathways to obtaining a midwifery qualification in Pakistan: become an LHV, or a nurse-midwife or a CMW.

In Pakistan, a two-year Post RN Midwifery degree programme has already started at a Public University, i.e. Dow University of Health Sciences, Karachi, and Private University Aga Khan University, Karachi; so far these programmes have produced more than 100 graduates in Pakistan (Lakhani et al., 2018).

Baccalaureate Studies of Midwifery Degree Programme

In September 2022, the PNMC with technical support of Midwifery Association of Pakistan (MAP), UNFPA and Health Services Academy (HAS), Islamabad accredited the first four-year BSM in Pakistan. This programme is undertaken in two public sector institutes: HSA in Islamabad & Fatima Jinnah Medical University FJMU in Lahore (UNFPA Pakistan, 2024). This

programme follows the ICM education standards (International Confederation of Midwives, 2021).

BSM started in February 2024 in HSA Islamabad with 50 student midwives. The curriculum is approved by the Higher Education Commission
(HEC), and the faculty members are being prepared through the online programme offered by Burnet University with the support of UNFPA.

Associate Midwives Degree Programme

Degree along with these above undergraduate and post-graduate programmes, the diploma/certificate courses for preparing Associate Midwives
will also be continued and will remain a mainstream programme in times to
come. For improving and strengthening the quality of teaching associate midwives, it is critical to equip their tutors with the skills required for enhanced
teaching (clinical and classroom).

National Midwifery Strategic Framework

PNMC with technical support of Midwifery Association of Pakistan developed the first-ever National Midwifery Strategic Framework (Ministry
of National Health Services, Regulations & Coordination, 2022). UNFPA
has supported the PNMC under umbrella of Ministry of Health, along with
World Health Organization and HSA. This Framework addresses the issues
of governance and leadership, nomenclature, scope of practice, structured
career pathway and acceptability of midwives as distinct health professionals. (UNFPA Pakistan, 2024). In other words, the Framework provides a
comprehensive and evidence-based roadmap for enhancing the scope and
quality of midwifery services in the country (Career Structure of Midwives).

CPD Programme for Midwives

One of the key gaps identified during the development of the National midwifery strategic framework was a plan for continuous professional development of the midwifery educators/tutors. To address this gap, UNFPA
provided its support to MoNHSR&C for designing a CPD for existing midwifery educators/tutors in Pakistan including BScM tutors.

TOT under this programme has done for all government midwifery tutors,
and step-down training is continuing.

Mentorship

The midwifery profession has gained significant recognition across Pakistan. This has necessitated a need for mentorship for all cadres of midwives.

Mentorship is a bond between two people, usually a senior and a junior, for the focused and skilled growth of the latter. It exists as:

A process where an experienced, well-regarded, understanding person (the mentor) helps another (usually younger) person (the mentee) in the development and rethinking of their ideas, learning, and personal and career growth. The mentor, who often (but not always) works in the same place or field as the mentee, does this by listening and/or talking in private to the mentee.

(Rehman et al., 2024)

Studies and reports highlight the inclusion of mentorship in midwifery programs to bridge theoretical and practical knowledge.

(Ashraf, 2020)

Types of Mentorship Models

- **One-on-One Mentorship:** Discuss traditional mentorship where an experienced midwife mentors a less experienced one.
- **Peer Mentorship:** Explore the benefits and challenges of peer mentorship, where midwives of similar experience levels support each other.
- **Group Mentorship and Training Programmes:** Explain group mentorship models, workshops, and formal training programmes offered to midwives in Pakistan.

In Pakistan, midwifery mentors are trained through structured formal and informal programmes that include both theoretical and practical components that have been implemented in accredited midwifery programmes. There are various mentorship models available each with their advantages and challenges, some are noted below:

- Government Mentorship Model
- PAIMAN and Takmil Model/MNCH Mentorship Model
- PPHI Mentorship Model (NGO)
- DUHS Mentorship Model (Govt/Public Institute)
- Aga Khan University Mentorship Model (Private Institute)
- Koohi Goth Mentorship Model (Private Institute)

Government Mentorship Model

The "buddy system," where experienced midwives guide novices and the supportive supervision model with mentorship, is particularly effective. Mentorship programmes that include regular feedback and performance evaluations also enhance the mentor-mentee relationship and promote professional growth (Nazia Ilyas, personal communication, November 18, 2024).

PAIMAN and Takmil Model/MNCH Mentorship Model

The PAIMAN mentoring framework for CMWs includes the following components:

1 **Training:** CMWs undergo comprehensive training focused on maternal and newborn health.
2 **On-the-Job Support:** Mentors offer guidance and assistance as CMWs implement their training in practical settings.
3 **Supervision and Feedback:** Mentors conduct regular evaluations to assess performance and provide constructive feedback.
4 **Peer Learning:** CMWs are given opportunities to collaborate and learn from one another.
5 **Continuous Development:** CMWs are encouraged to engage in ongoing education and professional development.

The overarching aim is to empower CMWs to provide exceptional care for mothers and their newborns (PDACP.163) (Kulsoom, personal communication, November 24, 2024).

PPHI Mentorship Model (NGO)

The primary objective is to empower CMWs to deliver exceptional care to mothers and newborns. PPHI mentoring model for CMWs at Basic Health Units (BHUs) (Sayani et al., 2017a) (PPHI SINDH – Karachi)

1 **Training Programme:** CMWs receive extensive training focused on maternal and newborn health.
2 **Practical Support:** Seasoned mentors guide CMWs in implementing their training in practical settings.
3 **Monitoring and Evaluation:** Mentors conduct regular assessments to review performance and provide constructive feedback.
4 **Collaborative Learning:** CMWs are encouraged to exchange experiences and best practices with their peers.
5 **Ongoing Education:** CMWs are motivated to seek additional education and training opportunities.

DUHS Mentorship Model (Govt/Public Institute)

Midwifery-Led Clinics: A Mentorship Programme

During clinical teaching to students of Two-Year Post RN BSM, Dow Institute of Nursing and Midwifery has launched Midwifery-Led Clinics within hospitals to provide practical training and mentorship opportunities. Important finding are as follows:

1 **Hands-On Mentorship:** Instructors supported students in handling both high- and low-risk cases pertaining to antenatal, postnatal, and delivery care.
2 **Skill Enhancement:** Students acquired valuable experience in clinical skills, decision-making, and evidence-based practices under the guidance of experienced professionals.
3 **Teacher Development:** This initiative also enabled educators to enhance their own skills while guiding the next generation of midwives.

This forward-thinking model improved the educational experience, ensuring that midwifery professionals are better equipped for their roles (Rukhsana Haroon, personal communication, December 5, 2024).

Aga Khan University Mentorship Model (Private Institute) Supported by UNFPA

A pilot mentorship training programme was developed to strengthen the skills and confidence of midwives. This initiative backed by organisations such as Aga Khan University and UNFPA, featured practical coaching and organised mentorship frameworks. Midwifery coaches offered support to midwives in rural clinics, helping them enhance the quality of care provided. The training focused on skill development and practical implementation, facilitating a smoother transition for midwives from academic education to clinical practice. The outcomes of this mentorship initiative have been encouraging, leading to an increase in midwives' knowledge, attitudes, and readiness to mentor their peers (Siyani et al., 2017b).

Koohi Goth Mentorship Model (Private Institute)

Empowering Midwifery: A Model of Excellence in Patient Care and Education

1 **Establishment of Midwifery-led Clinics and Hospital**
   Koohi Goth Hospital has introduced innovative Midwifery-led clinics and a Midwifery-led hospital, where midwives are at the forefront of patient care management.
2 **Role of Senior Midwives in Patient Care**
   Senior midwives are responsible for overseeing all operations, providing continuous education, and leading the care process for both high-risk and low-risk patients.
3 **Mentorship and Training for Student Midwives**
   Student midwives work under the guidance of senior midwives, gaining hands-on experience while actively participating in the running of these units, learning from day 1 of their education.

4 **Referral System for High-Risk Patients**
High-risk patients are identified and referred to doctors, ensuring that specialised care is provided, while low-risk patients are managed entirely within the Midwifery-led clinics.

5 **A Model of Effective Mentorship and Education**
The hospital's approach is a strong example of mentorship, where senior midwives effectively guide students, ensuring quality education and patient care throughout the entire training process (Noor Gul, personal communication, November 20, 2024).

Despite the recognised benefits of mentorship, several challenges hinder its implementation in Pakistan as is similar in other low-middle income countries and some could argue high-income countries, the first being around workforce, specifically retention and shortage. It is well known around the world that once qualified in a low-income country, the attract to move to a middle or high income is attractive. Pakistan is no different, some midwives, once registered leave thus reducing the workforce but also taking their acquired knowledge and skills specifically around mentorship. This leaves a gap of midwives who can then mentor the next generation. The next challenge is around culture and gender, as gender inequality and oppression are common in Pakistan. This can lead to institutional barriers, lack of funding, training, or support.

Here are some scenario-based activities designed to illustrate mentorship in midwifery in Pakistan. These activities incorporate real-life challenges and reflective questions that midwives may encounter, creating an opportunity for critical thinking, collaboration, and skills development.

REFLECTIVE ACTIVITY 1: NAVIGATING COMMUNITY RESISTANCE

A CMW, Mariam, is assigned to a rural village where she frequently faces resistance from family members and elders who disapprove of women working outside the home. Mariam's mentor, an experienced midwife who has worked in similar settings, helps her develop strategies to build trust and demonstrate the importance of skilled midwifery.

- Reflect on ways to introduce yourself and explain your role in a culturally sensitive manner.
- Role-play scenarios with a partner, practising how to address concerns respectfully and offer reassurance.
- After the role-play, discuss how different approaches could impact the acceptance of midwifery care within the community.

REFLECTIVE ACTIVITY 2: MANAGING HIGH-RISK CASES WITH LIMITED RESOURCES

In a small health facility, midwife Fatima is managing a labour case with complications. She lacks access to advanced medical equipment and relies on basic tools and her training. Her mentor, available by phone, guides her through decision-making steps to safely monitor and manage the labouring woman until emergency help arrives. This mentorship provides critical support, empowering Fatima to act confidently under pressure.

- List the essential steps to handle complications with limited resources.
- Engage in a discussion on how mentorship can enhance skills in such situations.
- Reflect on a previous experience where support from a mentor helped you manage a challenging situation.

REFLECTIVE ACTIVITY 3: DEVELOPING LEADERSHIP AND ADVOCACY SKILLS

Shabana, a newly trained midwife, is struggling with low self-confidence, especially when advocating for women's reproductive rights. Her mentor encourages her to develop leadership skills by gradually involving her in community education workshops and guiding her on handling difficult questions.

- Reflect on the role of a midwife as an advocate in maternal health.
- Work in small groups to develop an outline for a community workshop on reproductive health, focusing on culturally sensitive topics.
- Discuss ways mentorship could help overcome challenges related to advocacy and education.

Key Lessons from Pakistan's History

1 **Community Involvement:** The effectiveness of community-oriented midwifery programmes underscores the significance of involving local stakeholders in mentorship efforts.
2 **Global Partnerships:** Collaborations with entities such as WHO, UNICEF, and UNFPA have demonstrated success in implementing mentorship frameworks and should be expanded.
3 **Sustainability Issues:** Reliance on external funding sources has constrained the enduring impact of mentorship initiatives, highlighting the necessity for local financial support. Best Practices for Mentorship

Future Directions/Strategies to Improve Mentorship in Midwifery

1 **Institutionalising Mentorship:**

- Embed mentorship as a core component of midwifery education curricula.
- Develop national guidelines for midwifery mentorship programmes.

2 **Capacity Building for Mentors:**

- Train senior midwives in mentorship skills through workshops and CPD programmes.
- Provide financial and professional incentives to mentors.

3 **Leveraging Technology:**

- Expand e-mentorship initiatives to connect rural midwives with experienced mentors.

4 **Advocacy and Policy Support:**

- Engage policymakers to prioritise mentorship within maternal health strategies.
- Allocate dedicated resources for mentorship programmes in federal and provincial budgets.

5 **Monitoring and Evaluation:**

- Establish mechanisms to assess the impact of mentorship programmes on midwifery competencies and maternal outcomes. "It was evaluated that existing mentorship programs in midwifery and nursing schools. The findings suggest that regular assessments of mentorship effectiveness are essential for continuous improvement" (Rehman et al., 2024).

Conclusion

Pakistan has evolved as a country as has midwifery from informal apprenticeships to formal accredited educational programmes. The same applies to mentorship, which has become more structured. Together these have been influenced by healthcare policy changes and international organisations, with the aim of enhancing the quality of midwifery education in the country and improving the quality and safety of maternity care provision for women and babies.

Note

1 https://pnmc.gov.pk/wp-content/uploads/2023/09/PNC-Act-1973.pdf, https://pnmc.gov.pk/wp-content/uploads/2023/09/PNMC-Amended-Act-2023.pdf

References

Ali, S. A., Lakhani, A., Jan, R., Shahid, S., Baig, M., & Adnan, F. (2015). Enhancement of knowledge and skills of community midwives in Sindh, Pakistan. *Journal of Asian Midwives (JAM)*, 2(2), 36–56. https://ecommons.aku.edu/jam/vol2/iss2/5/

Ashraf, H. (2020). Strengthening midwifery education in Pakistan: A systematic review. *Journal of Midwifery and Women's Health*, 28(4), 302–313. https://iris.who.int/bitstream/handle/10665/368771/1020-3397-2022-2804-302-313-eng.pdf?sequence=1

Gul, N., personal communication, November 20, 2024. Senior Community Midwife. Koohi Goth Hospital. Karachi.

Haroon, R., personal communication, December 5, 2024. Lecturer in Dow Institute of Nursing and Midwifery, Dow University of Health Sciences, Karachi.

Hezekiah, J. (1993). The pioneers of rural Pakistan: The lady health visitors. *Health Care for Women International*, 14(6), 493–502. https://doi.org/10.1080/07399339309516079.

Ilyas, N., personal communication, November 18, 2024. Dept Director, Punjab Nursing and Midwifery Examination Board, Lahore.

International Confederation of Midwives. (2021). ICM Global Standards for Midwifery Education (revised 2021). ICM, Netherlands. https://internationalmidwives. org/resources/using-the-competencies-in-a-midwifery-curriculum/ https://internationalmidwives.org/resources/global-standards-for-midwifery-education/ (accessed January 10, 2025).

Kulsoom, personal communication, Director General Nursing and Midwifery. Nursing and Midwifery Examination Board, Quetta, November 24, 2024.

Lakhani, A., Jan, R., Baig, M., Mubeen, K., Ali, S. A., Shahid, S., & Kaufman, K. (2018). Experiences of the graduates of the first baccalaureate midwifery programme in Pakistan: A descriptive exploratory study. *Midwifery*, 59, 94–99. https://doi.org/10.1016/j.midw.2018.01.008

Ministry of National Health Services, Regulations & Coordination. (2022). National Vision and Strategic Framework For Midwifery - 2022 published by the Ministry of National Health Services, Regulations & Coordination Pakistan. https://www.scribd.com/document/683267116/National-Vision-and-Strategic-Framework-for-Midwifery-2022

Mubeen, K., Jan, R., Sheikh, S., Lakhani, A., & Badar, S. J. (2019). Maternal and newborn outcomes of care from community midwives in Pakistan: A retrospective analysis of routine maternity data. *Midwifery*, 79, 102553. https://doi.org/10.1016/j.midw.2019.102553 https://pakistan.unfpa.org/en/topics/sexual-and-reproductive-health-9

Rehman, R., Ali, T. S., Khalid, S., & Ali, R. (2024). The ongoing evolution of mentorship: Advancing the formal mentorship program at AKU-SONAM. *Pakistan Journal of Medical Sciences*, 40(3Part-II), 514. https://doi.org/10.12669/pjms.40.3.8212

Sayani, A. H., Jan, R., Lennox, S., Mohammad, Y. J., & Awan, S. (2017a). Evaluating the results of mentorship training for community midwives in Sindh, Pakistan. *British Journal of Midwifery*, 25(8), 511–518. https://doi.org/10.12968/bjom.2017.25.8.511 https://pphisindh.org/home/technical_resources.php?type=Maternal%20Health

Sayani, A. H., Jan, R., Lennox, S., & Mohammad, Y. J. (2017b). Development of mentorship module and its feasibility for community midwives in Sindh, Pakistan: A pilot study. *Journal of Asian Midwives (JAM)*, 4(1), 51–64. https://ecommons.aku.edu/jam/vol4/iss1/6/

Upvall, M. J., Sochael, S., & Gonsalves, A. (2002). Behind the mud walls: The role and practice of lady health visitors in Pakistan. *Health Care for Women International*, 23(5), 432–441.

USAID. (2012). *The Community Midwives Program in Pakistan*. Research and Development Solutions. Available from: https://www.academia.edu/6150955/Community_Midwives_CMW_in_Pakistan

20

MIDWIFERY MENTORSHIP IN SCOTLAND

Gail Norris

For this chapter, the following terms will encompass:

Mentor	A Nursing and Midwifery Council (NMC) mentor is a registrant who, following successful completion of an NMC-approved mentor preparation programme – or comparable preparation that has been accredited by an approved educational institute (AEI) as meeting the NMC mentor requirements – has achieved the knowledge, skills and competence required to meet the defined outcomes.
Midwife Mentor	A midwife who has successfully completed an NMC-approved mentor preparation programme and has been supervised signing off on three occasions.
Practice supervisor	Practice supervisors' role is to support and supervise nursing and midwifery students in the practice learning environment.
Practice assessor:	Practice assessors assess and confirm the student's achievement of practice learning for a placement or a series of placements.
Academic assessor:	Academic assessors collate and confirm the student's achievement of proficiencies and programme outcomes in the academic environment for each part of the programme
Midwifery practitioner	Midwives are skilled, autonomous practitioners who apply knowledge safely and effectively, to optimise outcomes for all women and newborn infants.

DOI: 10.4324/9781003533733-21

Midwifery Education in the UK

Since 1922, the United Kingdom (UK) has been made up of four countries: England, Scotland, Wales (which collectively make up Great Britain) and Northern Ireland (Le Var, 1997). Within these four countries, the United Kingdom Central Council (UKCC) had responsibility for the maintenance of a central register of nurses, midwives and health visitors; it was also empowered to set out rules governing the education and training requirements for admission to the register (Le Var, 1997). The UKCC operated through several committees, the membership of which included members of the four National Boards. The National Boards (one each for England, Scotland, Wales and Northern Ireland) and were required to ensure that appropriate training courses were provided to enable people to meet the standards necessary for admission to the register (Le Var, 1997). One of the major turning points in history was the establishment of the Nursing and Midwifery Council (NMC) in 2002, replacing the UKCC (United Kingdom Central Council for Nursing, Midwifery, and Health Visiting). Midwifery practice in the UK has since been regulated by the NMC, which has responsibility for setting the educational standards for promoting high education standards for nurses, midwives in the UK and nursing associates in England (Nursing and Midwifery Council (NMC), 2024a).

The landscape of nursing and midwifery legislation and education within the UK has recently undergone more significant changes because of the publication of new standards (as summarised in Table 20.1). These changes mark a shift towards a more structured and collaborative approach to supervision and assessment within midwifery education. For more details on mentorship in the UK, please see Chapter 13: Midwifery Mentorship in the UK.

This chapter will delve into the historical development of midwifery legislation and education, alongside the recent changes introduced by the NMC. Of particular focus will be the transition from the traditional mentor model to the introduction of practice supervisors, practice assessors and academic assessors, as outlined in the NMC Part 2: *Standards for Supervision and Assessment* and how these principles have been applied within a Scottish context.

Current Midwifery Legislation and Education Standards

After a two-year consultation, during which the NMC collaborated with midwives, student midwives, women, families, other healthcare professionals, charities and advocacy groups from all four UK nations, new standards were co-produced to fully equip future midwives. The *Standards of Proficiency for Midwives* were initially published in 2019 and later redesigned

TABLE 20.1 Realising Professionalism Standards

Part 1: Standards for Nursing and Midwifery Education (2018a: 2 republished 2023a)	These standards provide a framework for learning culture, education and governance and quality, student learning and empowerment, educators and assessors and curriculum.
Part 2: Standards for Student Supervision and Assessment (2018b: republished 2023b)	These standards set out the expectations for the support, supervision and assessment of students in the practice environment.
Part 3: Standards for Pre-registration Midwifery Programmes (2019: republished 2024b)	These standards set out the legal requirements for all pre-registration midwifery programmes.
Standards of Proficiency for Midwives (2019: republished 2024c)	These standards specify the knowledge, understanding and skills that midwives must demonstrate at the point of qualification, when caring for women across the maternity journey, newborn infants, partners and families across all care settings.

in 2024c. Alongside this, the NMC also released *Realising Professionalism: Standards for Education and Training.* These were set out in three parts (Table 20.1).

The development of the current *Standards of proficiency for midwives* (2024c) was led by the Scottish Professor Mary Renfrew. The standards of proficiency were developed in alignment with the International Confederation of Midwives' definition of the midwife:

A midwife is a person who has successfully completed a midwifery education programme that is based on the ICM Essential Competencies for Midwifery Practice and the framework of the ICM Global Standards for Midwifery Education.

(Nursing and Midwifery Council (NMC), 2024c, p. 4)

Professor Mary Renfrew also incorporated her own evidence-based definition of midwifery, alongside the framework for quality maternal and newborn care from *The Lancet* Series. This framework defines a midwife as:

A skilled, knowledgeable, and compassionate provider of care for childbearing women, newborn infants, and families across the continuum of care—from pre-pregnancy, through pregnancy, birth, postpartum, and the early weeks of life.

(Renfrew et al, 2014, p. 1130)

The new *Standards of proficiency for midwives* (2024c) are divided into six domains that are interrelated and build upon each other. These include:

Domain 1: Being an accountable, autonomous, professional midwife.
Domain 2: Safe and effective midwifery care: promoting and providing continuity of care and carer,
Domain 3: Universal care for all women and newborn infants,
Domain 4: Additional care for women and newborn infants with complications, Domain 5: Promoting excellence: the midwife as colleague, scholar and leader
Domain 6: The midwife as a skilled practitioner.

The context in which these standards and the Realising Professionalism: Standards for Education and Training are embedded differs between the four countries of the UK. For more details on mentorship in the UK, please see Chapter 13: Midwifery Mentorship in the UK and Chapter 14: Midwifery Mentorship in Ireland.

Setting the Scottish Context

In Scotland, there are three universities, Edinburgh Napier University (ENU), University of the West of Scotland (UWS) and Robert Gordon University (RGU), which are NMC Approved Educational Institutions (AEI) that provide midwifery education (Nursing and Midwifery Council (NMC), 2024b). Each university provides a pre-registration bachelor of midwifery programme, which is three years in length (minimum 4600 hours) in addition Edinburgh Napier University offers a two-year midwifery programme (minimum of 3600 hours) for students who are already registered with the NMC as a registered first level nurse (adult) but wishes to gain a midwifery qualification (Nursing and Midwifery Council (NMC), 2024b).

The number of student midwives recruited onto each programme each year is dependent upon the Scottish Government commissioned numbers. This is unique to Scotland where the Chief Nursing Officer Directorate of the Scottish Government makes recommendations to the Scottish Funding Council on the target number of pre-registration nursing and midwifery student places to be commissioned each year, based on workforce projections (NHS, Education for Scotland, 2021). Hence, the three appointed Lead Midwives for Education (LME) work closely with The Scottish Government, NHS Education Scotland, Royal College of Midwives and the Heads of Midwifery across the 14 Health Boards in Scotland to ensure a sustainable midwifery workforce (Nursing and Midwifery Council (NMC), 2024b). Scottish students do not pay university tuition fees, and nursing and midwifery students are supported by the Scottish Government with an annual non-mean-tested bursary to the sum of £10,000. Travel to and from clinical practice placements is also supported by the Scottish Government. Both student nurses and midwives have supernumerary status throughout the three-year programme (Nursing and Midwifery Council (NMC), 2024b).

It is widely recognised, learning in clinical practice provides the perfect opportunity for student midwives to achieve the skills necessary to become safe and competent practitioners (Saukkoriipi et al., 2020). As such all-midwifery programmes in the UK consist of an equal balance of 50 per cent theory and 50 per cent practice learning (Nursing and Midwifery Council (NMC), 2024b). During the three-year programme students are taught to provide safe and effective care for women and families across a variety of settings including hospitals, midwife-led units, birth centres and communities. Individuals are taught to understand and facilitate normal birth, identify and manage complications and develop the leadership and management skills embedded within the six NMC domains (Nursing and Midwifery Council (NMC), 2024c). Safe and effective midwifery care also encompasses fundamental components such as critical thinking, problem solving and positive role modelling (Nursing and Midwifery Council (NMC), 2024c).

It is imperative the clinical practice environment is conducive to learning with supportive guidance and supervision to enable students to develop these skills (Gray, 2018). Arguably, the quality of midwifery students graduating is the responsibility of both midwifery practitioners and educators, with the NMC setting standards to support learning and assessment in clinical practice (Amod & Mkhize, 2023). In essence this means that the practical and clinical preparation of student midwives is entrusted to midwifery practitioners to clinically prepare students for role-taking, enabling them to become competent, safe and independent practitioners (Mkhize, 2023). The underlying rationale for this is that students learn from skilled midwives in a safe supportive environment. Historically, midwife mentors were seen as professional role models that could enhance the student's skills development and provision of care to mothers and babies (Sheenan et al., 2022).

History of Mentoring in the UK

Pre-project 2000, the apprenticeship model of training that took place within Schools of Nursing and Midwifery located within the hospital setting, meant that students *"learnt on the job"* and were supervised within the hospital environment. Granted that while this offered students valuable hands-on experience, it also presented learning challenges. Historically, Andrews and Wallis (1999) reported that this often resulted in trained staff spending a limited amount of time supervising students. Only 65% of those students who started training became registered, with the remainder either discontinuing training or failing at examinations (Le Var, 1997). Students were often treated as team members rather than students with learning needs, with issues concerning the theory and practice gap identified (Amod & Mkhize, 2023).

In response, Project 2000 was introduced by the regulatory body United Kingdom Central Council for Nursing (UKCC) and led to the development of the document *Project 2000: A New Preparation for Practice (UKCC, 1986)*. Project 2000 was a joint exercise with the four national bodies, with a remit to determine the education and training required in preparation for the professional practice of nursing, midwifery and health visiting in the UK (Ousey, 2011).

Project 2000 established a move of students away from schools of nursing and midwifery into higher education. The main recommendations from Project 2000 included:

1 A three-year nursing programme with a common foundation programme of two years and one year in a chosen branch specialty.
2 Branches to include adult nursing, children's nursing, mental health nursing and learning disability nursing.
3 The total programme to lead to a Diploma in Higher Education
4 Midwifery was a separate three-year direct entry programme.
5 Full student status, with no contribution to rostered service (supernumerary status).
6 Improved educational facilities and the development of links with the higher education sector (Ousey, 2011).

The UKCC saw the implementation of Project 2000 as the means to develop nursing and midwifery programmes that intertwined both theory and practice (Ousey, 2011). The way that students were supervised in clinical practice was subsequently challenged by the introduction of Project 2000, and this became the main driver for ensuring students were supported by mentors in clinical practice (West et al., 2008). In response, the UKCC produced *Standards for the Preparation of Teachers of Nursing, Midwifery and Health Visiting* to ensure all mentors and teachers had appropriate skills to prepare students for the changing healthcare needs and to ensure student learning experiences and needs were fully supported and valued (UKCC, 2000).

When the United Kingdom Central Council for Nursing (UKCC) was replaced by the NMC in 2002, the *Standards for the Preparation of Teachers of Nursing, Midwifery and Health Visiting* were replaced with the *NMC (2006) Standards to support learning and assessment in practice (SLAIP),* with a second edition published in 2008.

The NMC (2008) clearly defined a mentor as:

An NMC mentor is a registrant who, following successful completion of an NMC approved mentor preparation programme – or comparable preparation that has been accredited by an AEI as meeting the NMC mentor requirements – has achieved the knowledge, skills and competence required to meet the defined outcomes.

(Nursing and Midwifery Council (NMC), 2008, p. 23)

Historically, on a national scale, there were inconsistencies in the approach to mentorship prior to the publication of these standards. The NMC (2008) role of the mentor aligned with the International Confederation of Midwives (ICM) definition of the midwife as the mentor organised and coordinated student learning activities in practice just as a midwife would coordinate care of the woman, supervised students in learning situations and provided them with constructive feedback on their achievements, set and monitored achievement of realistic learning objectives and assessed student performance including the compassionate attributes and behaviours outlined by the ICM (Nursing and Midwifery Council (NMC), 2008). Essentially, the foundation of the *Standards to Support Learning and Assessment in Practice (SLAIP) (2008)* was to ensure students were fit for practice at the point of registration with the responsibility for this entrusted to the midwifery mentor (West et al., 2008).

In response, NHS Education Scotland developed a *National Approach to Mentor Preparation for Nurse and Midwives* (2013) to fully support the implementation of these standards consistently across Scotland.

Mentorship in Scotland involves a direct relationship between the mentor (midwife) and the mentee (midwifery student), whereby students worked closely with mentors who assessed them against the NMC competencies, namely the essential skills clusters (Nursing and Midwifery Council (NMC), 2009). Mentor preparation programmes in Scotland were designed with learning outcomes consistent with Scottish Credit and Qualifications Framework (SCQF level 9) and included three modules including learning, professional accountability and relationships and a final unit (which in some countries maybe called modules or course) on student assessment (NHS Education, 2013). The programmes were developed to include a minimum of 10 days of notional learning with a minimum of 5 days of protected learning time, which included 2 days of face-to-face contact time. However, Veeramah (2012) reported that mentors often received very little or no protected time while on mentorship preparation programmes.

In addition to ensuring each student was supervised by a mentor, the NMC standards (2008) stipulated, all student midwives on the NMC-approved pre-registration midwifery education programmes could only be supported and assessed by mentors who had met the additional sign-off mentor criteria (Nursing and Midwifery Council (NMC), 2008). This criterion required that all sign-off mentors had a working knowledge of the pre-registration programme requirements, practice assessment strategies and be supervised on at least three occasions for signing off proficiency by an existing sign-off mentor before they could be entered into local databases as a sign-off mentor (Nursing and Midwifery Council (NMC), 2008). The expectation was that sign-off mentors were experienced mentors who could make a judgement about the student suitability to be placed on the professional register (Andrews et al., 2010). While it was recognised that sign-off mentors would need an additional one hour per week to undertake this role, there was no additional funding to ensure this (Andrews et al., 2010).

All practice placement providers in Scotland were responsible for ensuring that an up-to-date local register/database of mentors was maintained, with annotations of those who have met the NMC additional criteria for assessing proficiency (sign-off mentors) (Nursing and Midwifery Council (NMC), 2008).

The standards required that every student had a named sign-off mentor for each period of practice learning, who supervised them at least 40% of the time (Nursing and Midwifery Council (NMC), 2008). Despite this students' experiences of continuity of mentor varied significantly, making this requirement unrealistic in the reality of the clinical setting (Halla & Choucri, 2019). Scottish students reported similar inconsistencies in their mentorship experiences. Arguably, some students relished working with other midwives as it enhanced their practice learning (Cherney-Morris and NMC, 2014). Mandatory clinical practice grading was also introduced into the midwifery curricula by the NMC in 2009 with the rationale that it demonstrated equal value between theory and practice (Nursing and Midwifery Council (NMC), 2009). As a result, UK universities independently developed competency-based assessment scales to grade students' hands-on care. Several studies reported grading as being problematic with students who got on well with their mentors receiving a favourable grade and reports of grade inflation (Gray and Donaldson, 2009; Smith, 2007). To ensure continuity of assessment from each period of practice learning each student was required to carry an ongoing achievement record of achievement, which shared information from mentor to mentor on their achievement of competencies (Nursing and Midwifery Council (NMC), 2008). This system was well-received and accepted by Scottish students, contributing to a smoother transition between practice placements and ensuring that students met the required standards at each stage of their education.

Introduction of the Practice Supervisor, Practice Supervisor and Academic Assessor

Publication of the new standards *The Standards for Student Supervision and Assessment* witnessed the dissolution of the term mentor and saw the introduction of new roles namely the *practice supervisor, practice assessor* and *academic assessor* (Nursing and Midwifery Council (NMC), 2023b).

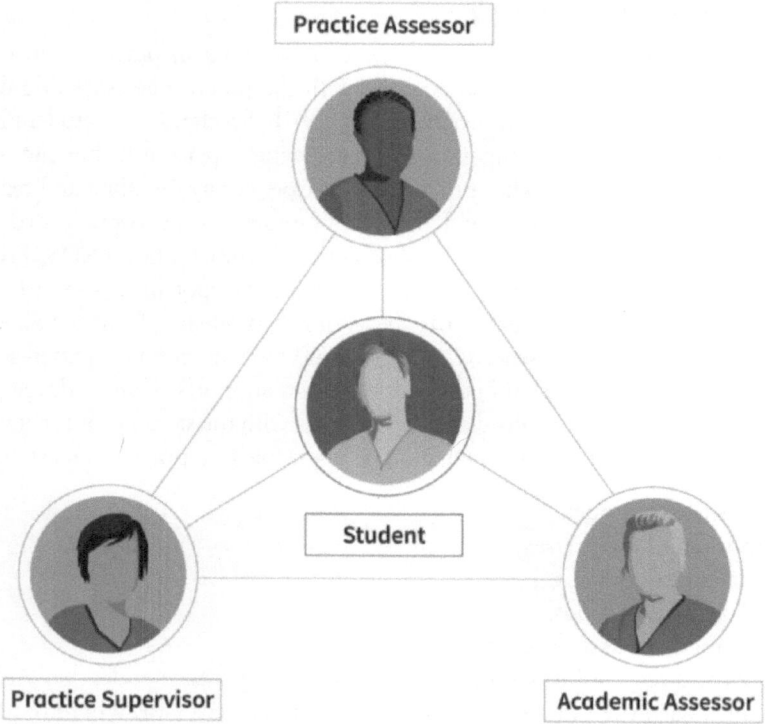

FIGURE 20.1 Regulatory roles for the supervision and assessment of nursing and midwifery students (reproduced by permission of NHS Education Scotland, 2019)

The current *Standards for Student Supervision and Assessment* (2023b) are outcome-focused and are designed to allow for local innovation in how each approved higher education institute (AEI) works in partnership with the clinical area to implement the practice supervisor, practice assessor and academic assessor roles to support student learning (Nursing and Midwifery Council (NMC), 2023b). In response, a Scottish national framework was developed providing guidance for the implementation of the practice supervisor, practice assessor and academic assessor roles (NHS, Education Scotland, 2019) (Figure 20.1).

REFLECTIVE ACTIVITY 1:

The NMC requirements should be considered when reading this next section. Please read the following: Standards for Student Supervision and Assessment

Each of these roles are now discussed in turn.

Role of the Practice Supervisor

The practice supervisor role supervises students learning in practice and is the main source of support for students along with the practice assessor and other staff (Figure 20.2 NHS Education Scotland, 2019). In Scotland, each student is assigned a nominated practice supervisor for each clinical placement but can work with and be supervised by other practice supervisors at any one time and regardless of the amount of time spent with the student, practice supervisors record their observations in the student's practice assessment documentation (NHS, Education Scotland, 2019). This provides students with the opportunity to work with different midwives and pick different aspects of role modelling from the different midwives (Hughes and Fraser, 2011). In Scotland the student's nominated supervisor conducts the student's initial orientation and supports them to develop an action plan of their learning need and agrees dates with the student for the interim and final performance review meetings. The main role of a practice supervisor:

- Acts as a role model,
- Supports and supervises,
- Provides feedback,
- Records observations,
- Contributes to assessments,
- Raises and respond to student conduct and competence concerns, and
- Engages with the practice assessor and academic assessor, where required (NHS, Education Scotland, 2019)

To fulfil this role the practice supervisor must have current knowledge and understanding of student proficiencies, programme outcomes and practice assessment document. In Scotland, a national pre-registration Midwifery Practice Assessment Document (MPAD) was developed to incorporate *Part 2: Standards for Student Supervision and Assessment* (Nursing and Midwifery Council (NMC), 2023b) and *the pre-registration midwifery proficiencies* (Nursing and Midwifery Council (NMC), 2024c).

Midwives at point of registration are expected to work in collaboration with the interdisciplinary and multiagency teams to provide midwifery care

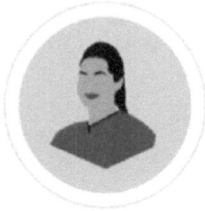

Practice Supervisor

FIGURE 20.2 Practice supervisor (reproduced by permission of NHS Education Scotland, 2019)

needed by women and newborn infants (Nursing and Midwifery Council (NMC), 2024c). Interprofessional practice learning experiences provide significant opportunities for student midwives to build these team working skills (Grace et al., 2016). The introduction of the new NMC standards, *The Standards for Student Supervision and Assessment* (Nursing and Midwifery Council (NMC), 2023b) recognises that interprofessional supervision by skilled practice supervisors can support students develop generic skills such as teamwork (Grace et al., 2016). In recognition of this The NMC *Realising professionalism standards* expect that nursing and midwifery students will experience interprofessional supervision from other registered health and social care professionals (Nursing and Midwifery Council (NMC), 2023b). However, practice supervisors must be registered with a professional regulator such as the Health Care Professionals Council (Nursing and Midwifery Council (NMC), 2023b) (see Table 20.2 as an example of how this can work).

At the point of registration the midwife must be able to demonstrate positive leadership and role modelling (Nursing and Midwifery Council (NMC), 2024c). Leadership development is therefore incorporated as part of the midwifery educational curricula with the recognition that interprofessional learning assists in leadership development (Nursing and Midwifery Council (NMC), 2024c; Van Diggele et al., 2020). For example, in Scotland, student midwives participate in multidisciplinary simulated obstetric emergency study days where they are involved in role play and immersive simulation. It has been widely recognised that mentors are crucial in the evaluation of the student's leadership and management competencies (Corbin et al., 2021).

Role of the Practice Assessor

In Scotland, student midwives must have registered midwives as their nominated practice assessors (NHS, Education Scotland, 2019). The role of a practice assessor (Figure 20.3 NHS Education Scotland, 2019) differs from the practice supervisor as their role is to assess the student's overall performance and confirm their achievement of practice learning. The practice assessor separates the responsibility for assessing the student from the practice supervisor with the hope of a more objective assessment of the student. The practice assessor is not required to supervise the student in practice but can contribute towards students' induction and orientation to the practice placement and may contributing to an initial meeting with the student, identifying student learning outcomes and agreeing dates for the interim and final performance review meetings (NHS, Education Scotland, 2019). To assess the student overall performance, the practice assessor must seek feedback from the practice supervisors regarding student conduct and performance (NHS, Education Scotland, 2019). Thus, regular communication between the practice supervisor and practice assessor is essential. Table 20.2 demonstrates how this can be achieved.

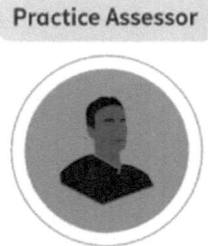

Practice Assessor

FIGURE 20.3   Practice Assessor (reproduced by permission of NHS Education Scotland, 2019)

Midwifery practice supervisors may also undertake the role of practice assessor; however, they cannot be a practice supervisor AND the nominated practice assessor for the same student (NHS, Education Scotland, 2019). Below is a summary of the role of the practice assessor:

- Seeks feedback from practice supervisors,
- Periodically observes students,
- Draws on evidence from other sources,
- Communicates and collaborates with the nominated academic assessor, and
- Makes and records objective, evidence-based assessments on student conduct, proficiency and achievement.

Academic Assessor Role

In Scotland, academic assessors are midwifery lecturers within an AEI who assess a student's learning for a part of the programme of education (NHS, Education Scotland, 2019). The academic assessor, in partnership with a nominated practice assessor, will communicate and collaborate to determine the student's achievement of proficiencies and programme outcomes for progression from one part of the programme to another (NHS, Education Scotland, 2019). The role of the academic assessor is summarised below:

- Communicates and collaborates with practice assessors,
- Makes and record objective, evidence-based assessments on student conduct, proficiency and achievement, and
- In partnership with the practice assessor, makes recommendations for progression for a part of the programme (NHS, Education Scotland, 2019).

Described below is the model used by Edinburgh Napier University.

- *The academic assessor may or may not be the personal development teacher for the student that they are confirming.*
- *A different academic assessor will be assigned to years 1, 2 and 3.*

Within the Scottish context, an example of how a student (Anna) can be best supported by practice supervisor, practice assessor and academic assessor throughout her eight-week clinical placement is noted in Table 20.2.

TABLE 20.2 Example of How a Student Can Be Supported in Clinical Practice By Practice Supervisor, Practice Assessor, and Academic Assessor (adapted from NHS, Education Scotland, 2019)

Week 1	Practice supervisor Karen and practice assessor Fiona undertake student orientation and induction to practice placement. Both the practice supervisor and practice assessor can agree dates for interim review and final assessment and records this in the MPAD. Both agree how they will communicate and collaborate for this student. Throughout the practice placement – the practice assessor, where possible, creates opportunities to observe Anna, such as during handovers, team meetings and/or when providing nursing or midwifery care and seeks feedback from practice supervisors
Week 2	Practice supervisors Karen, Elaine, Michelle and Diane supervise Anna the student, observe clinical skill and proficiency development and record in MPAD.
Week 3	Practice supervisors Elaine and Diane supervise Anna the student, observe communication and professional conduct development and record in MPAD.
Week 4	Practice supervisors Karen, Elaine and Michelle observe Anna develop clinical skills and proficiency. The practice assessor Fiona and/or the nominated practice supervisor Karen undertake the student's interim review meeting and records this in the MPAD
Week 5	Practice supervisors Karen, Elaine, Michelle and Diane supervise Anna the student, observe communication and professional conduct development and record in MPAD
Week 6	Practice supervisor Georgia supervises the student Anna, contributing towards the assessment and planning of midwifery care, and then Anna is allocated the afternoon to work with the paediatrician to develop her skills in examination of the newborn.
Week 7	Practice supervisors Elaine and Michelle observe the student develop clinical skills and proficiency.
week 8	Towards the end of the practice placement – the practice assessor Fiona draws on evidence from other sources (nominated practice supervisor/ supervisors) and their own observations to undertake a fair and objective assessment of the student's conduct, proficiency and achievement of their learning outcomes and records this in the MPAD. Practice assessor Fiona and academic assessor Stephanie collaborate to evaluate evidence of the students conduct and performance and make recommendations for the student.

TABLE 20.3 NHS Education for Scotland (NES): The Preparation for Practice Supervisors and Practice Assessors Preparation Programme

Unit 1	Roles and responsibilities
Unit 2	Learning theory
Unit 3	Creating a positive learning environment
Unit 4	Feedback
Unit 5	Assessment
Unit 6	Supporting learners

Preparation of the practice supervisor, practice assessor and academic assessor

The preparation of midwife practitioners is imperative to support midwifery students practice learning experience (Amod & Mkhize, 2023). Practice supervisor preparation is implemented in the final year of the pre-registration programme as all midwifery students at point of registration must be able to support and supervise students in the provision of midwifery care (Nursing and Midwifery Council (NMC), 2024c). In Scotland the NHS Education for Scotland (NES): The Preparation for Practice Supervisors and Practice Assessors preparation programme is utilised for this and consists of Units 1–6 outlined in Table 20.3. Available via the digital platform namely TURAS.

Practice Assessor Preparation

The preparation for the practice assessor appears to be less prescriptive now than previously. To develop knowledge, skills and experience to prepare for the practice assessor role individuals must complete a reflective self-assessment, which essentially involves reflecting on the role of the practice assessor and self -identification of areas for development. See Table 20.4 for example of self-assessment template. There are a variety of resources that can be utilised to upskill including face-to-face Preparation of Practice Assessor workshops and resources outlined at the end of this chapter.

REFLECTIVE ACTIVITY 2

If you are currently a practice assessor (mentor), reflect on your own self-assessment and areas for development OR

If you are currently a student, think of a time when you have been assessed by a practice assessor (mentor) in the clinical environment or within the university's clinical lab reflect on your perception of how they performed using the practice assessor template noting any areas for development.

TABLE 20.4 Practice Assessor Preparation: Reflective self-assessment (reproduced by permission of NHS Education for Scotland, 2019)

The NMC *practice supervisor and practice assessor requirements (What do I need to be able to do?)*	*Transferable skills (What knowledge, skills and experience do I currently have?)*	*Areas for development (What knowledge, skills and experience do I need to consolidate, enhance or develop?)*
Practice assessors • Conduct assessments to confirm student achievement of proficiencies and programme outcomes for practice learning • Assessment decisions are informed by feedback sought and received from practice supervisors • Make and record objective, evidence-based assessments on conduct, proficiency and achievement, drawing on student records, direct observations, student self-reflection and other sources • Maintain current knowledge and expertise relevant for the proficiencies and programme outcomes they are assessing • In partnership with the nominated academic assessor evaluate and recommend the student for progression for each part of the programme, in line with programme standards and local and national policies		

Preparation of the Academic Assessor

For midwifery lecturers without prior experience, preparation must include a selection or all the following:

• Undertake a reflective self-assessment to consider what knowledge, skills and experience referring to the academic assessor role and undertake development activities related to the academic assessor role (see Table 20.5). These activities can form the basis of conversation with line managers and provide evidence for revalidation purposes (Nursing and Midwifery Council (NMC), 2021).
• Work towards a teaching qualification and/or recognition as a Fellow from the UK Professional Standards Framework for teaching and supporting learning in higher education. (NHS Education for Scotland, 2019).

TABLE 20.5 Example of a Reflective Self-assessment Template for Transition to the Academic Assessor Role (reproduced by kind permission from NHS, Education Scotland, 2019)

The NMC academic assessor role (What do I need to be able to do?)	Transferable skills (What knowledge, skills and experience do I currently have?)	Areas for development (What knowledge, skills and experience do I need to consolidate, enhance or develop?)
• collate and confirm student achievement of proficiencies and programme outcomes in the academic environment for each part of the programme • make and record objective, evidence-based decisions on conduct, proficiency and achievement and recommendations for progression, drawing on student records and other sources • maintain current knowledge and expertise relevant for the proficiencies and programme outcomes they are assessing and confirming		

Continuity of Care/Carer in Scotland

Student midwives must demonstrate the ability to provide continuity of midwifery care/carer across the whole continuum of care (Nursing and Midwifery Council (NMC), 2024c). The Scottish Government (2017) *The Best Start Policy* principles are used as a driver to support the student experience of case loading (Table 20.6).

TABLE 20.6 Best Start Principles

- All mothers and babies are offered a truly family-centred, safe and compassionate approach to their care.
- Fathers, partners and other family members are actively encouraged and supported to become an integral part of all aspects of care.
- Women experience real continuity of care and carer across the whole maternity journey, with vulnerable families being offered any additional tailored support they may require.
- Services are redesigned using the best available evidence, to ensure optimal outcomes and sustainability, and maximise the opportunity to support normal birth processes and avoid unnecessary interventions.
- Staff are empathetic, skilled and well supported to deliver high quality, safe services every time.
- Multi-professional team working is the norm within an open and honest team culture, with everyone's contribution being equally valued.

Despite the NMC not prescribing a case-loading model for students, different continuity of care models (case loading/team midwifery) are in operation across Scotland. For example, the pre-registration midwifery programme at Edinburgh Napier University purposes:

1 *A minimum caseload should be two clients with a maximum of five.*
2 *It is also recognised that not all students will be able to provide intra-partum care – and that this will be dependent upon when clients go into labour and individual student commitments.*

To support students in these environments, the practice supervisor, practice assessor and academic assessor model are embedded.

REFLECTIVE ACTIVITY 3

Please read the following scenario

Scenario 1

Sarah is a first-year student midwife who has been assigned to the Willow community team of midwives for her first clinical placement.
   You are **Sarah's nominated practice supervisor. In, preparation for Sarah's first clinical placement can you :**

1 Identify the practice learning experiences available for her
2 Consider what links you have with other practice learning environments that would provide Sarah with a varied learning experience (e.g. charities, third sector).

Post-Registration Students

The Scottish practice supervisor, practice assessor and academic assessor framework was developed to support, supervise and assess both pre-registration and post-registration nursing and midwifery students. For post-registration students, the framework provides a structured approach to mentorship and assessment, which is crucial for ensuring consistent quality in continuing professional development. The evolving nature of its application with post-registration students will likely address challenges such as the differing needs of post-registration students, who may require more specialised support and assessment tailored to their advanced roles. With the continued use of this framework and student feedback adjustments are likely to refine the process, ensuring that it remains fit for purpose.

Summary

In summary, the chapter has explored the role of the midwifery mentor within the UK context, beginning first by tracing the historical development of the role and how this has evolved into the practice supervisors, practice assessors and academic assessors, particularly in Scotland. The chapter outlines how these roles are formalised within the UK's midwifery legislative framework, focusing on how midwives are developed for these roles and their significance in supporting both pre- and post-registration midwives to meet their learning needs.

SUPPORTING RESOURCES

Please use the following resource links:

- https://learn.nes.nhs.scot/45749/future-nurse-and-midwife/practice-supervisors-and-practice-assessors-learning-resource
- https://www.nmc.org.uk/globalassets/sitedocuments/education-standards/student-supervision-assessment.pdf
- https://learn.nes.nhs.scot/44454
- https://www.nmahpdevelopmentframework.nes.scot.nhs.uk/
- https://learn.nes.nhs.scot/735/flying-start-nhs
- https://www.nmc.org.uk/standards/standards-for-midwives/standards-of-proficiency-for-midwives/

ACTIVITY 3 POTENTIAL ANSWERS

Scenario 1

1 As Sarah's nominated practice supervisor, you are responsible for Sarah's initial orientation and should support her to develop an action plan of her learning needs at the appropriate academic level of the programme. You can review the students assessment document to guide you with this and ask Sarah to identify some of her own learning outcomes that she wishes to achieve with you. You can direct Sarah to read around some of the topics related to her learning plan. Plan learning activities that will help Sarah achieve her learning outcomes, e.g. attendance at an antenatal clinic affords the opportunity to observe the midwife's communication skills, practice clinical skills,

e.g. BP, abdominal palpation. You could arrange for Sarah to observe some postnatal visits and breastfeeding support offered to breastfeeding women. This placement also gives Sarah the opportunity to participate in postnatal examinations of both mother and baby. As the nominated practice supervisor you need to agree dates with Sarah for the interim and final performance review meeting. Her nominated practice assessor might want to be present at Sarah's orientation and help support the development of her action plan.

2 You could arrange time for Sarah to visit breastfeeding peer support groups, local charity groups, e.g. Dads Rock (fathers postnatal and toddler group) Sure Start Services (in Scotland, this is a social development group that supports the development of early relationships between parents and children, good parenting skills, family functioning and early identification and support of children with emotional, learning or behavioural difficulties). Consider arranging time with other healthcare professionals, e.g. GP. Health Visitor, community mental health team or community physiotherapist. This will give Sarah the opportunity to understand other roles within the multidisciplinary teams.

References

Amod, H., & Mkhize, S. W. (2023). Supporting midwifery students during clinical practice: Results of a systematic scoping review. *Interactive Journal of Medical Research*, 12(1), e36380.

Andrews, M., Brewer, M., Buchan, T., Denne, A., Hammond, J., Hardy, G., Jacobs, L., McKenzie, L., & West, S. (2010). Implementation and sustainability of the nursing and midwifery standards for mentoring in the UK. *Nurse Education in Practice*, 10(5), 251–255.

Andrews, M., & Wallis, M. (1999). Mentorship in nursing: A literature review. *Journal of Advanced Nursing*, 29(1), 201–207.

Chenery-Morris, S., & NMC (2014). Exploring students' and mentors' experiences of grading midwifery practice. *Evidence Based Midwifery*, 12(3), 101.

Corbin, A., Darling, E., Pearce-Kelly, T., & Wise, K. (2021). The application of health leadership competencies around the world to the Canadian midwifery profession: A scoping review: L'Application à la Profession de sage-femme au Canada de compétences en Leadership de la santé provenant du monde entier: examen de la portée. *Canadian Journal of Midwifery Research and Practice*, 20(1), 18–30.

Grace, S., McLeod, G., Streckfuss, J., Ingram, L., & Morgan, A. (2016). Preparing health students for interprofessional placements. *Nurse Education in Practice*, 17, 15–21.

Gray, M. (2018). Midwifery mentorship: What do we know about the mentors' perspective of the role? *Australian Midwifery News*, 18(1), 50–51.

Gray, M. A., & Donaldson, J. (2009). *Exploring Issues in the Use of Grading in Practice: Literature Review*. Edinburgh Napier University, Edinburgh.

Hallam, E., & Choucri, L. (2019). A literature review exploring student midwives' experiences of continuity of mentorship on the labour ward. *British Journal of Midwifery*, 27(2), 115–119.

Hughes, A. J., & Fraser, D. M. (2011). "There are guiding hands and there are controlling hands": Student midwives experience of mentorship in the UK. *Midwifery*, 27(4), 477–483.

Le Var, R. M. (1997). Project 2000: A new preparation for practice—has policy been realized? Part I. *Nurse Education Today*, 17(3), 171–177.

NHS Education for Scotland (NES). (2019) *A National Framework For Practice Supervisors, Practice Assessors And Academic Assessors in Scotland*. https://www.nes.scot.nhs.uk/media/fxdd4d01/scottish_approach_to_student_supervision_and_assessment_interactive.pdf

NHS Education for Scotland (NES) (2021) *The Midwifery Workforce and Education Review for Scotland*. https://www.nes.scot.nhs.uk/media/kmnod1av/the-midwifery-workforce-and-education-review-for-scotland.pdf

NHS Education Scotland. (2013). *National Approach to Mentor Preparation for Nurse and Midwives Core Curriculum Framework* (2nd ed.). NES.

Nursing and Midwifery (2024c). *Standards of Proficiency for Midwives*. NMC.

Nursing and Midwifery Council (NMC) (2008). *Standards to Support Learning and Assessment in Practice*. NMC.

Nursing and Midwifery Council (NMC). (2009). *Standards for pre-Registration Midwifery Education*. NMC.

Nursing and Midwifery Council (NMC). (2021). *What is revalidation?* https://www.nmc.org.uk/revalidation/overview/what-is-revalidation/

Nursing and Midwifery Council (NMC). (2023a). *Part 1: Standards Framework for Nursing and Midwifery Education*. NMC.

Nursing and Midwifery Council (NMC). (2023b). *Part 2: Standards for Student Supervision and Assessment*. NMC.

Nursing and Midwifery Council (NMC). (2024a). *Nursing and Midwifery Council* https://www.nmc.org.uk/

Nursing and Midwifery Council (NMC). (2024b). *Part 3: Standards for pre-Registration Midwifery Programmes*. NMC.

Ousey, K. (2011). The changing face of student nurse education and training programmes. *Wounds UK*, 7(1), 70–75. ISSN 1746-6814

Renfrew, M. J., McFadden, A., Bastos, M. H., Campbell, J., Channon, A. A., Cheung, N. F., Delage, D., Downe, S., Powell, K., McCormick, F., & Declercq, E. (2014). Midwifery and quality care: Findings from a new evidence-informed framework for maternal and newborn care. *The Lancet*, 384(9948), 1129–1145.

Saukkoriipi, M., Tuomikoski, A., Sivonen, P., Kärsämänoja, T., Laitinen, A., Tähtinen, T., Kääriäinen, M., Kuivila, H., Juntunen, J., Tomietto, M., & Mikkonen, K. (2020). Clustering clinical learning environment and mentoring perceptions of nursing and midwifery students: A cross-sectional study. *Journal of Advanced Nursing*, 76(9), 2336–2347.

Scottish Government. (2017). *The best start: five-year plan for maternity and neonatal care*. https://www.gov.scot/publications/best-start-five-year-forward-plan-maternity-neonatal-care-scotland/

Sheehan, A., Elmir, R., Hammond, A., Schmied, V., Coulton, S., Sorensen, K., Arundell, F., Keedle, H., Dahlen, H., & Burns, E. (2022). The midwife-student mentor relationship: Creating the virtuous circle. *Women and Birth*, 35(5), e512–e520.

Smith, J. (2007). Assessing and grading students' clinical practice: midwives' lived experience. *Evidence-Based Midwifery*, 5(4), 112–119.

United Kingdom Central Council for Nursing, Midwifery and Health Visiting. (2000). *Standards for the Preparation of Teachers of Nursing, Midwifery and Health Visiting*. UKCC.

United Kingdom Central Council for Nursing, Midwifery and Health Visiting. Education Policy Advisory Committee. Project Group. (1986). *Project 2000: A New Preparation for Practice*. United Kingdom Central Council for Nursing, Midwifery and Health Visiting.

Van Diggele, C., Burgess, A., Roberts, C., & Mellis, C. (2020). Leadership in healthcare education. *BMC Medical Education, 20,* 1–6.

Veeramah, V. (2012). Effectiveness of the new NMC mentor preparation course. *British Journal of Nursing, 21*(7), 413–418.

West, S., Clark, T., & Jasper, M. (2008). *Enabling Learning in Nursing and Midwifery Practice*. John Wiley & Sons.

21

MIDWIFE MENTORING IN THAILAND

*Bootsakon S. Guyot, Saisamorn Chaleoykitti,
and Daniel K. Guyot*

Thailand and Midwifery Care

Thailand, a geographically small country, has diverse environments ranging from tropical beaches and small islands to bustling metropolitan regions. Thailand's population of 66 million people has distinct regional dialects. The people are 92% Buddhist, 5% Muslim, and 1% Christian. Births in Thailand have been declining over the last decade, from 776,370 births in 2013 to 517,934 births in 2023 (Bureau of Registration Administration, 2023) his long-term decline is linked to increasing educational levels, prosperity, and an immensely popular condom campaign begun in the 1970s by Mechai Viravaidya (Bristol, 2008; Harris & Thaiprayoon, 2022). Births per year are expected to continue to decline to a projected 491,000 births in 2040 (Ministry of Public Health, 2024).

Traditional midwifery practice in Thailand was local, holistic, and provided by midwives (*Maw-Tam-Yae Thai*) who had experiential knowledge but little formal training (Boonterm et al., 2024). These women provided prenatal counselling, supported pregnant women to give birth in their own homes, and supported the health of mothers and newborns through counselling, food recommendations, and herbs. Today, a few traditional midwives practice in rural and mountainous areas particularly along the Thai-Myanmar border (Kruekaew & Kritcharoen, 2018).

In 1985, the Thai Nursing and Midwifery Council gained government recognition as the nursing accrediting agency and kept the initial role of midwifery as forming central competencies for all RNs. Thus, the authority belongs to the nursing profession to shape and continue to reshape the modern practice of midwifery, precepting, and mentoring (Vlerick et al., 2024;

DOI: 10.4324/9781003533733-22

Thamsrisawat, 2016). Recognition of the accrediting agency also led to the integration of nursing and midwifery education qualifications with all Thai Nurses also being qualified midwives (TNMC, 1997). Midwifery education is explained further in the next section.

In 2014, the Ministry of Public Health stipulated that childbirth should take place at hospitals, except in emergencies when the mother could not reach a public or private hospital in time (Ministry of Public Health, 2024; Weckend et al., 2022). In 2019, privately operated nurse-led clinics were authorised by the National Health Security Office and the Thai National Nursing and Midwifery Council (TNMC, 1997). For Thai citizens, all services at these clinics are paid for through Thailand's universal healthcare system. Any nurse-midwife can open a clinic to provide essential care for childbearing women covering health education, and prenatal and postnatal care. However, labour and birth care are not permitted. During the Covid-19 pandemic, an exception allowed midwife births for expecting mothers in mountainous areas where travel to a hospital could take six to nine hours. The "Safe Birth for All" project was launched via a public-private partnership between the Thai Ministry of Public Health, United Nations, and the Recliff Corporation (Ministry of Public Health, 2024). These limited and crucial exemptions provide roles for non-Thai midwives and midwifery mentors to work directly for aid agencies such as the United Nations, the Red Cross, and Doctors Without Borders.

In 2023, the Thai government reimbursed 22,067,700 Baht for services across 22,750 cases, at 186 nurse-led clinics (TNMC, 2023). Economic incentives as well as cultural incentives, such as the freedom to create your own work environment, could prompt rapid growth in the number of nurse-led clinics, thus creating the need for mentoring in community-based midwifery and in midwifery management. It is important to underscore the helpful role the Ministry of Public Health continues to play through constant monitoring of and support for nurse-led clinics. The ministry, which receives electronic data on every billed health service, constantly monitors trends in healthcare delivery and also rolls out new health promotion programmes and campaigns. They also act as a clearing house for professional development opportunities (Sirisomboon et al., 2024; Srisaeng et al., 2020). Further, they do all the media, advertising, and promotion for nurse-led clinics. In fact, clinics are not allowed to put up their own signage. Signage is provided and continually updated by the Ministry of Public Health.

Midwifery Education in Thailand

All Thai Nurses are also trained midwives as midwifery education is integrated into the 3rd and 4th year of all nursing curricula and is covered in the licensing process. Thailand has accredited 87 nursing-midwifery educational institutions, with an additional 22 institutions approved to open new faculties of nursing. The tuition cost for a four-year bachelor's in nursing-midwifery science ranges from 281,000 Baht at Kasetsart University (Thai language programme) to 690,000 Baht at Assumption University (English language programme) (Assumption University, 2024). Other universities with English language international programmes in nursing and midwifery science include Asia-Pacific International University, Chiang Mai University, Huachiew Chalermprakiet University, Shinawatra University, Saint Louis College, and St. Theresa University.

Midwifery Curricula

The nurse-midwifery curricula and licensure requirements are set by the Thai Nursing and Midwifery Council (TNMC) which was established in 1985, by the Nurses' Association of Thailand. As noted earlier, during the third year of the educational programme, students spend 30 weeks (240 hours) in a hospital maternity ward to translate theory into practice. Moreover, they have provided practicing preparation of antenatal care and obstetric simulation for increasing their confident and selves efficacy of midwifery care at labor room (Kuesakul et al., 2024). It is not until their fourth year that there are specific requirements around a minimum number of high-risk births that a student must attend. In essence each nurse/midwife student is required to take care of pregnant women in the antenatal care clinic for a total of ten women (five women who experience a normal pregnancy, and five women who experience a high-risk pregnancy), at least two women who experience normal physiological labour and birth, as well as five women who experience birth complications (e.g., forceps-assisted birth/vacuum-assisted birth/cesarean birth)(Liblub et al., 2020)In the postnatal period a student nurse-midwife must care for five women (two who experience normal postnatal care and at least three women who experience common postpartum complications). Nurse-midwifery students' educational programmes are divided into eight areas of care: (1) obstetric nursing; (2) maternal and child nursing; (3) pediatric nursing; (4) adult nursing; (5) geriatric nursing; (6) mental health and psychiatric nursing; (7) community health nursing and primary medical care; and (8) the law for professional nursing and midwifery (Boonterm et al., 2024; TNMC, 1997; WHO, 2020).

Midwifery Preceptors and Undergraduate Nurse-Midwife Education

In Thailand the term preceptor is reserved for teachers of undergraduate nurse-midwifery students. Midwifery preceptors must have an active nursing license, a Bachelor of Nursing Science with at least two years' experience in midwifery practice, have completed the 30-hour preceptor training course, and have passed the certificate exam from TNMC.

The role of a preceptor in Thailand is to support and educate undergraduate nurse-midwifery students and to help the new nurse-midwife gain confidence in their skills in clinical settings (Pezaro, et al., 2024; Pongboriboon, 2018). Students are not permitted to undertake any clinical care without a preceptor present; however, they can visit the women assigned to them in the birth room and in the postpartum care department. Additionally, they can provide knowledge about HIV/AIDS prevention during pregnancy to reduce newborn infection and maintain good maternal and child health (Harris & Thaiprayoon, 2022). A preceptor can integrate the nursing processes based on the essential five techniques for helping nurse-midwifery students including: (1) nursing assignment; (2) clinical teaching bedside education; (3) nurse-midwifery conferences; (4) nurse-midwifery rounds; and (5) evidence-based practice (Hanucharurnkul, 2022; Pongboriboon, 2018; Thamsrisawat, 2016; TNMC, 1977). They focus on basic midwifery skills during clinical teaching and work alongside a maximum of eight nurse-midwifery students for an eight-hour shift. Preceptors facilitate students in developing skills in eight areas:

1 Caring for pregnant women, newborns and families during pregnancy, childbirth, and the postnatal period, adapting to each woman's needs.
2 Screening for health risks and make appropriate referrals.
3 Assisting in normal deliveries and perform episiotomy and repair.
4 Effectively promoting breastfeeding.
5 Assisting a physician in performing obstetric procedures.
6 Providing family planning services within the scope of the nursing profession.
7 Teaching, advising, and educating women on safe sex, marriage preparation, preparation for becoming parents, childbirth preparation, and care of mother during pregnancy, labour, and care of newborns.
8 Promoting bonding among fathers, mothers, newborns, and family members during the pregnancy, birthing process, and postnatal period (Buakhai & Rithpho, 2019; Hanucharurnkul, 2022; Pongboriboon, 2018; Thamsrisawat, 2016; TNMC, 1997).

Mentorship in Thai Hospitals

Some previous studies revealed that the mentorship system was the key to filling the gaps of nursing and midwifery shortage in the fields of nurse-midwife in clinical practice and education (Mala et al., 2024; Amod et al., 2024; Bradford et al., 2022; Hanucharurnkul, 2022; Nertprasertkul & Jansoontraporn, 2021; Thamsrisawat, 2016). The term mentor is used for those who guide/

educate registered nurse/midwives and graduate students (Sarnkhaowhom & Suwathanpornkul, 2018; Proctor, 2001). Nurses can specialise in midwifery by obtaining advanced clinical supervision and earning an advanced degree (Bampenphon, 2023; Nantsupawat et al., 2019; Benner, 1983;) Well respected universities offer a Master of Nursing Science in Advanced Midwifery Practice, or in a related field. PhD programmes are offered in Advanced Midwifery/Maternal and Child Health Nursing or a related field. A new degree is now offered, the Doctor of Nursing Practice in Advanced Midwifery, DNP (TNMC, 2024).

Midwifery mentors are registered nurse-midwives with a master's degree in midwifery nursing or related fields with approximately 3,000 hours of midwifery experiences. Mentors do not need the preceptor's certificate, rather there is an educational programme (course), which once successfully completed results in the nurse-midwife becoming a certified mentor. The nurse-midwives are registered into the programme though nursing administrator selection or self-selection. Self-selection involves an Individual Development Plan (IDP) relevant to the department the nurse-midwife is working in to receive a full scholarship for a master's degree in a nursing science programme in mentorship. This master's in advanced midwifery is run by nursing departments and costs approximately 450,000–500,000 Baht for the two years' programme. Coursework earns 24 credits and a research thesis 12 credits. The essential competencies of mentors include:

1 following the standards of professional nursing and midwifery set by the TNMC,
2 transferring tacit and explicit knowledge of nursing and midwifery skills to support mentees,
3 taking administrative leadership to improve the quality of nursing management, and
4 using effective communication to develop the nursing care system and around 3000 hours of clinical practice (Hanucharurnkul, 2022; Thamsrisawat, 2016; TNMC, 1997).

Upon completion of the Master's qualification, one can apply for the qualifying examination of advanced practice nurse (APN) from TNMC by submitting three case studies, research publications, and an oral presentation to the TNMC's committees.

Advanced Practice Nurses in Midwifery

To help readers understand how an APN functions within Thailand, we have included a scenario of a day in the life of a midwifery APN.

SCENARIO

An APN in midwifery was assigned by the head of hospital nursing department as mentor for eight postgraduate nurse-midwifery students. She worked alongside all of them, applying the nursing process and care for childbearing women in a ward environment. She provided bedside teaching about electronic fetal monitoring (EFM), the Leopold maneuver to evaluate the fetal position, and applying an antocodynamometer on the fundus. She allocated the students to appropriate women supporting them to achieve proficiency in all outcome-based standards of midwifery education. The APN as mentor of new midwives was also a role model for new nurse-midwives as mentees. She provided support while new graduates gained clinical experience and confidence in professional skills. The APN worked in partnership with the mentee, providing important information. Then she provided an opportunity for the mentee to do more self-study and self-learning in government Universities based on her confirmation and reflection of what was good or what should be improved to become more proficient and competent in specific skills. After the mentees finished their practice, the mentor provided feedback to her mentees.

Hospital-based APN midwives oversee individualised care for women throughout pregnancy to serve the mother and newborn as individuals, families, and communities. Home visits are a crucial aspect of this care and allow for both observation of, and health promotion education about potential risk factors such as addiction or smoking (Guyot & Tungtrongvisolkit, 2024) (Therefore, the midwifery APN is a specialist in maternity care, including newborn care Hanucharurnkul, 2022; Pongboriboon, 2018; Thamsrisawat, 2016).

Non-Thai Registered Nurse-Midwives

The TNMC awards licensure to non-Thai registered nurses who graduated outside of Thailand only if they pass the Thai language nursing and midwifery licensure examination. Although a few non-Thai RNs work at international hospitals catering to foreign passport holders, the authors were unable to identify any non-Thai nurse-midwives.

The Future of Midwifery Mentorship in Thailand

In Thailand, as throughout the developing world, traditional midwifery remains only in rural and remote regions. As modernisation spreads into remote areas, the current trend is for nurse-midwives to work in hospitals where doctors are the ultimate decision makers (Bradford et al., 2022). Thai nurse-midwives work in institutions designed for doctors, confining their roles as assistants to doctors. The current requirement that all births should take place in hospitals with a doctor ultimately in charge of care decisions, diminishes the role of the midwife in the decision-making process.

The innovation of nurse-run clinics has created two expansive, essential, and exciting roles for nurse-midwives and hence two new strong roles for mentors (Amonprompukdee et al., 2020) They are community-based nursing/midwifery and community clinic management. Because the demand for the clinics comes from low-income communities, the new nurse/midwives will have to learn how to transfer their hospital skills to a clinic without standard hospital equipment and into homes with few amenities (Kanopthummakul & Roonpho, 2024).

New faculties of nursing/midwifery can bring fresh ideas and draw on the best evidence-based practices from around the world to support Thailand midwifery curriculum development. Further the influence of international midwives into the Thai maternity system will help shape future maternity care and education. Kasetsart University is one of the top 5 public universities in Thailand racing to hire the best faculty and become a center of excellence, already has over 2600 applicants vying for 70 spots in its inaugural class starting May 2025. At KU-Nurse the department of Maternal & Child Health Nursing and Midwifery is striving to become a national leader in midwifery education for undergraduates, preceptors, and mentors with Thailand's first center for clinical midwifery simulation and biofeedback-based resiliency training.

Decades of shortages in nurse-midwives continue to cause crowding at government hospitals. Staff shortages are further exacerbated by nurse-midwife "burnout". In the short term, implementation of effective resilience training with mindfulness and biofeedback learning (Khazan, 2019; Lehrer et al., 2020) can help mitigate the erosion of this workforce by stanching the exodus of staff. Over a longer period, two recent developments to address nurse-midwife shortages have the potential to positively impact midwifery mentorship and leadership in innovations in maternal and child health care delivery in Thailand. First, to reduce to volume of visits to hospitals, nurse-midwives are now empowered to open their own primary care clinics, where they have the freedom to implement advances in integrative medicine such as biofeedback therapy for stress reduction during childbirth. Second, to meet the demand for more nurses in public and private institutions across Thailand, there is a demand for more Bachelor of Nursing & midwifery science programmes (22 new programmes approved in 2024). New programmes create space for innovations such as incorporating resiliency training in the core curricula. Taken together, we believe these developments create the environment for great advancements in midwifery mentorship and midwifery care in Thailand.

REFLECTIVE ACTIVITY 1

Fostering growth and resilience is at the heart of the restorative function of clinical supervision. In *"Resilience training that can change the brain"*, Tabibnia and Radecki (2018) describe 15 strategies that boost resilience. (Figure 21.1 Resilience training that can change the brain [Adapted from Tabibnia & Radecki, 2018]). The diagram shows 15 strategies that can increase resilience and lead to long-term change in the nervous system. Cognitive pathways are shown on the left. Behavioral pathways are shown on the right. Three mindset factors (concentric blue circles) can improve learning and implementation of these resilience-boosting strategies. Thin arrows from these strategies converge in a thicker arrow illustrating the additive effect of using multiple strategies. As the arrows pass through the concentric circles representing the mindset factors they grow in thickness depicting the additive effects on neuroplasticity and resilience. For your convenience we have included the 15 strategies in a figure Resilience training that can change the brain, reproduced from the original article. However, we encourage you to read the original article. It could possibly change the life of your brain

- Choose three strategies to increase your resilience. As you learn to implement these strategies, teach them to a friend, a student, or a co-worker.

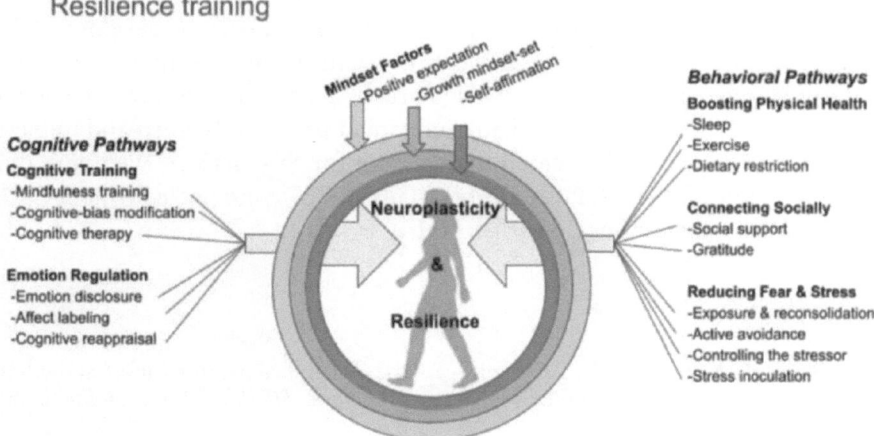

FIGURE 21.1   Resilience training that can change the brain (Adapted from Tabibnia & Radecki, 2018)

REFLECTIVE ACTIVITY 2

Biofeedback learning boots resilience through changes in the brain and the peripheral nervous system. Heart rate variability biofeedback improves emotional and physical health and performance (Leher et al., 2020). Increasingly biofeedback is used to improve the performance of individuals and teams, including teams of astronauts, elite US military units, Olympians, and college athletes and performing artists (Khazan, 2019; Thompson & Thompson, 2021). See https://aapb.org/ for more information.

After familiarising yourself with biofeedback learning, consider the following questions.

- Could biofeedback learning be used as a complementary strategy for fostering the growth and resilience of midwifery students, midwives, and their mentors?
- Why or why not?
- Would you consider listing biofeedback as a 16th strategy for resilience training?
- Can you think of any other strategies for resilience training that might be added to Tabinia and Radecki's (2018) list?

Acknowledgements

We thank the Thailand Nursing and Midwifery Council for developing the public-private partnership framework to grant all nurse-midwives the opportunity to create their own nurse-led primary care clinics to promote better health for all people. We also thank individual pregnant women and nursing students who provided essential information for this chapter. We thank our parents, James F. Guyot, PhD, Dorothy Guyot, PhD, and uncle William Carlson, MD for suggestions on earlier drafts.

References

Amod, H. B., Ndlovu, L., & Brysiewicz, P. (2024). Clinical mentorship of midwifery students: The perceptions of registered midwives. *Health SA Gesondheid*, 29, 2492.

Amonprompukdee, A., Junprasert, T., & Surakarn, A. (2020). Nursing supervision: A scoping review. *Nursing Journal of The Ministry of Public Health*, 30(3), 144–157.

Assumption University. (2024). Approximate fees for International Students in undergraduate programs. https://admissions.au.edu/wp-content/uploads/2024/10/TUITION-FEES-EN8.png

Bampenphon, S. (2023). The effect of clinical supervision model in nursing care process for nurses. *Hua Hin Medical Journal, 3*(3), 57–71.

Benner, P. (1983). *From Novice to Expert: Excellence and Power in Clinical Nursing Practice* (pp. 13–34). Addison-Wesley.

Boonterm, B., Kamdangyodtai, Y., & Chuthaputti, A. (2024). History, present and prospect of Thai traditional medicine. In *History, Present and Prospect of World Traditional Medicine* (pp. 703–760).

Bradford, H., Hines, H. F., Labko, Y., Peasley, A., Valentin-Welch, M., & Breedlove, G. (2022). Midwives mentoring midwives: A review of the evidence and Best practice recommendations. *Journal of Midwifery & Women's Health, 67*(1), 21–30.

Bristol, N. (2008). Mechai Viravaidya: Thailand's "Condom King". *The Lancet, 371*(9607), 109.

Buakhai, P., & Rithpho, P. (2019). Reflections of positive experiences in midwifery and nursing of maternal-newborn education in Thailand: Lessons learned from Naresuan university. *Journal of Health and Caring Sciences, 1*(2), 110–117.

Bureau of Registration Administration. (2023). *Official statistics registration systems.* https://www.bora.dopa.go.th/.

Guyot, B. S., & Tungtrongvisolkit, N. (2024). The development of nursing model for promoting optimal birth outcomes in pregnant women with secondhand smoke exposure. *Journal of The Royal Thai Army Nurses, 25*(1), 374–382.

Hanucharurnkul, S. (2022). Advanced practice nursing: Importance and development. *Thai Journal of Nursing and Midwifery Practice, 9*(1), 5–20. Retrieved from https://he02.tci-thaijo.org/index.php/apnj/article/view/257491.

Harris, J., & Thaiprayoon, S. (2022). Common factors in HIV/AIDS prevention success: Lessons from Thailand. *BMC Health Services Research, 22*(1), 1487.

Kanopthummakul, V., & Roonpho, P. (2024). Factors influencing intentions to resign among personnel: A case study of public health professionals in warm community nursing clinics (Doctoral dissertation, Silpakorn University).

Khazan, I. (2019). *Biofeedback and Mindfulness in Everyday Life: Practical Solutions for Improving Your Health and Performance* (p. 386). W.W. Norton, & Company.

Kruekaew, J., & Kritcharoen, S. (2018). Thai Traditional midwifery care. *Journal of Research in Nursing-Midwifery and Health Sciences, 38*(1), 103–110.

Kuesakul, K., Nuampa, S., Pungbangkadee, R., Ramjan, L., & Ratinthorn, A. (2024). Evaluation of antenatal simulation-based learning on satisfaction and self-confidence levels among Thai undergraduate nursing students during the COVID-19 pandemic: A mixed-method study. *BMC Nursing, 23*(1), 161.

Lehrer, P., Kaur, K., Sharma, A., Shah, K., Huseby, R., Bhavsar, J., & Zhang, Y. (2020). Heart rate variability biofeedback improves emotional and physical health and performance: A systematic review and meta analysis. *Applied Psychophysiology and Biofeedback, 45*, 109–129.

Liblub, S., Gum, L., & Bazargan, M. (2020). How do pregnant women perceive the role of the midwife in Thailand? A descriptive study. *Journal of Asian Midwives (JAM), 7*(2), 33–47.

Mala, O., Forster, E. M., & Kain, V. J. (2024). Thai nurses' and midwives' perceptions regarding barriers, facilitators, and competence in neonatal pain management. *Advances in Neonatal Care, 24*(2), 26–38.

Ministry of Public Health. (2024). The 2nd National Reproductive Health Development Policy and Strategy (2017–2026) on the Promotion of Quality Birth and Growth. https://rh.anamai.moph.go.th/th/download-03/download?id=39713&mid=31985&mkey=m_document&lang=th&did=13761.

Nantsupawat, A., & Sngounsiritham, U. (2019). Mentoring system and nursing professional development. *Nursing Journal*, *46*(3), 232–238.

Nertprasertkul, V., & Jansoontraporn, P. (2021). The development of competency scale for nurses mentors in Vajira Hospital. *Journal of The Royal Thai Army Nurses*, *22*(3), 313–321.

Pezaro, S., Zarbiv, G., Jones, J., Feika, M. L., Fitzgerald, L., Lukhele, S., & Hardtman, P. (2024). Characteristics of strong midwifery leaders and enablers of strong midwifery leadership: An international appreciative inquiry. *Midwifery*, *132*, 103982.

Pongboriboon, U. (2018). Being the preceptor: The challenge of nurse's self-efficacy. *Journal of the Royal Thai Army Nurses*, *19*(Supplement).

Proctor, B. (2001). Training for the supervision alliance attitude, skills and intention. In J.R. Cutcliffe, T. Butterworth, & B. Proctor (Eds.), *Fundamental Themes in Clinical Supervision* (pp. 25–46). Routledge.

Sarnkhaowhom, C., & Suwathanpornkul, I. (2018). The clinical supervision process of nurse preceptors in Thailand: A meta-ethnography research. *Walailak Journal of Science and Technology (WJST)*, *17*(5), 423–429.

Sirisomboon, R., Nuampa, S., Leetheeragul, J., Sudphet, M., Pimol, K., Sirithepmontree, S., & Silavong, L. (2024). Enhancing the competencies of obstetrical nurses and midwives in high-risk pregnancy management through simulation-based training in Lao people's democratic republic: A pilot study. *Midwifery*, *137*, 104132.

Srisaeng, P., & Upvall, M. J. (2020). Looking toward 2030: Strengthening midwifery education through regional partnerships. *Journal of Advanced Nursing*, *76*(2), 715–724.

Tabibnia, G., & Radecki, D. (2018). Resilience training that can change the brain. *Consulting Psychology Journal: Practice and Research*, *70*(1), 59.

Thailand Nursing and Midwifery Council. (1997). Profession nursing and midwifery Act, B.E.2528*(1997); Revision of the Act B.E.2540 (1997). Retrieved July 20, 2024, from https://www.tnmc.or.th/images/userfiles/files/Professional%20Nursing%20and%20Midwifery%20Act%202528%20Revision%202540.pdf.

Thailand Nursing and Midwifery Council. (2024). The Educational institutions provide the Bachelor of Nursing Science program that has been certified by the Nursing and Midwifery Council; graduates have the right to apply for an exam to register and receive a professional license. https://www.tnmc.or.th/images/userfiles/files/Newsletter2565/11.pdf

Thamsrisawat, J. (2016). The competencies of nurse preceptors for new nurses at a private hospital in Chonburi province. Unpublished master's thesis, Christian University, Thailand.

Thompson, M., & Thompson, L. (2021). Neurofeedback with biofeedback for stress management. In P.M. Lehrer, & R.L. Woolfolk (Eds.), *Principles and Practice of Stress Management* (pp. 214–263). Guilford Publications.

Vlerick, I., Kinnaer, L. M., Delbaere, B., Coolbrandt, A., Decoene, E., Thomas, L., & Van Hecke, A. (2024). Characteristics and effectiveness of mentoring programmes for specialized and advanced practice nurses: A systematic review. *Journal of Advanced Nursing*, *80*(7), 2690–2714.

Weckend, M., Davison, C., & Bayes, S. (2022). Physiological plateaus during normal labor and birth: A scoping review of contemporary concepts and definitions. *Birth*, *49*(2), 310–328.

World Health Organization. (2020). Regional Strategic Directions for strengthening Midwifery in the South-East Asia Region 2020–2024.

22

MIDWIFERY MENTORSHIP

Australian Cultural Considerations

Stacey Butcher and Linda Deravin

Introduction

The *National Aboriginal and Torres Strait Islander Health Workforce Strategic Framework and Implementation Plan 2021–2031* (Australian Government Department of Health, 2022) acknowledges that investment in the First Nations health workforce will increase Australia's ability to "close the gap in health and life outcomes and ensure a culturally safe and responsive health sector" (2022, p. 6). Yet, the representation of a First Nations midwifery workforce is critically low. Several factors contribute to this underrepresentation, and strategies to increase this workforce have had limited success. Further discussion is provided later in this chapter.

Internationally, mentoring is acknowledged as a key strategy for supporting the retention and career development of individuals from underrepresented groups, such as First Nations midwives, in the workplace (Hayward, 2024) However, this has not been demonstrated to the same level of success in Australia (Biles et al., 2023; Schwartz, 2019). In a study by Hildebrand et al. (2023), styles of clinical supervision across a range of health professions within regional and rural Australia were reviewed. Hildebrand et al. (2023) discovered that programmes were only focused on General Practitioners and nurse practitioners. There was a lack of clinical supervision models that focused on midwifery. Even though the models and styles reviewed had valuable components, there was not a single model that was wholly appropriate for midwives, let alone First Nations midwives working in remote health practice.

DOI: 10.4324/9781003533733-23

REFLECTIVE ACTIVITY 1

Can you identify what may be some of the key reasons why First Nations people do not enter the midwifery profession? Create a short list now and revisit your list at the end of the chapter. Did you add anything to your list?

Challenges Faced by First Nations Midwives

First Nations people's health staff make positive differences in the cultural safety of health service experiences for First Nations Australian peoples. However, there is a requirement for more First Nations people's health workforce as it is currently well below population parity. The burden of disease for First Nations peoples is 2.3 times more than for non-Indigenous Australians. While the workforce is growing, the current growth rate is not fast enough to substantially change this situation. Nationally, in 2023, approximately 490 First Nations midwives represented 1.69% of the total midwifery workforce (Department of Health and Aged Care, 2023), a slight increase from 1.33% ($n = 350$) in 2019 (Australian Institute of Health and Welfare, 2019). This rate remains far below parity for First Nations women's most recently reported birthing rate of 5% in 2021 (Australian Institute of Health and Welfare, 2023). Assuming First Nations birth and population rates remain static, along with university completion rates, an additional 1270 midwives (birth population) are required to reach the midwifery workforce and birth rate parity (Hartz et al., 2025; Fleming et al., 2020).

The inability to retain and support First Nations midwives in mainstream healthcare is directly associated with poorer health outcomes for First Nations women (Hayman et al., 2009; West et al., 2013). In 2017, the "Closing the Gap" report revealed a significant increase in First Nations students attending universities. However, despite this growth, First Nations students' success and completion rates remain low compared to their non-Indigenous peers (Fleming et al., 2020).

Racism and Discrimination

The challenges facing First Nations midwives have long been recognised, with high levels of individual racism and low levels of Cultural Safety (Biles et al., 2023; Burnett et al., 2020). At an organisational level, workforce attrition among First Nations midwives affects staff retention and ultimately compromises the delivery of safe and quality healthcare for First Nations women and families (Biles et al., 2021; 2023). Factors such as these have created an environment where the First Nations midwifery workforce is in crisis (Biles et al., 2023). Given this current landscape, there is a pressing need to meaningfully address cultural safety within Australian healthcare organisations and improve working conditions for First Nations midwives.

Racism has been institutionalised within healthcare since its inception and is rooted in colonialism. This is evident in Australia, New Zealand, the United States (US), and other Western countries. A prime example of this is Florence Nightingale as a famous non-Indigenous nurse who, in 1860, founded the first formal training school for nurses in London, which only accepted European women of the "right caliber" (Waite & Nardi, 2019).

In Australia, a review of mainstream healthcare services during 2017–2019 found that ~25% of NSW Health employees experienced racism in the workplace (Public Service Commission, 2019). The *Australian National Scheme Aboriginal and Torres Islander Health and Cultural Safety Strategy 2020–2025* (AHPRA, 2020) illustrated the importance of ensuring culturally safe and respectful practice; health practitioners must not only acknowledge colonisation and systemic racism, social, cultural, behavioural, and economic factors that impact individual and community First Nations Peoples health. The mentor and mentee in a mentorship partnership need to ensure they individually reflect on racism, their own biases, assumptions, stereotypes, and prejudices, and provide mentorship that is holistic, free of bias and racism. This relationship then fosters a safe working environment through leadership to support the rights and dignity of First Nations people.

First Nations midwives and students need to feel safe and empowered to speak out against racism. The structural, individual, and ideological racism in healthcare shows that racism is rarely called out, named, or openly discussed. Midwifery educators often seem more concerned with preserving a façade of harmony and homogeneity, never to be "upset" by opening the proverbial "can of worms" of racism (Burnett et al., 2020). Iheduru-Anderson (2021) states that when there is any mention of "Whiteness", "White privilege", "White guilt", "White fragility", or even "White supremacy", it almost guaranteed to induce anger, defensiveness and resistance among many non-Indigenous academics, students and clinicians. Even though this is an American researcher, the evidence is transcribed over into the Australian environment easily.

REFLECTIVE ACTIVITY 2

Birthing on Country is a significant initiative that supports First Nations women to birth in a culturally safe environment.

- If a First Nations woman is not able to birth on country, as a student midwife what other culturally appropriate supports could be provided to birthing mothers in your care?
- What makes your suggestions culturally appropriate or safe?

Mentoring First Nations Midwives in Australia

First Nations midwifery workforce is vital to ensure best practice and culturally relevant, evidence-based maternity care is provided to First Nations women and families (Hickey et al., 2018). It is highlighted throughout this text and within contemporary research that the effectiveness of mentoring is well documented in maintaining the workforce (Biles et al., 2023). However, there is minimal research and evidence on mentorship among First Nations midwives in Australia.

The benefits of any mentoring relationship include developing a culture of support within the workplace, increasing confidence in skills and ability, and improving the retention of an existing workforce and the graduation of students (Bradford et al., 2022; Mills et al., 2007). This is even more pertinent for First Nations midwives who are entering environments that may be perceived as hostile, unfriendly, unfamiliar, and culturally unsafe (Biles et al., 2021).

Currently, programmes for First Nations Midwives are uncommon in Australia. One state within Australia has implemented a pilot project called the New South Wales (NSW) Health – *Deadly Aboriginal and Torres Strait Islander Nursing and Midwifery Mentoring (DANMM) Programme*. In this mentoring programme both mentors and mentees undergo an education programme to enhance their cultural awareness and humility. Mentors and mentees are matched and work with each other for a period of 12 months. Hayward (2024) highlights that mentorship programmes like DANMM can facilitate the development of professional networks and opportunities for First Nations midwives, connecting mentees with other midwifery professionals.

What Mentoring Looks Like in a Culturally Safe Space

Culturally safe learning and teaching environments, academics, and health professionals in clinical settings are paramount to supporting the success of First Nations students and midwives (Fleming et al., 2020). Culturally safe mentoring should be seen as a tool to build workforce retention and the wider workforce's cultural capability (Biles et al., 2023). Recognising culture is significant and imperative when implementing mentorship programmes (Biles et al., 2023). Mentorship requires exploring culture, as it is imperative in building relationships and partnerships to grow and gain ongoing mentoring (Biles et al., 2023).

It is important the mentee feels physically, spiritually, socially, and emotionally safe within the space. Therefore, cultural safety is a large component of mentoring, as well as its effectiveness. A culturally safe mentoring programme ensures that the mentor critically reflects on knowledge, skills, attitudes, behaviours, and power differentials between the mentor and mentee. The mentee is able to cultivate support within the health workforce that builds trust and establishes a culturally safe workplace. The depth and breadth of the mentoring relationships facilitates feelings of being culturally safe impacts the ability for sensitive topics like racism to be explored (Biles et al., 2021).

Mentoring programmes can support not only the learning of the mentee but also the learning of mentors. Fleming et al. (2017) demonstrated value in formalised mentorship for both First Nations peoples and non-Indigenous clinicians due to the learning through the two-way learning model. When mentors have a positive experience, this may enhance their understanding of culture and what it means to be a mentor, leading to improved workplace culture.

Yarning

Fleming et al. (2020) identified yarning as an appropriate way to explore culture. Yarning is a form of relaxed storytelling that facilitates discussion about a key topic (Biles et al., 2021). Yarning for First Nations Peoples is an integral part of their lives and a way to make sense of the lived experience (Geia et al., 2013, 2020). It is not a static process; it begins and progresses through loud and raucous engagement, which then moves into contemplation and silence (Geia et al., 2013).

Yarning is a decolonising approach that reflects First Nations People's epistemology ways of being, knowing and doing (Fleming et al., 2020). The power of yarning is held by the participant who guides the focus of the discussion (Biles et al., 2021). Yarning enables a "sense of belonging" in a safe environment and enables participants to challenge cultural misconceptions, biases, assumptions, and values (Biles et al., 2023; Fleming et al., 2020). Yarning circles can provide safety and security for an individual to ask questions.

Peer Mentoring

There are a number of different ways to provide mentoring, as you have seen throughout this text. However, research has illustrated the importance of peer-to-peer mentoring for students and new graduate midwives. Hogan et al. (2017) illustrated that 80% of mentors and mentees assisted with clinical placement and assisting with communication skills and confidence. This is supported by Mckellar & Kempster (2015) that 80% of mentees increase their motivation to complete their first year at university. However, there is minimal research that fully focuses on First Nations Students and midwives in this space.

REFLECTIVE ACTIVITY 3

Donna is a First Nations woman and an experienced midwife with over 20 years of working in both midwifery group practices and in acute care health facilities. Donna has an undergraduate student midwife, Natasha, who works with her on the evening shift. Julie, a full-term primip, presents to the birthing suite and is imminently about to give birth. Julie only asks her questions to Natasha as she is lighter skinned like Julie. Natasha is feeling very uncomfortable and deflects these questions to Donna, who is the skilled and experienced midwife, who calmly and patiently answers all of Julie's questions.

What should Natasha and Donna do in this instance?
Do the rights of the labouring woman supersede discriminatory behaviour?

   After the successful birth, Donna and Natasha debriefed about this event. Donna seems angry about how she was treated, and Natasha fears that she will get an unfavourable assessment as the birthing mother refuses to speak to Donna.

What might Natasha consider saying to support Donna?
Should Donna be silent, and what strategies might she use in the future to manage situations like these?
In this situation, who is the mentor, and who is the mentee?

Mentoring in Future

For First Nations midwives to remain within the health workforce, ongoing programmes that acknowledge and cultivate support in a culturally appropriate and safe way can make a difference towards future recruitment and retention (Biles et al., 2021)

Cultural Safety workplaces and mentoring programmes are seen as tools to not only build workforce retention but also build cultural capability within the wider workforce and need to be long-term commitments for organisations. Therefore, targeted mentorship programmes should not be ad hoc and in the long-term strategy.

Summary

Establishing a mentoring relationship that supports the novice midwife is an essential tool for supporting the midwifery workforce into the future. This is even more relevant and needed if we are to successfully build a First Nations midwifery workforce. Barriers to midwives staying within the profession include racism, discrimination, the whiteness of colonialised health care systems. Ways to address these barriers include providing culturally safe spaces not only for First Nations midwives but also all midwifery staff and students regardless of cultural background or geographical location. Opportunities for mentors and mentees to learn from one another in a two-way learning mentorship model should be supported, encouraged, and implemented. Successful mentoring can bring many benefits to both midwives and the woman, babies and families that they care for.

REFLECTIVE ACTIVITY 4

1 What government policy prevents initiatives such as Birthing on Country from being universally adopted across Australia?
2 What are some of the key cultural considerations that should be adopted when entering a mentoring relationship between the mentor and mentee?
3 What impact does racism have on increasing a First Nations midwifery workforce?

Acknowledgement

The authors of this chapter wish to acknowledge the traditional custodians and owners of the sovereign lands upon where they are located and pay their respects to Elders both past and present, recognising that connection to Country is as strong now as it always was and always will be.[1]

Note

1 Note on terminology – The term First Nations, which is used throughout this chapter, is a collective term that refers to Indigenous Australian and Aboriginal and Torres Strait Islander peoples of Australia. First Nations peoples will refer to themselves by any of these terms and may also identify through language groups. This term is used in acknowledgement that First Nations peoples have the right of self-determination to identify however they choose to do so.

References

Australian Bureau of Statistics. (2021). *Estimates of Aboriginal and Torres Strait Islander Australians*. Australian Bureau of Statistics. Retrieved 13 March from https://www.abs.gov.au/statistics/people/aboriginal-and-torres-strait-islander-peoples/estimates-aboriginal-and-torres-strait-islander-australians/latest-releasehttps://www.abs.gov.au/statistics/people/aboriginal-and-torres-strait-islander-peoples/estimates-aboriginal-and-torres-strait-islander-australians/latest-release

Australian Government Department of Health. (2022). *National Aboriginal and Torres Strait Islander Health Workforce Strategic Framework and Implementation Plan 2021–2031*. Department of Health. https://www.health.gov.au/sites/default/files/documents/2022/03/national-aboriginal-and-torres-strait-islander-health-workforce-strategic-framework-and-implementation-plan-2021-2031.pdf:

Australian Institute of Health and Welfare. (2019). *Factsheet, Nursing and Midwifery 2019*. Department of Health. https://hwd.health.gov.au/resources/publications/factsheet-midw-2019.pdf

Australian Institute of Health and Welfare. (2023). *Australia's Mothers and Babies 2021: Web Report*. Australian Government. https://www.aihw.gov.au/getmedia/bf03fda0-6d37-46f3-8ba6-9c3ebadc26f8/australia-s-mothers-and-babies.pdf?v=20240115130043&inline=true

Biles, J., Deravin, L., McMillan Am, F., Anderson, J., Sara, G., & Biles, B. (2023). Aboriginal and Torres strait Islander nurses and midwives culturally safe mentoring programmes in Australia: A scoping review. *Contemporary Nurse*, 59(2), 173–183. https://doi.org/10.1080/10376178.2023.2175700

Biles, J., Deravin, L., Seaman, C. E., Alexander, N., Damm, A., & Trudgett, N. (2021). Learnings from a mentoring project to support Aboriginal and Torres Strait Islander nurses and midwives to remain in the workforce. *Contemporary Nurse*, 57(5), 327–337. https://doi.org/10.1080/10376178.2021.1991412

Bradford, H., Hines, H. F., Labko, Y., Peasley, A., Valentin-Welch, M., & Breedlove, G. (2022). Midwives mentoring midwives: A review of the evidence and Best practice recommendations. *Journal of Midwifery & Womens Health*, 67(1), 21–30. https://doi.org/10.1111/jmwh.13285

Burnett, A., Moorley, C., Grant, J., Kahin, M., Sagoo, R., Rivers, E., Deravin, L., & Darbyshire, P. (2020). Dismantling racism in education: In 2020, the year of the nurse & midwife, "it's time". *Nurse Education Today*, 93, 104532. https://doi.org/10.1016/j.nedt.2020.104532

Department of Health and Aged Care. (2023). *Nurses & Midwives Dashboard: Midwives 2022*. Department of Health and Aged Care. Retrieved 12 March from https://hwd.health.gov.au/nrmw-dashboards/index.html

Fleming, T., Creedy, D. K., & West, R. (2020). The influence of yarning circles: A cultural safety professional development program for midwives. *Women Birth*, *33*(2), 175–185. https://doi.org/10.1016/j.wombi.2019.03.016

Fleming, T., Creedy, D. K., & West, R. (2017). Impact of a continuing professional development intervention on midwifery academics' awareness of cultural safety. *Women Birth*, *30*(3), 245–252. https://doi.org/10.1016/j.wombi.2017.02.004

Geia, L., Baird, K., Bail, K., Barclay, L., Bennett, J., Best, O., Birks, M., Blackley, L., Blackman, R., Bonner, A., Bryant Ao, R., Buzzacott, C., Campbell, S., Catling, C., Chamberlain, C., Cox, L., Cross, W., Cruickshank, M., Cummins, A., & Wynne, R. (2020). A unified call to action from Australian nursing and midwifery leaders: Ensuring that Black lives matter. *Contemporary Nurse*, *56*(4), 297–308. https://doi.org/10.1080/10376178.2020.1809107

Geia, L. K., Hayes, B., & Usher, K. (2013). Yarning/Aboriginal storytelling: Towards an understanding of an Indigenous perspective and its implications for research practice. *Contemporary Nurse*, *46*(1), 13–17. https://doi.org/10.5172/conu.2013.46.1.13

Hartz DL, Coleman R, Butcher S, McGrath L, Buzzacott C, Williams K, Coe A, Kosiak M. (2025) What are the experiences of Aboriginal and/or Torres Strait Islander midwifery students and midwives? A scoping review. *Women Birth*, *38*(1), https://doi.org/10.1016/j.wombi.2024.101856

Hayman, N. E., White, N. E., & Spurling, G. K. (2009). Improving Indigenous patients' access to mainstream health services: The Inala experience. *Medical Journal of Australia*, *190*(10), 604–606. https://doi.org/10.5694/j.1326-5377.2009.tb02581.x

Hayward, A. (2024). *Exploring and defining an ideal mentorship model for newly registered indigenous midwives in Manitoba*. https://www.midwives.mb.ca/document/6020/exploring-and-defining-mentorship-model-indigenous-midwives.pdf

Hildebrand, F., Gray, M., & McCullough, K. (2023). Models of clinical supervision of relevance to remote area nursing & primary health care: A scoping review. *Australian Journal of Rural Health*, *31*, 826–838. https://doi.org/10.1111/ajr.13038

Hickey, S. D., Maidment, S. J., Heinemann, K. M., Roe, Y. L., & Kildea, S. V. (2018). Participatory action research opens doors: Mentoring Indigenous researchers to improve midwifery in urban Australia. *Women Birth*, *31*(4), 263–268. https://doi.org/10.1016/j.wombi.2017.10.011

Hogan, R., Fox, D., & Barratt-See, G. (2017). Peer to peer mentoring: Outcomes of third-year midwifery students mentoring first-year students. *Women Birth*, *30*(3), 206–213. https://doi.org/10.1016/j.wombi.2017.03.004

ICM. (2020). *Mentoring Guidelines for Midwives*. https://internationalmidwives.org/resources/mentoring-guidelines-for-midwives/

Iheduru-Anderson, K. C. (2021). The White/Black hierarchy institutionalizes White supremacy in nursing and nursing leadership in the United States. *Journal of Professional Nursing*, *37*(2), 411–421. https://doi.org/10.1016/j.profnurs.2020.05.005

McKellar, L., & Kempster, C. (2015). We're all in this together: Midwifery student peer mentoring. *Women and Birth*, *28*. https://doi.org/10.1016/j.wombi.2015.07.156

Mills, J., Francis, K., & Bonner, A. (2007). The accidental mentor: Australian Rural nurses developing supportive relationships in the workplace. *Rural Remote Health*, *4*(7). https://pubmed.ncbi.nlm.nih.gov/18069907/https://pubmed.ncbi.nlm.nih.gov/18069907/

Public Service Commission. (2019). NSW public sector aboriginal employment strategy 2019–2025: NSW working together for a better future. https://www.psc.nsw.gov.au/assets/psc/documents/2022-Aboriginal-Employment-Strategy-refresh.pdf

Schwartz, S. (2019). *Educating the Nurse of the Future—Report of the Independent Review into Nursing Education.* Commonwealth of Australia. Retrieved from https://www.health.gov.au/sites/default/files/documents/2019/12/educating-the-nurse-of-the-future.pdf

Waite, R., & Nardi, D. (2019). Nursing colonialism in America: Implications for nursing leadership. *Journal of Professional Nursing, 35*(1), 18–25. https://doi.org/10.1016/j.profnurs.2017.12.013

West, R., Usher, K., Buettner, P. G., Foster, K., & Stewart, L. (2013). Indigenous Australians' participation in pre-registration tertiary nursing courses: A mixed methods study. *Contemporary Nurse, 46*(1), 123–134. https://doi.org/10.5172/conu.2013.46.1.123

23

MIDWIFERY MENTORSHIP IN AUSTRALIAN CURRICULA

Fiona Arundell

Introduction

In Australia, pre-registration midwifery education is offered at undergraduate and postgraduate levels. All students undertake practice experience or Work-integrated Learning (WIL), and are supported by an experienced midwife. The terminology used to describe this support midwife is not generic, and there are many terms applied throughout Australia including mentor, preceptor, clinical supervisor, facilitator and buddy midwife. Various models of midwifery student support in Australia have been described, such as preceptorship (Griffiths et al., 2020; Licqurish & Seibold, 2008; Thomas et al., 2023), mentorship (Dewar et al., 2020; Jefford et al., 2021; Sheehan et al., 2022; 2023) and clinical facilitators (McKellar et al., 2018). Regardless of nomenclature, a commonality is that many midwives have not received any formal education to assist them to undertake the responsibility of supervising student development in the practice setting. In this chapter, the term mentoring will be used to describe an experienced midwife supporting the development of a midwifery student in the practice setting, in place of other terms such as preceptor, supervisor and facilitator.

Australian universities are required to meet the challenge of educating midwifery students who can attain the philosophical and applied requirements of midwifery practice. To assist this process, they are guided by global and national standards for midwifery education.

The International Confederation of Midwives (ICM) revised their Global Standards for Midwifery Education (ICM, 2021). The standards set international benchmarks for the development, implementation and evaluation of midwifery programmes and engagement with quality improvement and reporting.

DOI: 10.4324/9781003553733-24

Global Standards for Midwifery Education

The Global Standards for Midwifery Education (ICM, 2021) provide foundation expectations for midwifery education programmes. The standards provide a framework for curriculum development, ensuring the ICM Essential Competencies for Midwifery Practice (ICM, 2024) are addressed. Internationally these standards have been adapted by registering bodies of countries; in the case of Australia, they have been modified in the development of national education standards. The ICM Global Standards for Midwifery Education (ICM, 2021) suggest that midwifery programmes should be comprised of a minimum of 40% theory and 50% practice; this ratio emphasises the significance of acquiring theoretical and practical knowledge to ensure midwives provide optimal care. To ensure midwifery students meet competency, the ICM (ICM, 2022) has developed a companion document for the ICM Global Standards for Midwifery Education specifically focused on the implementation of practical/clinical experience. The companion document titled Guidance for meeting the ICM Global Standards for Midwifery Education (ICM, 2022) covers many topics such as location of placements, experience with a variety of models of care and student safety. The document emphasises the impact of positive and negative support on midwifery student development (ICM, 2022). The document also specifically directs midwifery educators to consider if midwives who support students have welcoming attitudes and behaviours, and if there are processes in place for student support if they are demeaned or inappropriately criticised whilst on placement (ICM, 2022). The document articulates the terms to describe midwives who support midwifery students on practice as midwifery preceptor/clinical teacher to emphasise the assessment expectations of the role. A midwifery preceptor/clinical teacher is defined as,

> An experienced midwife engaged in the practice of midwifery who is competent and willing to teach students in the clinical setting. A preceptor/clinical teacher works closely with the student midwife to provide guidance, training, support, assessment evaluation and constructive feedback and serves as a role model for the student midwife.
>
> *(ICM, 2022, p. 10)*

These abilities are very specific and not the skill set of a midwife, therefore, to be able to fulfil the support requirements of midwifery students, midwives need to be supported to meet these expectations. For an Australian academic responsible for curriculum development, this document provides the most detailed outline of the expectations of a midwife responsible for supporting student development in the practice setting.

Midwifery Education in Australia

There are several forms of pre-registration midwifery programmes in Australia including a direct entry Bachelor of Midwifery, combined Bachelor of Midwifery/Bachelor of Nursing and postgraduate programmes for registered nurses, at Graduate Diploma or Masters level (DoHA, 2019). Alumni of these programmes meet the Midwife Standards for Practice (NMBA, 2018) as stipulated by the Nursing and Midwifery Board of Australia (NMBA).

In Australia, the Australian Nursing and Midwifery Accreditation Council (ANMAC) oversees the accreditation of pre-registration midwifery programmes. Education providers are guided in the development of a programme by the Midwife Accreditation Standards (Australian Nursing and Midwifery Accreditation Council, 2021). Once accredited by ANMAC the programme must be approved by the NMBA prior to being eligible for implementation. Five standards comprise the Midwife Accreditation Standards (Australian Nursing and Midwifery Accreditation Council, 2021), which include:

- Safety to the public,
- Governance,
- Programme of study,
- Student experience, and
- Student assessment.

The standards are all supported with criteria however the focus of the document is the overall governance of the programme and strategies to reduce risk. The previous version of the Midwife Accreditation Standards published in 2014 clearly stated that programmes were to be comprised of 50% theory and 50% practice experience; however, the 2021 version does not stipulate a percentage. There is one reference in the document that acknowledges the education providers responsibility for the preparation and support of midwives (referred to as preceptors) who support students on midwifery practice experience, the form and extent of the preparation is not elaborated.

The Midwife Standards for Practice (NMBA, 2018) is comprised of seven standards with a focus on the provision of safe knowledgeable midwifery care. The seven standards include:

- Promotes health and wellbeing through evidence-based midwifery practice,
- Engages in professional relationships and respectful partnerships,
- Demonstrates the capability and accountability for midwifery practice,
- Undertakes comprehensive assessments,

- Develops plans for midwifery practice,
- Provides safety and quality in midwifery practice and
- Evaluates outcomes to improve midwifery practice (NMBA, 2018).

The standards are comprised of 38 criteria which describe the actions and behaviours of midwives to fulfil the seven standards. Only one of these criteria 3.4 specifies the role of the midwife in relation to the educational support of others, *Contribute to a culture that supports learning, teaching, knowledge transfer and critical reflection* (NMBA, 2018, p. 5).

Thus, the two Australian documents that guide midwifery education in Australia, the Midwife Accreditation Standards (Australian Nursing and Midwifery Accreditation Council, 2021) and Midwife Standards for Practice (NMBA, 2018) provide minimal direction for education providers in relation to the mentoring support of midwifery students whilst undertaking clinical practice experience. The ICM (2022) document does at least provide a brief outline of the role expectations of a midwife preceptor.

In Australia, most of the responsibility for the provision of practice education for midwifery students and the development of knowledge and skills has been assigned to clinical midwives. These midwives have a significant role in integrating practice and theoretical knowledge for midwifery students. However, as well as supporting midwifery students, clinical midwives have a primary responsibility to meet the needs of the women and babies they are caring for, leaving minimal time for student support. There are no national guidelines on the preparation of midwives to provide support for midwifery students in the practice setting. In Australia, some midwives may have undertaken training within their hospital such as a preceptorship or mentorship course. These courses are often of short duration ranging from a few hours to a few days, and course completion is not linked to assessment.

This contrasts with the UK, for example, who in 2006 developed national standards for student mentorship in the practice setting (Nursing and Midwifery Council, 2006). The Standards to Support Learning and Assessment in Practice (Nursing and Midwifery Council, 2008) clearly articulates the role of a mentor. The document details the expectations of a mentor in relation to personal development and the development of others which is discussed further in Chapter 12. However, post-implementation of the UK model did raise the question: Should mentorship only be undertaken by those who have undertaken further qualifications or should mentorship be a role undertaken by all midwives? Please go to Section II, *Mentorship, Leadership and Education: A Global Perspective,* where country-specific chapters detail how midwifery mentorship is undertaken.

REFLECTIVE ACTIVITY 1

Reflecting on your personal experience of mentorship, answer the below question:

• Should Australia develop a specialised national post-registration mentorship programme, or should education providers embed mentorship within pre-registration courses, thus preparing all future midwives for the role of mentor?

Currently, there is not a consistent approach to the inclusion of teaching mentorship in pre-registration midwifery programmes in Australia. For some programmes, there is no mentorship content; for other programmes, mentorship is addressed but as a topic within a subject and then in some institutions, there are standalone subjects that are focused on mentorship. Mentorship is also taught in some post-registration midwifery programmes as part of a clinical education specialisation pathway.

Case Study Implementation of Mentorship Into a Midwifery Programme

In this part of the chapter, the Bachelor of Midwifery at Western Sydney University (WSU) Australia will be used an example that has been designed with mentorship included and to provide midwifery students with 50% theory and 50% practice experience. When planning for the current curriculum, it was agreed to develop and implement a subject that highlighted the important role of the midwife in supporting the development of midwifery students, women and peers. It was agreed amongst academics there is currently an inconsistency in the provision of knowledgeable, timely and salient support of midwifery students on midwifery practice experience; this inconsistent support reduces the potential for students to develop. The subject is titled, Midwife as Facilitator of Learning and is taught in the final semester of the three-year programme. It was decided to place the subject in the last semester of the programme because students would have experienced many hours of practice experience and be cognisant of what works well and not so well in relation to student support. Instead of waiting in the hope that in the future these students may reciprocate positive support and meaningful education that they had received, we wanted to develop a subject that provided background, context and skills necessary for the successful mentorship of midwifery students on practice experience. There is a similar subject at Southern Cross University and University of the Sunshine Coast.

REFLECTIVE ACTIVITY 2

- Have you been expected to provide mentorship to a midwifery student?
- How confident were you to undertake this role?
- What were your strengths?
- Which areas needed more development?

At WSU, the subject introduced the theoretical understanding of adult learning principles and learning styles; the intention was that providing students with greater insight into their own learning styles would assist them to support others more effectively. The major content of the subject focused on mentorship of midwifery students on practice experience and was supported from the findings of an appreciative inquiry study that was focused on the role of the midwife in providing positive experiences for midwifery students on practice experience (Arundell et al., 2024a, 2024b). The study generated three distinct and sequential practices of midwives; these were forming a relationship, introducing the student to the community of practice and sharing craft knowledge, which are summarised below.

Forming a Relationship

Central to successful mentorship is the relationship formed between a mentor and mentee, a successful relationship developed from trust, challenge and support. The mentor also generated effective relationships with women and their practice was woman-centred. These two characteristics mirror Titchen's Critical Companionship Framework (Titchen, 2000). Titchen's (2000) framework was designed to enable an experienced nurse to share their craft knowledge with a less experienced nurse and reflect a model of care in which the nurse and patient form an effective relationship. In the midwifery setting, this model reflects woman-centred care. A successful relationship requires the four components of particularity, reciprocity, graceful care and mutuality.

Introducing Students to the Community of Practice

Lave and Wenger (1991) argue that a novice should not be situated in a workplace setting and assume learning will occur, for learning to occur the novice needs to join the community of practice. Midwifery students are novices in the discipline of midwifery; midwives can provide students an opportunity to develop knowledge and skills through legitimate peripheral participation. Joining the community of practice involves acculturation, which is facilitated through the novice being provided meaningful peripheral opportunities which lead to legitimate members of the community (Lave & Wenger, 1991); in this case, the mentor provides the opportunity for a midwifery student.

Sharing Craft Knowledge

The concepts of saliency and temporality when effectively supporting students were explained. Strategies to support student development were explored including role modelling, articulation of craft knowledge, listening and questioning, problematisation, moderating support, reflection, self-reflection and critique.

The Midwife as Facilitator of Learning subject was structured as a combination of online learning and on-campus workshop activities. Online lectures, readings and activities provided theoretical context that could then be practically applied in workshops. The two and a half years of practice experience prior to undertaking the subject enabled students to bring real-life experiences to the workshops. Workshops were designed to focus on what had previously worked well instead of focusing negative experiences on placement. Recalling and reflecting on positive experiences was very inspiring and encouraged an "I want to be like this" mindset.

REFLECTIVE ACTIVITY 3

Recall a positive mentoring experience as a midwifery student.

- What were the skills, strengths and qualities that the mentor brought to the experience?
- Do your skills link with the three distinct and sequential practices of midwives found in the Arundell et al. (2024b) study: Forming a relationship, Introducing the student to the community of practice and Sharing craft knowledge?

Conclusion

This chapter focused on midwifery mentorship in Australian curricula yet is applicable in any country that teaches midwifery. Currently, there are minimal national and international guidelines to support the inclusion of mentorship in midwifery curricula; despite this lack of guidelines, several Australian institutions have included content relating to mentorship in curricula.

The significance of the positive impact of a successful mentor/mentee relationship has been demonstrated; however, the art of mentorship is not inherent to midwives resulting in inconsistent experiences of mentorship for mentor and mentee. The inclusion of mentorship education in all midwifery pre-registration curricula in Australia would foster the development of midwives who are confident and competent to fulfil the role of mentor.

References

Arundell, F., Peters, K., & Sheehan, A. (2024a). Professional identity: Students' learning from the attributes and behaviours of midwives on clinical placement. *Women and Birth*, 37(5), 101657.

Arundell, F., Sheehan, A., & Peters, K. (2024b). Strategies used by midwives to enhance knowledge and skill development in midwifery students: An appreciative inquiry study. *BMC Nursing*, 23(1), 137.

Australian Nursing and Midwifery Accreditation Council (2021). *Midwife Accreditation Standards 2021*. ACT.

Dewar, B., Stulz, V., Buliak, A., Connolly, L., McLaughlin, K., Newport, K., Rebolledo, S., Stephenson, L., MacBride, T., Lennon, K., & Drayton, N. (2020). Exploring and developing student midwives' experiences (ESME) – An appreciative inquiry study. *Midwifery*, 91, 102844.

DoHA. (2019). *Australia's Future Health Workforce Report – Midwives*. Australian Government.

Griffiths, M., Gamble, J., & Creedy, D. (2020). Midwifery student evaluation of practice: The MidSTEP tool -perceptions of clinical learning experiences. *Women and Birth*, 33(5), 440–447.

ICM. (2021). ICM Standards for Midwifery Education global-standards-for-midwifery-education_2021_en.pdf (internationalmidwives.org).

ICM. (2022). *Guidance for Meeting the ICM Global Standards for Midwifery Education (2021): Practical/clinical Experience*. International Confederation of Midwives.

ICM. (2024). *ICM Essential Competencies for Midwifery Practice*. The Hague: International Confederation of Midwives.

Jefford, E., Nolan, S., Munn, J., & Ebert, L. (2021). What matters, what is valued and what is important in mentorship through the appreciative inquiry process of co-created knowledge. *Nurse Education Today*, 99, 104791.

Lave, J., & Wenger, E. (1991). *Situated Learning: Legitimate Peripheral Participation*. Cambridge University Press.

Licqurish, S., & Seibold, C. (2008). Bachelor of midwifery students' experiences of achieving competencies: The role of The midwife preceptor. *Midwifery*, 24(4), 480–489. http://search.ebscohost.com/login.aspx?direct=true&db=rzh&AN=105602588&site=ehost-live

McKellar, L., Fleet, J., Vernon, R., Graham, M., & Cooper, M. (2018). Comparison of three clinical facilitation models for midwifery students undertaking clinical placement in South Australia. *Nurse Education in Practice*, 32, 64–71.

NMBA (2018). *Midwife Standards for Practice*. NMBA.

Nursing and Midwifery Council (2006). *Standards to Support Learning and Assessment in Practice: NMC Standards for Mentors, Practice Teachers and Teachers*. Nursing and Midwifery Council.

Nursing and Midwifery Council (2008). *Standards to Support Learning and Assessment in Practice: NMC Standards for Mentors, Practice Teachers and Teachers*. Nursing and Midwifery Council.

Sheehan, A., Dahlen, H., Elmir, R., Burns, E., Coulton, S., Sorensen, K., Duff, M., Arundell, F., Keedle, H., & Schmied, V. (2023). The implementation and evaluation of a mentoring program for Bachelor of Midwifery students in the clinical practice environment. *Nurse Education in Practice, 70.* https://doi.org/10.1016/j.nepr.2023.103687

Sheehan, A., Elmir, R., Hammond, A., Schmied, V., Coulton, S., Sorensen, K., Arundell, F., Keedle, H., Dahlen, H., & Burns, E. (2022). The midwife-student mentor relationship: Creating the virtuous circle. *Women & Birth, 35*(5), e512–e520.

Thomas, K., Yeganeh, L., Vlahovich, J., & Willey, S. (2023). Midwifery professional placement: Undergraduate students' experiences with novice and expert preceptors. *Nurse Education Today, 131,* Article 105976. https://doi.org/10.1016/j.nedt.2023.105976

Titchen, A. (2000). *Professional Craft Knowledge in Patient Centred Nursing and the Facilitation of Its Development.* Ashdale Press.

24

MIDWIFERY MENTORSHIP IN PRACTICE

An Organisational Perspective

Kelley Lennon and Olivia Tierney

Introduction

The evolution of midwifery practice in Australia has consistently highlighted the critical role of mentorship in developing and sustaining a skilled, confident workforce. As healthcare continues to grow in complexity, the intersection of mentorship and leadership becomes increasingly vital for organisational success and professional development. Australian healthcare system's unique challenges, including geographical diversity and varying practice settings, make effective mentorship programmes essential for maintaining high standards of midwifery care and professional development.

In recent years, the importance of structured mentorship has gained increased recognition within healthcare as crucial to supporting the attraction and retention of our midwifery workforce (Homer et al., 2024; Wissemann et al., 2022). Acknowledgement of the importance of mentorship reflects a growing understanding that effective mentorship programmes contribute to individual professional growth, organisational resilience, and improved service efficiencies. Mentoring between midwives and midwifery students is valued, improves experiences, supports the transition of new-to-practice midwives, enables midwives to practice to their full potential, and aids in leadership development (Jefford et al., 2021; Newton et al., 2022; Sheehan et al., 2022; 2023). This chapter explores how midwifery leaders can effectively foster, implement, and sustain mentorship programmes that benefit both individual midwives and affect organisations. Although this chapter has a primary focus within the Australian healthcare context, what is discussed can be applied within a global healthcare context.

DOI: 10.4324/9781003533733-25

Regulatory and Professional Framework

Understanding the regulations and frameworks that govern midwifery practice in Australia is fundamental to underpin developing and implementing effective mentoring programmes. The intricate web of legislation, professional standards, and ethical obligations creates the foundation for successful mentorship programmes. These frameworks guide practice and establish clear lines of accountability and responsibility. The Nursing and Midwifery Board of Australia (NMBA) regulatory frameworks define the professional standards of practice and behaviours for midwives. This includes registration standards, standards for practice, professional codes, and guidelines (NMBA). These standards are informed by the International Confederation of Midwives (ICM) definition of a midwife. All midwives in Australia are governed by the Midwife Standards for Practice, which outline that all midwives must "Contributes to a culture that supports learning, teaching, knowledge transfer and critical reflection" (Standard 3.4). This goes a step toward ensuring all midwives receive and give professional development support to each other. Mentoring is one way of enabling midwives and midwifery students a programme of support that can enable reciprocal learning.

The regulatory framework encompasses several key elements:

- Professional Standards: The NMBA's professional practice framework outlines specific requirements for continuing professional development and peer support (NMBA).
- Ethical Obligations: The Code of Ethics for Midwives in Australia emphasises the professional responsibility to support colleagues and contribute to the profession's development (NMBA).
- Accountability Mechanisms: Clear lines of responsibility and accountability are established through various professional and organisational frameworks.

The ICM recognises mentoring as professional support that encourages reflective practice, quality improvement, life-long learning, and teamwork among midwives (International Confederation of Midwives, 2020). The ICM defines mentoring as support for midwives as "A reciprocal learning relationship in which a mentor and mentee agree to a partnership where they work together toward achievement of mutually defined goals that will develop a mentee's skills, abilities, knowledge and/or thinking" (International Confederation of Midwives, 2020). In Australia, it has been identified and recommended not only to maintain but also to build a midwifery workforce into the future; the government should invest in and support quality mentoring programmes (Homer et al., 2024).

Healthcare System Integration

Translating mentorship from concept to practice within complex healthcare systems requires strategic planning, clear vision, organisational commitment, and leadership. Healthcare leaders must navigate various organisational structures, resources, and priorities while maintaining focus on the value that structured mentorship brings to workforce development and the development of woman-centred midwifery practice. Successful and sustained integration of mentorship programmes for the midwifery workforce within healthcare systems will benefit from a comprehensive understanding of organisational dynamics and leadership principles. Leadership in healthcare organisations must recognise mentorship as a strategic investment rather than an optional addition to professional development. This perspective requires leaders to support, role model, and champion mentorship at all levels, from clinical leaders to executive management, and the recognition that all midwives have a role to play in leadership, ensuring that programmes receive adequate support and resources to thrive.

Midwifery leaders are pivotal in fostering successful mentorship programmes by enabling environments that value and prioritise professional development. This includes establishing clear organisational strategies that support time for mentorship activities, developing formal recognition systems for mentors, and integrating mentorship into career development pathways. This is outlined in the case study example in Section 4 of this chapter. Leaders must also demonstrate their commitment through role modelling, visible support and active participation in mentorship initiatives. Several factors can influence the successful implementation of mentorship programmes. Workforce shortages and high clinical demands often compete with mentorship activities for time and attention (Wissemann et al., 2022). Geographic distances in rural and regional settings can complicate traditional mentorship models, necessitating innovative approaches such as virtual mentoring platforms. Cultural and organisational resistance to change may also impede programme implementation. Adopting an approach of determining what works well and discovering adaptable models and methods will aid in overcoming barriers and enable sustained integration into the healthcare system.

Resource allocation represents a critical component of successful mentorship integration. Organisations must commit to providing adequate resources, protected time, and management support to ensure programme sustainability. This includes investing in mentor training, developing support materials, and establishing evaluation frameworks to measure programme effectiveness.

Successfully integrating mentorship programmes within healthcare systems depends on their alignment with organisational and leadership goals and values. When mentorship is viewed as integral to achieving key organisational objectives such as workforce attraction and retention, contemporary practice and clinical excellence, it can be effective to justify and sustain the necessary resource investments. Healthcare leaders must regularly evaluate and adjust mentorship programmes to ensure they meet organisational needs and the evolving requirements of the midwifery workforce.

By addressing these various aspects of system integration thoughtfully and systematically, healthcare organisations can create robust mentorship programmes that contribute meaningfully to professional development and midwifery success. The key lies in maintaining a balanced approach that acknowledges both the challenges and opportunities while remaining focused on the ultimate goal of supporting excellence in midwifery practice.

The Model for Change, Mentorship in Midwifery: A Case Study

Effective mentorship requires a structured, evidence-based approach that can be consistently applied while remaining flexible enough to adapt to various healthcare contexts. The NSW Health Mentoring in Midwifery (MiM) model presents a framework specifically designed for the Australian midwifery context, incorporating both traditional mentoring principles and innovative approaches to professional development.

Case Study

NSW Health developed the MiM programme using Appreciative Inquiry (AI) principles to facilitate opportunities for connection, learning and growth for midwifery students and midwives. The programme's key objectives are to support the midwifery profession, develop leadership at all levels and help retain a strong, confident, and skilled midwifery workforce. The NSW Nursing and Midwifery Office (NaMO) established a working group with membership that included midwifery leaders, students, and educators to co-create and implement a MiM programme across all health services in the state. At the core of the MiM programme is relationship-centred practice, which is central to promoting learning in the workplace. The three relationship-based frameworks include Caring Conversations, The Senses Framework, and the AI Grounding Statements (Nolan et al., 2006) underpin the programme function interchangeably to enable people to acknowledge achievements, encourage better listening, and make space for the contributions of self and others to enhance the quality of learning and development for all.

This initiative included piloting the programme at four health services to evaluate the experience of midwifery leaders in co-creating and implementing the programme before implementing it across the state. The programme was implemented over two years to facilitate the engagement of midwives at the workplace and ensure a successful and sustainable model. The NSW NaMO continuously engaged with midwifery leadership across the state to plan and implement sustainable solutions tailored to meet local needs, extending beyond the two-year structured implementation period. The programme format proved to be readily adaptable to meet individual requirements of maternity services according to available resources and in response to workforce needs. Since commencing in 2022, more than 30% (1180) of the midwifery workforce has engaged in mentoring.

Following the pilot phase, a staged implementation strategy commenced utilising MiM facilitators to train and support incoming facilitators, progressing to a state-wide Community of Practice. The Community of Practice membership continues to expand to include local champions to continue supporting the programme and ensure sustainability following the structured implementation phase. Evaluation of this programme found that leadership skills were enhanced for all those involved in the co-creation and implementation of the programme. Participants identified three themes related to their experience: Connection; Learning; and Growth. Using AI tools supported people in their confidence in engaging with and communicating with others, facilitating learning in the workplace, and advocating for change. It has been reported that being involved in the co-creation and implementation of the programme has enabled leadership development, which is transferable to other initiatives and leadership roles.

Sustaining A Mentorship Culture

The vision outlined in the NSW Health MiM programme case study was to develop and implement an innovative, sustainable mentoring programme that can be embedded into midwifery practice, where mentoring others wasn't another thing to do, but rather, a way of doing things differently.

At the core of this programme is the concept that what we focus on, grows and expands, to build positive work environments that are realised together. The MiM programme is readily transferable across all midwifery training and clinical facilities to become a part of the midwifery culture in NSW.

The MiM programme provides access to innovative training that focuses on the power of relationships, emphasising working with, rather than on people, ultimately keeping women and their families at the centre of safe, compassionate, and effective midwifery care. Establishing mentorship as a core organisational value requires more than just implementing programmes – it demands cultural transformation. Organisations must create environments where mentorship is valued, supported, and integrated into daily practice, becoming part of the professional identity of every midwife.

The MiM programme is a key strategy in strengthening the midwifery workforce in NSW Health. Enabling attraction and retention, diversity, and quality in the midwifery workforce is crucial to providing safe and effective maternity care. Chapters 25 and 27 discuss MiM's further.

REFLECTIVE ACTIVITY 1

Reflect on the maternity unit/service in which you currently work.

- Is your midwifery workforce at capacity? Or do you have a staff shortage, or skill mix discrepancy?
- Do you have a formal mentoring programme where new staff, less experienced staff and/or students are mentored by those with the skills and capacity to support professional development?

  - Or does ad hoc mentoring occur? If so, who does it and what might happen if those staff members left?

- Who is responsible to develop, implement, and ensure sustainability of a mentoring programme?
- How might *you* support a mentoring programme that could improve attraction and retention, diversity, and quality in the midwifery workforce?

Leadership Development Through Mentorship

Mentorship is a powerful catalyst for leadership development, creating a pipeline of confident, competent midwifery leaders. The development of strong midwifery leadership is fundamental to the advancement of the profession and the improvement of perinatal outcomes (Pezaro et al., 2024) and is discussed in Chapter 3: Midwifery Leadership in Healthcare: theories and models. Investment and engagement in mentorship programmes can result in multiple returns, from improved clinical outcomes to enhanced organisational capability and succession planning. The International College of Midwives (2022) emphasises that effective midwifery leadership is essential across all healthcare system levels to drive change and support the development of safe, high-quality maternity services. This leadership extends beyond traditional management roles to encompass clinical leadership, research leadership, and educational leadership positions which is discussed in Chapters 3 and 28. Through structured mentorship programmes, emerging leaders can develop the complex skills to navigate these diverse leadership pathways (Adcock et al., 2022).

Developing compassionate midwifery leadership requires a multifaceted approach that combines formal learning with experiential development opportunities. Mentorship programmes provide a safe space for current and future leaders to explore their leadership styles, challenge assumptions, and develop skills and capabilities. This was evident in the

NSW Health case study. This approach enables emerging and current midwifery leaders to learn from experienced mentors who can share insights, guide them through complex situations, and offer support during challenging transitions. This mentorship fosters reciprocal learning, and mutual growth, allowing leaders to learn and develop their skills collectively.

Investment in leadership development through mentorship must be strategic and sustained. For the midwifery workforce to successfully develop effective leadership pipelines, implementing mentoring programmes with development pathways, regular evaluation points, and opportunities for practical leadership experience is required (Homer et al., 2024). These mentoring programmes should align with organisational goals while remaining flexible enough to accommodate individual career aspirations and learning needs. The return on investment in leadership development through mentorship can be measured through various metrics, including improved staff retention rates, increased leadership capability, and enhanced organisational performance indicators. However, the most significant returns often come through developing a more engaged, confident, and capable midwifery workforce that can drive innovation and improvement in maternity services.

By fostering a culture of mentorship with an explicit focus on leadership development, organisations can create sustainable pathways for professional growth while building the leadership capacity necessary for the future of midwifery practice. This investment in leadership development through mentorship is crucial for ensuring the continued evolution and excellence of maternity services.

Conclusion and Future Directions

As healthcare and midwifery workforce evolves around the world, so must our approach to mentorship in midwifery practice. Drawing together the key themes explored throughout this chapter, we recognise that effective mentorship programmes are fundamental to developing effective midwifery leadership for all and ensuring excellence in maternity care. Mentorship programmes must be implemented and adapted to be flexible and accessible for all.

The call to action is clear: healthcare organisations must prioritise and invest in structured mentorship programmes supporting all midwives' leadership development and professional growth. By fostering a culture of mentorship, we can build a resilient midwifery workforce capable of meeting future challenges while maintaining the woman-centred care central to our profession. The future of midwifery leadership depends on the actions we take today to support and develop the next generation of midwifery leaders.

References

Adcock, J. E., Sidebotham, M., & Gamble, J. (2022). What do midwifery leaders need in order to be effective in contributing to the reform of maternity services? Women and Birth : Journal of the Australian College of Midwives, 35(2), e142–e152. https://doi.org/10.1016/j.wombi.2021.04.008

Homer, C. S. E., Small, K., Warton, C., Bradfield, Z., Baird, K., Fenwick, J., Gray, J. E., & Robinson, M. (2024). Midwifery Futures – Building the Future Australian Midwifery Workforce. A Research Project Commissioned by the Nursing and Midwifery Board of Australia. Burnet Institute, Curtin University and the University of Technology Sydney.

International Confederation of Midwives. (2020). Mentoring Guidelines for Midwives. https://internationalmidwives.org/resources/mentoring-guidelines-for-midwives/

International College of Midwives. (2022). Midwifery Leadership: Guide. https://internationalmidwives.org/resources/guide-for-midwifery-leadership/

Jefford, E., Nolan, S., Munn, J., & Ebert, L. (2021). What matters, what is valued and what is important in mentorship through the Appreciative Inquiry process of co-created knowledge. Nurse Education Today, 99, 104791. https://doi.org/10.1016/j.nedt.2021.104791

Newton, M., Faulks, F., Bailey, C., Davis, J., Vermeulen, M., Tremayne, A., & Kruger, G. (2022). Continuity of care experiences: A national cross-sectional survey exploring the views and experiences of Australian students and academics. Women and Birth, 35(3), e253–e262. https://doi.org/10.1016/j.wombi.2021.05.009

Nolan, M. R., Brown, J., Davies, S., Nolan, J., & Keady, J. (2006). The senses framework: improving care for older people through a relationship-centred approach. Getting Research into Practice (GRiP) Report No. 2 Project Report. University of Sheffield. https://shura.shu.ac.uk/280/1/PDF_Senses_Framework_Report.pdf

Nursing and Midwifery Board of Australia. (2023). Retrieved 27th March 2024 from https://www.nursingmidwiferyboard.gov.au

Pezaro, D. S., Zarbiv, G., Jones, J., Feika, M. L., Fitzgerald, L., Lukhele, S., McMillan-Bohler, J., Baloyi, O. B., Maravic da Silva, K., Grant, C., Bayliss-Pratt, L., & Hardtman, P. (2024). Characteristics of strong midwifery leaders and enablers of strong midwifery leadership: An international appreciative inquiry. Midwifery, 132, 103982. https://doi.org/10.1016/j.midw.2024.103982

Sheehan, A., Dahlen, H. G., Elmir, R., Burns, E., Coulton, S., Sorensen, K., Duff, M., Arundell, F., Keedle, H., & Schmied, V. (2023). The implementation and evaluation of a mentoring program for bachelor of midwifery students in the clinical practice environment. Nurse Education in Practice, 70, 103687. https://doi.org/10.1016/j.nepr.2023.103687

Sheehan, A., Elmir, R., Hammond, A., Schmied, V., Coulton, S., Sorensen, K., Arundell, F., Keedle, H., Dahlen, H., & Burns, E. (2022). The midwife-student mentor relationship: Creating the virtuous circle. Women and Birth: Journal of the Australian College of Midwives, 35(5), e512–e520. https://doi.org/10.1016/j.wombi.2021.10.007

Wissemann, K., Bloxsome, D., De Leo, A., & Bayes, S. (2022). What are the benefits and challenges of mentoring in midwifery? An integrative review. Women's Health, 18. https://doi.org/10.1177/17455057221110141

25

MIDWIFERY MENTORSHIP

Mentee Perspective

Virginia Stulz and Nicola Drayton

Introduction

Midwifery students can flourish in supportive learning environments in the complex workplace of midwifery practice. There are opportunities the midwifery workforce can embrace to support the next generation of midwives. This chapter provides insight into the exploration of midwives' and midwifery students' experiences of learning to be a midwife in the complex world of midwifery practice and the support strategies that might assist the professional development of the next generation of midwives.

The Study

The Exploring Midwifery Students' Experiences study (Dewar et al., 2019) was an appreciative inquiry study that generated an experience-based understanding of what was working well in relation to Australian midwifery students' experiences of learning to be a midwife, and co-creating with midwives and students, how to enhance and enrich learning experiences. This study was commissioned by the New South Wales (NSW) Health (Nursing and Midwifery Office) and was a collaboration with NSW Health, University of the West of Scotland, School of Nursing and Midwifery, Centre for Nursing and Midwifery Research, Nepean Hospital, Western Sydney University and three other local health districts including South Eastern Sydney (St George hospital), Western Sydney (Blacktown hospital), and Hunter New England (John Hunter) to progress improving the experiences of midwifery students (Dewar et al., 2019).

DOI: 10.4324/9781003533733-26

Appreciative Inquiry

Appreciative inquiry was developed by Cooperrider and Srivasta in 1987 as part of the business discipline (Van Der Haar & Hosking, 2004) and further developed by Dewar in the area of nursing and midwifery (Dewar, 2012). The approach provided evidence so that midwifery students could move towards a future where they could feel valued and supported, which is crucial to attracting midwifery students to this area of work and to retain the future midwifery leaders (Dewar et al., 2020). Appreciative inquiry is a methodology that uncovers a 'positive core' within an organisation and seeking out 'the life' of those within and the organisation itself (Cooperrider et al., 2005; Sharp et al., 2017).

Appreciative inquiry has four phases of inquiry that include Discover, Envision, Co-create, and Embed, offering an opportunity for learning in clinical practice (Dewar et al., 2017). The *Discovery* phase enquires about what is working well in practice, what is valued, and what matters in the current working environment. This phase assists with the next phase of *Envision* which involves envisioning a desired future which leads into the next phase which is to *Co-create* and discusses thoughts about possible ways of doing this. Small prototypes or trials are then formulated to try to envision possibilities. Meaningful ways to implement successful developments are devised. The *Embed* phase follows which is about these developments becoming normal routine practice and contemplating what is required to continue flourishing and learning (Dewar et al., 2020).

The Senses Framework

The Senses Framework was developed by Nolan et al. (2006) and the data that we collected on this project were mapped to this Framework. We used the Senses Framework as it provided a theoretical and analytical lens that focused on gaining a greater appreciation for what midwives and midwifery students valued as important components of enriched learning environments (Dewar et al., 2020). This enabled a more nuanced specific set of signifiers for the senses which had meaning for those involved in assisting midwifery students, mentors, and midwives to participate in achieving optimal learning experiences where the senses were met for everyone (Dewar et al., 2019).

Data were aligned to the Senses Framework, and for the purpose of this chapter, we are going to focus on five out of the six senses which relate to mentoring which include security, purpose, continuity, achievement, and significance. Analysing the data against the Senses Framework enabled refinement of the meaning of all senses within the context of the midwifery students' and midwives' experiences of learning and working together. All the senses do overlap and interrelate with each other despite being discrete (Dewar et al., 2020).

Mentorship and Midwifery Student Learning

Mentorship is designed to assist midwifery students' learning in clinical environments and has been identified as heralding both positive and negative experiences. A successful relationship between a midwifery student and a mentor can promote positive experiences in clinical placement areas and contribute to quality learning experiences and subsequently confident practitioners in the future (Gray, 2018). The support of a midwifery mentor during the new graduate's year has been identified as a valuable asset in culminating confidence and keeping new graduates in the workforce (Cummins et al., 2016; 2017; Dixon et al., 2015). A closer exploration and understanding of specific behaviours supporting learning between the mentor and mentee relationship would assist in sharing what is valued (Dewar et al., 2020). Being matched formally to a mentor has shown that new graduates can establish more meaningful relationships with the midwife. However, if new graduates choose their own mentor, this has also been shown to develop trusting relationships with a more experienced midwife. (Cummins et al., 2017). The aim of Dewar and colleagues' study in 2020 was to work collaboratively with midwifery students and midwives to generate experience-based understanding of what was working well for midwifery students' learning (Dewar et al., 2020).

Methods Used in the Study

Emotional Touchpoints

Individual emotional touchpoint interviews were carried out with midwifery students and midwives to explore how they felt about mentorship. The 'touchpoints' refer to neutral points in the experience so, for example, 'working with my mentor', and 'support' were used as the touchpoints. Using emotional touchpoints provides some structure and guidance in capturing the stories and experiences of women, staff, and students. They can be used on an individual basis or group setting. They can be supported with a variety of tools such as words, cards, or other imagery. Participants were then asked to select from a range of both positive and negative emotional words (for example awkward, let down, frustrated, heard, involved, supported) that sum up what the experience felt like, then explain why they felt this way. The information found can be used to make improvements to the topic being explored.

Photoelicitation

Individuals were asked to select a photo image that explained how they were feeling about an experience, for example, being supported in the unit, and why they selected that particular photo. Creative approaches such as painting, photo elicitation, creative writing, music, and dancing can be used to help engage our senses and express feelings and experiences that might be difficult to put in words (Drayton, 2022).

Findings

Sense of Security

Midwifery students did not want to feel incompetent, but they also did not wish for inferior care of the women if they were left to attend to tasks for which they felt unprepared. They valued feedback from their mentors and valued environments where they felt safe to receive feedback. Mentors for the midwifery students meant they could work to the best of their ability without feeling judged, and to have the physical and emotional demands of their role acknowledged.

Midwifery students valued receiving timely and specific feedback from their mentors, especially in the moment: "I felt safe in my practice because the midwife I was working with made the experience good. She gave me good feedback in the moment." This feedback in the moment contributed to the sense of security that people felt and highlighted the importance of giving and receiving feedback as a reciprocal process (Dewar et al., 2020). Midwifery students valued the time mentors provided, showing them how to do things and encouraging them to 'give it a go' themselves. Midwives also shared they need to feel safe with what they did not know. One midwife was surprised that she had never learnt about how to be a mentor in the workplace. Midwifery students spoke about the importance of being supported in the workplace as everyone working together to help them get through this learning experience (Dewar et al., 2019). A sense of security in the relationship as well as the environment was important for midwifery students.

Sense of Purpose

Mentors provided opportunities for midwifery students to be able to fulfil their obligations and aspirations. Taking a chance to support someone to develop these was valued enormously: "I like it when the midwife says this is your woman for the day and I get to look after her myself – with the midwife in the background there to ask any questions. It makes me feel she trusts me."

A sense of purpose also aligned with balancing feeling comfortable with uncertainty and knowing the daily routine of how things were done in that particular work environment. This overlaps with the sense of security where feeling incompetent was uncomfortable. Midwifery students valued mentors taking the time to 'show them the ropes' (Dewar et al., 2020).

Sense of Continuity

A sense of continuity related to the midwifery student making valued connections with their mentor. This was seen as building on what was already known as well as valuing consistency in various approaches to learning and development for everyone. Some midwifery students felt the consistency of mentor was important to support the identification of strengths: "It is helpful if we have the same midwife supporting us or group of midwives – they get to know your strengths." There were different views about how to support the building of strengths of each other in the midwifery student/mentor relationship and this was important for a sense of continuity. Others recommended a team approach to mentoring (Dewar et al., 2020).

Sense of Achievement

A sense of achievement related to receiving feedback from the mentor, being supported to learn about things that mattered to the student, and setting realistic goals to achieve (Dewar et al., 2020). As this student reported:

> My mentor giving me positive feedback in the moment made me feel comfortable and supported. For me, being honest and realistic helps to give me a sense of achievement and a clear view of the direction I need to travel. I feel like you always want to achieve everything you want to but sometimes this is not possible as a student midwife. So being realistic is key. We as individuals don't always realise our strengths so I like to have that reinforcing feedback.
>
> *(Dewar et al., 2019)*

The timing of the feedback was seen as important and many of the midwifery students spoke about feedback and appreciation in the moment:

> I think it is important to provide feedback contemporaneously, saying things like 'you should feel proud of yourself'. Her saying to me at that point was so important, if she had said that to me two weeks later, it would not have meant anything to me.
>
> *(Dewar et al., 2020)*

An awareness about the mentor–mentee relationship helped midwifery students understand and appreciate the midwife even more as this student reports: "I really value it when the midwife takes the time to explain things especially in a chaotic situation" (Dewar et al., 2019).

Sense of Significance

Midwifery students valued feeling cared for in the mentor relationship. Students wanted to be heard by their mentors and felt their contribution mattered. A sense of significance was realised when the mentor valued the midwifery student's learning in clinical practice as a priority. Language was another important aspect that helped the students feel that they mattered (Dewar et al., 2020). As these students reported: "Using respectful language that values us as people" and "The language that the mentor uses when letting you do tasks makes a big difference, because it is important for us to develop understanding and learning, ..." and "I have been thinking about our language in giving feedback and how it is so important, maybe we could say "I would appreciate if you could ..." We could then provide the purpose for doing it this way. I don't like being told "you should have done," wouldn't it be better to say – "it would be lovely if you are able to... "I feel that this would help people share and feel comfortable to give and receive feedback" (Dewar et al., 2019).

Working with a Mentor

Midwifery students were asked about what was important about a mentor in their learning journey and it was thought that years of experience as a midwife was not the most important aspect and that the mentor being able to ask the student questions to assist them in processing things and reflecting was important. The following quotes are recommendations from midwifery students about what it looks like from a mentee's perspective.

When the midwife is here it makes me feel more confident. When I have support, I feel I can ask questions. Good mentors talk and show interest in you, others you just follow around and I feel a bit stupid.

It would be great if all student midwives could have a week of just observing. We have already seen midwives arrive and leave three months later. To have a permanent mentor or mentors where you work with them continually would be excellent. And working their shifts would help also. As a student midwife, I value the midwife's transfer of knowledge and wisdom.

I am curious about how we can facilitate continuity of midwifery mentor and if this is the best way to go? Perhaps consistency of approach is the best way to go.

The midwife's wealth of experience was amazing and her suggestions were really helpful for my learning about what it means to be a midwife.

What if a key feature of preparation to be a student midwife and a midwife mentor was resilience training and self-care training? – Imagine if we nurtured each other the same way we nurtured our women – safe, quality, caring.

My mentor is fantastic, she knows my strengths.

REFLECTIVE ACTIVITY 1

• Using the principles of emotional touch points and reflecting on working with your mentor, think about the words that come to mind and why you chose those words?

Discussion

Irrespective of geographical location or model of care successful relationships between mentors and midwifery students enabled thriving, nurturing learning environments that increased students' capacity for knowledge, and the opportunity to promote future inquiry (Dewar et al., 2020). Mentoring approaches increase the diversity of the midwifery workforce (Valentin-Welch, 2016), especially with a national and international shortage of midwives. It is vital that midwifery mentors are provided preparation and education with the same students so they can build familiarity with students' skills and abilities and be able to appropriately monitor their progress and learning (Gray & Downer, 2021). Timing and availability of a mentor have been shown to be vital to provide sufficient support whenever it is needed (Hopkinson et al., 2023).

Other studies (Gray, 2018; Pryjmachuk & Richards, 2008) have also identified that interpersonal relationships and successful learning experiences also contributed to students transitioning into the workforce as confident health practitioners. Mentoring programmes could prevent early attrition from the workforce, build confidence, build resilience, and increase skill acquisition. Mentoring programmes could also contribute to an increasing and sustainable workforce (Bradford et al., 2022; Thomas, 2022). Peer mentoring programmes offer an alternative to mentor programmes, mentees report feeling comfortable asking a peer questions relating to how to communicate with midwives, completing necessary documentation, and clarifying concerns (Hogan et al., 2017; McKellar & Kempster, 2017). Hogan et al.'s (2017) study on a peer mentoring programme shows they have the capacity to enhance the student's experience, building confidence, time management, and clinical decision-making skills along with leadership development.

Midwifery students in our Australian study identified that a team approach to mentoring is important (Dewar et al., 2020). Similarly, a United Kingdom study demonstrated their peer mentoring programme for final university midwifery students transitioning into health professionals in their first year of practice, promoted the development of teamwork and communication skills (Fisher & Stanyer, 2018). Midwifery students in our study valued feedback from their mentors in a non-judgmental way. A recent American review (Bradford et al., 2022) showed that midwifery mentees also valued feedback from the mentor and their non-judgmental attitudes, identifying these as important personal attributes in a mentor.

Midwifery students in our study also identified they were able to feel comfortable about being uncertain and valued the mentors 'showing them the ropes'. Jefford et al. (2021) also used an appreciative inquiry approach with midwifery students to explore what was important about mentorship. They found that students valued feeling safe and having a sense of belonging when the mentor took the time to assist the student to learn and flourish in the clinical environment (Jefford et al., 2021). Jefford et al. (2021) also found that trust was an overarching theme that resonated between the midwifery student, and the mentor and affected the woman's quality care. The midwifery students in our study also felt it was valuable when the mentor trusted the student in caring for the woman for the day, knowing, that the mentor was in the background if needed. Setting realistic goals was important for midwifery students in our study and this resonates with other research which identified being open, honest, and reflective as important attributes when students were setting goals (Jefford et al., 2021; Saukkoriipi et al., 2020). Being valued as a midwifery student in our study meant that the mentor felt that the student's contribution mattered. Other research has shown that midwifery students value the feedback, planning, and continuity from their mentor (Moran & Banks, 2016).

Conclusion

The changing global landscape of the midwifery profession requires enabling environments and support systems that prevent burnout and stress and encourage retention and professional development of midwives. As stated by an Australian midwifery student, "What if a key feature of preparation to be a student midwife and a midwife mentor was resilience training and self-care training? – Imagine if we nurtured each other the same way we nurtured our women – safe, quality, caring." To work and learn effectively, midwives around the world, like midwifery students, rely on environments that generate a sense of belonging and achievement of goals. It is important therefore for both midwives and midwifery students to have the capacity to build safe, trusting relationships, where they can address personal and professional issues and build an understanding of the role of the midwife. They need access to resources and an enabling environment that can provide leadership, strategies, and tools to meet their professional development goals. Midwifery mentoring, at all levels in the health service context, can help shape an enabling environment.

Acknowledgements

We would like to acknowledge the other ESME colleagues who worked on this project with us: Belinda Dewar, Alexa Buliak, Louise Connolly, Karen McLaughlin, Katie Newport, Susan Rebolledo, Lorraine Stephenson, & Tamsin MacBride, and the Ministry of Health for providing this opportunity for this important work.

References

Bradford, H., Findletar Hines, H., Labko, Y., Peasley, A., Valentin-Welch, V., & Breedloves, G. (2022). Midwives mentoring midwives: A review of the evidence and Best practice recommendations. *Journal of Midwifery & Women's Health*, 67, 21–30. DOI: 10.1111/jmwh.13285.

Cooperrider, D., & Whitney, D. D. (2005). *Appreciative Inquiry: A Positive Revolution in Change*. Berrett-Koehler Publishers.

Cummins, A. M., Denney-Wilson, E., & Homer, C. S. E. (2016). The challenge of employing and managing new graduate midwives in midwifery group practices in hospitals. *Journal of Nursing Management*, 24(5), 614–623.

Cummins, A. M., Denney-Wilson, E., & Homer, C. S. E. (2017). The mentoring experiences of new graduate midwives working in midwifery continuity of care models in Australia. *Nurse Education in Practice*, 24, 106–111.

Dewar, B. (2012). Using creative methods in practice development to understand and develop compassionate care. *International Practice Development Journal*, 2(1), 1–11. http://www.fons.org/library/journal.aspx

Dewar, B., Sharp, C., Barrie, K., MacBride, T., & Meyer, J. (2017). Caring conversation framework to promote person centred care: Synthesising qualitative findings from a multiphase programme of research. *International Journal of Person Centred Medicine*, 7(1), 21–35.

Dewar, B., Stulz, V., Buliak, A., Connolly, L., Mc Laughlin, K., Newport, K., Rebolledo, S., Stephenson, L., MacBride, T., Lennon, K., & Drayton, N. (2020). Exploring and developing student Midwives' experiences (ESME) – An appreciative inquiry study. *Midwifery*, 91, 102844. https://doi.org/10.1016/j.midw.2020.102844

Dewar, B., Stulz, V., Drayton, N., Buliak, A., Connolly, L., McLaughlin, K., Newport, K., Rebolledo, S., Stephenson, L., & MacBride, T. (2019). *"Exploring Student Midwives' Experiences (ESME study): an appreciative inquiry"* prepared on behalf of the Nursing and Midwifery Office, New South Wales.

Dixon, L., Calvert, S., Tumilty, E., Kensington, M., Gray, E., Lennox, S., Campbell, N., & Pairman, S. (2015). Supporting new zealand graduate midwives to stay in the profession: An evaluation of the midwifery first year of practice programme. *Midwifery*, 31(6), 633–639. https://doi.org/10.1016/j.midw.2015.02.010

Drayton, N. (2022). Creating a symbol of hope for 2021. *International Practice Development Journal*, 12(1), [10]. https://doi.org/10.19043/ipdj.121.010

Fisher, M., & Stanyer, R. (2018). Peer mentoring: Enhancing the transition from student to professional. *Midwifery, 60*, 56–59. https://doi.org/10.1016/j.midw.2018.02.004

Gray, M. (2018). Midwifery mentorship; What do we know about the mentors' perspective of the role? *Australian Midwifery News, 18*, 50–51. https://doi.org/10.1016/j.midw.2020.102844 ISSN: 1446-5612.

Gray, M., & Downer, T. (2021). Midwives' perspectives of the challenges in mentoring students: A qualitative survey. *Collegian, 28*, 135–142. https://doi.org/10.1016/j.colegn.2020.05.004

Hogan, R., Fox, G., & Barratt-See, G. (2017). Peer To Peer mentoring: Outcomes of third-year midwifery students mentoring first-year students. *Women and Birth, 30*, 206–213. http://dx.doi.org/10.1016/j.wombi.2017.03.004

Hopkinson, D., Gray, M., George, K., & Kearney, L. (2023). Nurturing our new midwives: A qualitative enquiry of mentor's experiences of supporting new graduate midwives working in continuity of care models. *Women and Birth, 36*(4), 357–366.

Jefford, E., Nolan, S., Munn, J., & Ebert, L. (2021). What matters, what is valued and what is important in mentorship through the appreciative inquiry process of co-created knowledge. *Nurse Education Today, 99*, 104791. https://doi.org/10.1016/j.nedt.2021.104791

McKellar, L., & Kempster, C. (2017). We're all in this together: Midwifery student peer mentoring. *Nurse Education in Practice, 24*, 112–117. http://dx.doi.org/10.1016/j.nepr.2015.08.014

Moran, M., & Banks, D. (2016). An exploration of the value of the role of the mentor and mentoring in midwifery. *Nurse Education Today, 40*, 52–56. http://dx.doi.org/10.1016/j.nedt.2016.02.010

Nolan, M. R., Brown, J., Davies, S., Nolan, J., & Keady, J. (2006). *The Senses Framework: Improving Care for Older People Through a Relationship-Centred Approach.* University of Sheffield. http://shura.shu.ac.uk/280/.

Pryjmachuk, S., & Richards, D. A. (2008). Predicting stress in pre-registration midwifery students attending a university in Northern England. *Midwifery, 24*, 108–122. https://doi.org/10.1016/j.midw.2020.102844

Saukkoriipi, M., Tuomikoski, A. M., Sivonen, P., Kärsämänoja, T., Laitinen, A., Tähtinen, T., Kääriäinen, M., Kuivila, H. M., Juntunen, J., Tomietto, M., & Mikkonen, K. (2020). Clustering clinical learning environment and mentoring perceptions of nursing and midwifery students: A cross-sectional study. *Journal of Advanced Nursing, 76*, 2336–2347. DOI: 10.1111/jan.14452.

Sharp, C., Dewar, B., Barrie, K., & Meyer, J. (2017). How being appreciative creates change – Theory in practice from health and social care in Scotland. *Action Research, 16*, 1–21. https://journals.sagepub.com/doi/full/10.1177/1476750316684002

Thomas, C. (2022). Coaching and mentoring skills: A complement to the professional midwifery advocate role. *British Journal of Midwifery, 30*(5), 290–296.

Valentin-Welch, M. (2016). Evaluation of a national e-mentoring program for ethnically diverse student nurse-midwives and student midwives. *Journal of Midwifery & Women's Health*, 759–767. DOI: 10.1111/jmwh.12547.

Van Der Haar, D., & Hosking, D. M. (2004). Evaluating appreciative inquiry: A relational constructionist perspective. *Human Relations, 57*(8), 1017–1036.

26

THE ROLE OF SUPPORTING MENTORSHIP IN MIDWIFERY

Terri Downer

Definition Responsibilities and Qualities of a Mentor

A midwifery mentor is an experienced midwifery practitioner who facilitates learning, supervises, and assesses students in clinical settings, creating an environment conducive to learning. The International Confederation of Midwives (ICM) defines mentoring as:

> A reciprocal learning relationship in which a mentor and mentee agree to a partnership where they work together toward achievement of mutually defined goals that will develop a mentee's skills, abilities, knowledge and/ or thinking.
>
> *(International Confederation of Midwives (ICM), 2020)*

Key responsibilities of midwifery mentors include facilitating learning opportunities, role modelling, supporting reflective practice, and advocating for mentees (Amod et al., 2024; NSW Ministry of Health, 2024; Sheehan et al., 2022). According to the ICM (2020) guidelines, effective mentors facilitate the mentees' learning experiences by actively involving them in clinical decision-making processes and promoting critical thinking skills. This involves creating a safe learning environment where students feel safe to express their concerns and ask questions. Furthermore, mentors nurture and advocate for the students by liaising with the educational institutions regarding clinical learning goals to support student learning needs and to help the student/ mentee develop confidence (Amod et al., 2024; Sheehan et al., 2022). As can be seen from the description above, this is an enormous role with much responsibility.

DOI: 10.4324/9781003533733-27

Effective mentoring in midwifery requires a unique combination of personal attributes, professional expertise, and interpersonal skills, which is discussed further in Section 1 Mentorship History & Theory Chapter 5 Midwifery Mentorship: Professional and Personal Attributes. Research has identified several key characteristics of successful midwifery mentors:

- Clinical competence: An experienced mentor with a strong foundation of up-to-date midwifery knowledge and skills is essential for guiding mentees effectively (Bradshaw et al., 2019; Hill et al., 2022).
- Patience and support: Understanding the challenges faced by mentees and providing support is important for building confidence (Nolan et al., 2022).
- Communication skills: Clear, open, and respectful communication nurtures trust and facilitates effective feedback (Jefford et al., 2021; Panda et al., 2021).
- Adaptability: Tailoring mentoring approaches to individual mentees' learning styles and needs enhances the effectiveness of the mentoring process (International Confederation of Midwives (ICM), 2020).
- Effective leadership: Creating a positive learning environment, supporting work-life balance (Thumm & Flynn, 2018).
- Reflective practice: Mentors who reflect on their practice and experiences enhance their effectiveness and encourage lifelong learning (NSW Ministry of Health, 2023).

Through these qualities and attributes, mentors enable their students to recognise their potential not only to grasp complex concepts but also to succeed and become mentors themselves in the future.

Preparing to Become a Mentor

The journey to becoming an effective midwifery mentor requires a combination of formal education, professional experience, and personal development. This section explores the key components of mentorship preparation and provides examples of mentorship preparation programmes, which compliments the chapters in Section 2 Mentoring, leadership, and education in midwifery – Global.

Preparation Programmes for Mentors in Midwifery

According to the Nursing and Midwifery Council (NMC) (2023) in the UK, mentors must possess post-registration experience in midwifery and complete the Standards for Student Supervision and Assessment (SSSA) training programme accredited by the NMC. This training equips mentors with the skills to support, assess, and guide midwifery students in clinical settings (Nursing and Midwifery Council (NMC), 2023). These programmes of study typically include a minimum period of post-registration clinical experience. They usually include teaching and assessment strategies, communication skills, and education about supporting students with diverse learning needs. Additionally, mentors are required to engage in continuous professional development (CPD) to stay updated with the latest practices and maintain their registration. Gaining experience as a midwifery mentor by shadowing experienced mentors would provide insights into best practices. Ongoing professional development is also crucial to maintain mentorship status, including regular updates and participation in mentor support networks (Edwards et al., 2005). This is discussed further in Chapter 12: Midwifery Mentorship in the United Kingdom.

Stefaniak and Dmoch-Gajzlerska (2021) also emphasise the importance of dedicated mentor training programmes, which have been shown to enhance the mentoring skills of midwives and improve the overall quality of clinical education. Further noting midwifery mentors play an important role in shaping the next generation of midwives, and their preparation is essential for effective mentorship. Education and training requirements for midwifery mentors have been developed to meet the changing needs of the profession. Educational institutions for midwifery, such as the Medical University of Warsaw have also established specific mentor training programmes (Stefaniak & Dmoch-Gajzlerska, 2021).

Several Australian institutions have developed comprehensive mentor preparation programmes tailored to midwifery practice. Several studies have highlighted the need for training in mentorship prior to undertaking the role of a mentor (Sheehan et al., 2022; Stefaniak & Dmoch-Gajzlerska, 2021; Tuomikoski et al., 2020). Sheehan et al. (2022) explore the developing relationship between mentors and mentees participating in a structured midwifery mentoring programme in New South Wales (NSW). The study recognises the importance of good mentoring for the students' adjustment to learning in the clinical environment, emphasising the mutual benefits for both mentors and mentees. In NSW, the Mentoring in Midwifery (MiM) programme has been developed by the Nursing and Midwifery Office (NaMO) of the NSW Ministry of Health (2024). The programme aims to develop reciprocal learning relationships that expand opportunities for connection, learning, and growth for midwives and midwifery students. The programme is open to midwives who would like to further develop and enhance their mentoring skills. The programme includes workshops and resources based on Appreciative Inquiry, Caring Conversations, and the Senses Framework which is discussed in Chapters 24, 25 and 27 (please see country-specific resources at the end of the chapter and other chapters in this section of the book).

Building Effective Mentor–Mentee Relationships

The foundation of successful midwifery mentoring lies in the quality of the relationship between mentor and mentee. This partnership plays a crucial role in shaping the mentee's professional development and, ultimately, the quality of care provided to women and their families. This section explores the key aspects of building and maintaining a successful mentor–mentee relationship in midwifery.

Building Trust

Establishing trust and rapport is essential for a productive mentor–mentee relationship. Trust allows mentees to feel safe in sharing their concerns through authentic presence, asking questions, and taking risks in their learning (Kramer, 2024). To build trust, mentors should create a welcoming environment, demonstrate consistency, practice active listening, and maintain confidentiality. Gray and Downer (2021) highlight in their qualitative survey that mentors often face challenges in building these relationships, particularly when dealing with students who lack confidence or struggle with communication. They suggest that mentors who invest time in getting to know their mentees personally and professionally are better equipped to overcome these challenges.

Effective communication is essential to successful mentoring. Mentors should employ various strategies to facilitate clear, constructive, and supportive communication. In their mentoring guidelines, the ICM (2020) emphasise the importance of establishing trust and mutual respect and using open-ended questions to encourage reflection and critical thinking. They also stress the need for providing specific, timely, and balanced feedback that focuses on behaviour rather than personality. Adapting communication style to the mentee's preferred learning approach can significantly enhance the effectiveness of the mentoring relationship and ensure a supportive and productive mentoring environment, ultimately benefiting both the mentor and mentee (Bradford et al., 2022).

Setting Expectations

Setting clear expectations and goals provides structure and direction for the mentoring relationship. In their Mentoring Toolkit, the NSW Government recommend setting agreed expectations including well-defined goals and setting ground rules. Collaboratively setting Specific, Measurable, Achievable, Relevant, and Time-bound (SMART) goals that align with the mentee's learning needs and professional aspirations can provide a clear roadmap for the mentoring relationship (; South Eastern Sydney Local Health District (SESLHD), 2020). Frequent check-ins and formal and informal progress reviews are important for maintaining support and addressing any challenges. By setting clear expectations and goals, mentors can provide structured guidance, while mentees can focus their efforts on targeted areas of improvement, leading to a more effective and rewarding mentorship experience (SESLHD, 2020).

Managing Expectations

Managing expectations is essential for maintaining a positive mentor-mentee relationship. Gray and Downer (2021) found that mentors often struggle with balancing their clinical responsibilities with mentoring duties. They suggest that being realistic about what can be achieved within the constraints of the clinical environment and gradually increasing the mentee's independence can help manage expectations effectively. Addressing misalignments promptly and collaboratively problem-solving when issues arise is essential for maintaining a healthy mentoring relationship. By managing expectations effectively, being patient and honest, mentors can create a positive learning environment that promotes growth and development for mentees (Dragon, 2019; Mathope et al., 2023).

The inherent power imbalance in mentor–mentee relationships can impact the learning experience and must be carefully navigated. Acknowledging the power differential and creating a collaborative environment where mentees are encouraged to share their knowledge and experiences can help mitigate this imbalance (Hill et al., 2022). Sheehan and colleagues (2023) refer to flattening the hierarchy and encouraging a sense of belonging through shared social encounters. Encouraging a culture of mutual respect is important when mentoring, particularly in acknowledging and valuing the mentee's background, culture, and individual learning journey. Professional boundaries must be maintained throughout the mentoring relationship, with clearly defined boundaries, roles, and expectations established early on (Hill et al., 2022).

Developing a strong mentor–mentee relationship is an important aspect of effective mentoring in midwifery. By focusing on building trust, employing effective communication strategies, setting clear expectations and goals, and addressing power dynamics, mentors can create a supportive learning environment. This nurturing relationship not only facilitates the mentee's professional growth but also enhances the mentor's development and advances the midwifery profession (Hill et al., 2022).

ACTIVITY 1: REFLECTION ON MENTORING EXPERIENCE

As you read about the responsibilities of building effective mentor–mentee relationships, reflect on your own experiences either as a mentor or mentee. Make some notes that describe a significant mentoring interaction you have had. Consider:

- What made it effective or ineffective?
- How did it align with or differ from the best practices discussed in this chapter so far?
- How might you apply the insights gained from your reflection to future midwifery mentoring relationships with students?

Assessment and Support

Assessment and support are essential components in the role of the midwifery mentor, ensuring mentees develop the necessary skills, knowledge, and competencies to provide safe and high-quality woman-centre care. Assessment that is fair and equitable plays an important part in maintaining professional standards and accountability within the midwifery profession.

Methods of Assessment

Methods of assessment in midwifery mentoring have evolved to include a more holistic approach. Bradshaw and colleagues (2019) highlight the importance of using a variety of assessment methods to capture the comprehensive nature of midwifery practice. These methods may include direct observation of clinical skills, case-based discussions, reflective writing, ePortfolios, and simulation-based assessments.

Ensuring fairness and objectivity in assessment remains a key concern for midwifery mentors. Hill and colleagues (2022) emphasise the importance of clear assessment criteria and rubrics aligned with professional competency standards. The Australian Midwifery Standards Assessment Tool (AMSAT) is one such tool that is instrumental in achieving this by providing a standardised and consistent framework for assessing midwifery practice against established criteria. The AMSAT promotes transparency and reduces bias through its structured approach, enabling mentors to evaluate students' performance objectively and fairly (Sweet et al., 2019). Resources such as video case studies for midwifery mentors who use this tool are freely available on the Australian College of Midwives website (ACM, 2021).

Supporting Struggling Students

Supporting struggling students is an essential aspect of the mentor's role in assessment and evaluation. Effective techniques include the implementation of early feedback, which provides opportunities for reflection, goal setting, and setting a learning or action plan that is clear for the student (Power & Jewell, 2018). Hughes and Fraser (2011) also propose a structured approach to identifying and supporting students who are not meeting expected competencies. This approach involves early identification of concerns, collaborative goal setting with the student, ensuring feedback is objective, implementation of targeted support strategies, and regular review of their progress, both informally and formally. The authors stress the importance of maintaining open communication and providing constructive feedback throughout the placement and recommend that it should not be left until the end of the placement.

It has been recognised in the literature there is an issue with failing to fail underachieving students (Houghton, 2016). There are many reasons mentors may find it challenging with failing students such as a lack of support and guidance, time-consuming, failing students provokes emotional issues, mentors have a lack of confidence, and may give students the benefit of the doubt (Houghton, 2016). Failing to fail is of concern to midwifery practice, and mentors need to be aware of the consequences and issues relating to safety for women and their families and learn how to seek support for student's who are causing concern (Houghton, 2016).

Cultural Sensitivity

Cultural sensitivity in assessment has also emerged as an important consideration in midwifery mentoring. West et al. (2016) highlight the need for culturally sensitive assessment practices that recognise and value diverse perspectives and approaches to midwifery care. In their scoping review, Biles and colleagues (2023) discuss creating an inclusive environment to promote retention in the midwifery workforce. Midwifery mentors must engage in ongoing cultural education to effectively support their mentees, ultimately improving maternal and infant health outcomes within Indigenous communities which is discussed further in Chapter 22. Emphasising cultural safety is essential for effective mentorship and equitable healthcare delivery (Biles et al., 2023).

Assessment and evaluation in midwifery mentoring continue to evolve, embracing more holistic and culturally responsive approaches. By ensuring fairness and objectivity, supporting struggling students, continuously improving programmes based on feedback, and integrating evidence-based practice, mentors can effectively assess and evaluate mentees' progress to help them develop as competent and compassionate midwives.

ACTIVITY 2: CASE STUDY ANALYSIS

Take a moment to reflect on what you have learnt so far in this chapter and analyse the following case study:

A student midwife is struggling with confidence in clinical skills despite theoretical knowledge. The mentor observes inconsistent performance.

Consider the following:

- How would you approach this situation as a mentor?
- What strategies could you apply?
- How would you balance support with the need for objective assessment?
- Development of an action plan for this student, considering the various aspects of mentoring discussed in this chapter.

Challenges and Emerging Trends in Midwifery Mentoring

Midwifery education and practice is continuously evolving, presenting both challenges and opportunities for mentoring in midwifery. This section explores current issues, emerging trends, and suggests future directions for research in midwifery mentoring.

Current Issues in Midwifery Mentorship

Increasing student numbers and fewer registered midwives undertaking mentorship training are placing considerable strain on mentors' ability to support students on midwifery practical experience placements (Chenery-Morris & Divers, 2024). A key issue is the imbalance between the number of trained mentors and student enrollment in midwifery programmes, which can lead to inadequate supervision and concerns there will be too few mentors to support students (Greatbatch, 2016). Increasing the number of students, while promising for the future of the profession, necessitates a re-evaluation of current mentoring capacities and strategies. Additionally, balancing the workload of mentors with their clinical responsibilities can be challenging, potentially impacting the time and attention they can dedicate to their mentees (Stafaniak et al., 2021).

Another issue facing midwifery mentoring is the struggle many mentors face in achieving a healthy work-life balance (Wissemann et al., 2022). Midwives report difficulty in mentorship when juggling their clinical responsibilities with their mentoring duties. This balancing act often leads to increased stress and potential burnout among mentors, which can negatively impact the quality of education and support they provide to the students (Bradford et al., 2022).

Other challenges to mentoring include the lack of standardised mentorship training programmes and the challenge of maintaining a consistent practice, leading to variability in the quality of mentorship provided (Wissemann et al., 2022). The use of ongoing training for mentors and preceptors is recommended throughout the literature (Panda et al., 2021; Stefanil & Dmoch-Gajzlerska, 2020; Wissemann et al., 2022).

Technological Advancements

Technology is playing an increasingly pivotal role in reshaping midwifery mentoring, offering both new opportunities and challenges including the use of virtual mentoring, ePortfolios, and the use of artificial intelligence (AI). The COVID-19 pandemic served as a catalyst for the rapid adoption of virtual mentoring (Abou-Zamzam et al., 2023). Virtual mentoring can be described as pairing a novice midwife or student with an educator or midwife with extensive experience, who interact using the internet (Clement, 2014). Virtual mentoring connects mentors and mentees from any location that has access to the Internet, enabling real-time feedback. Virtual digital tools have opened new possibilities for remote support, mentorship, and guidance. For example, in their Helping Babies Breathe (HBB) project Abou-Zamzam and colleagues (2023) used trainers based in the United States to provide virtual mentorship to participants in Madagascar thus opening all kinds of mentorship possibilities.

The use of ePortfolios in midwifery has become popular and offers an efficient way to document and evaluate students' clinical learning (Downer & Slade, 2019). ePortfolios also provide students with a centralised platform to store evidence of their midwifery practice experiences which mentors then sign (Gray et al., 2019). Although there is no agreed national format for recording the information required in the ePortfolio, the integration of digital portfolios and competency tracking systems is streamlining the assessment process (Gray et al., 2020). Downer and Slade (2019) highlight how these electronic tools are not only making the evaluation process more efficient but also providing richer, more comprehensive data on student progress in meeting the Australian Nursing and Midwifery Accreditation Council (ANMAC) requirements. This information enables mentors to tailor their support and guidance more effectively to individual student learning needs whilst they are on clinical placement.

Looking to the future, artificial intelligence (AI) holds significant promise for enhancing mentoring. In their scoping review, Kranz and Abele (2024) analyse the opportunities and challenges and how emerging AI technologies have been integrated into midwifery education preparing midwifery students for a future where AI plays a significant role. O'Connor et al. (2022) report that AI has the potential to support clinical decision-making processes; however, the authors (2023) raise concerns about accountability if AI systems are used due to the potential for misinformation. The World Health Organization (WHO) (2021) also raises similar concerns regarding ethical challenges and risks when using AI for health care. While still in its early stages, AI could change how mentoring is conducted, offering data-driven insights into student performance during simulations, immediate individualised feedback, and learning support (Kranz & Abele, 2024).

Recommendations

To continue advancing the field of midwifery mentoring, future research should focus on several key areas. Promoting diversity and inclusion within midwifery, as highlighted by West and colleagues (2016), is essential for creating a culturally competent workforce. Evaluating the long-term impact of different mentorship models on practice and outcomes for students supporting women and their families can offer valuable insights into the most beneficial approaches to mentorship. Additionally, investigating the effectiveness of technology-enhanced mentoring, including AI, may transform skill development and assessment processes. Furthermore, exploring strategies that support mentors in maintaining a healthy work-life balance to prevent burnout may help reduce attrition in the midwifery workforce. This research is crucial for ensuring the sustainability of mentoring programmes and the well-being of mentors themselves. Researching these innovations through evidence-informed practice, will ensure that mentors continue to develop competent, compassionate, and confident midwifery practitioners.

Conclusion

This chapter explored the role of mentoring in midwifery. Effective mentors combine clinical expertise, interpersonal skills, and a commitment to life-long learning to nurture mentees' professional growth. The chapter emphasises the importance of supportive learning environments, reflective practice. Key challenges, such as time constraints and increasing student numbers, are acknowledged alongside innovative solutions such as the integration of technology. The importance of ongoing professional development for mentors is highlighted along with fair assessment practices.

Looking ahead, emerging trends are identified, including technological advancements and the growing emphasis on cultural competence. Mentoring remains central to midwifery education, shaping competent and compassionate future practitioners. The ongoing need for research and innovation in mentoring is recognised, and its vital role in maintaining high standards of care is important for promoting positive outcomes for women and their families. Looking to the future, mentoring will continue to be an important aspect in developing the midwifery workforce and supporting a new generation of skilled practitioners ready to meet the challenges and opportunities of contemporary midwifery practice. The integration of AI in the future may further enhance mentoring by providing innovative tools for personalised learning and feedback to support the growth of midwifery students.

Country-Specific Resources

Website

NSW Government (2024). Mentoring in Midwifery (MiM) Programme: https://www.health.nsw.gov.au/nursing/culture/Pages/mentoring-in-midwifery.aspx

Resources

Programme outline: https://www.health.nsw.gov.au/nursing/culture/Publications/mentoring-program-outline.pdf

Resource book: https://www.health.nsw.gov.au/nursing/culture/Publications/mentoring-resource-book.pdf

Facilitators guide: https://www.health.nsw.gov.au/nursing/culture/Publications/mentoring-facilitators-guide.pdfrs guide

Website

NSW Government (2024). Mentorship: A Guide for Mentors: https://www.seslhd.health.nsw.gov.au/mentorship-a-guide-for-mentors

Resources

Guidelines for Mentorship: Guidelhttps://www.seslhd.health.nsw.gov.au/sites/default/files/groups/Nursing_and_Midwifery/Nightingale Challenge/Mentorship/GUIDELINES FOR MENTORING 2020.docines for Mentorship

Getting Started: A guide for your first meeting: Gehttps://www.seslhd.health.nsw.gov.au/sites/default/files/groups/Nursing_and_Midwifery/Nightingale Challenge/Mentorship/KEY ACTIVITIES FOR ESTABLISHING THE MENTORING RELATIONSHIP 2020.pdftting Started: A guide for your first meeting

SESLHD Mentoring Toolkit (People & Culture 2020): SEShttps://www.seslhd.health.nsw.gov.au/sites/default/files/groups/Nursing_and_Midwifery/Nightingale Challenge/Mentorship/SESLHD Mentoring Toolkit Feb 2020.pdfLHD Mentoring Toolkit (People & Culture 2020)

Enabling & Appreciative Questions: https://www.seslhd.health.nsw.gov.au/sites/default/files/groups/Nursing_and_Midwifery/Nightingale Challenge/Mentorship/Enabling and Appreciative-Questions.pdf

Website

Government of Western Australia Department of Heal Nursing and Midwifery Office (2017) Preparing for Mentoring Sessions: Prephttps://www.health.wa.gov.au/-/media/Files/Corporate/general-documents/nursing-and-midwifery/PDF/NMO-Mentor-Network-Factsheet-2--Mentee-Preparing-for-the-Mentoring-sessions.pdfaring for Mentoring Sessions

References

Abou-Zamzam, A., McCaw, J., Niarison, H. R., Ravelojaona, V. A., & Shilkofski, N. (2023). Cross-sectional study in Madagascar demonstrates efficacy of virtual mentoring and flipped classroom modifications of neonatal resuscitation programme helping babies breathe. *Acta Paediatrica*, 112(8), 1783–1789. https://doi.org/10.1111/apa.16819

Amod, H. B., Ndlovu, L., & Brysiewicz, P. (2024). Clinical mentorship of midwifery students: The perceptions of registered midwives. *Health SA Gesondheid*, 29(4), 2492–2492. https://doi.org/10.4102/hsag.v29i0.2492

Australian College of Midwives (ACM). (2021). *Australian Midwifery Standards Assessment Tool*. https://midwives.org.au/Web/Web/Professional-Development/AMSAT/Australian_Midwifery_Standards_Assessment_Tool.aspx

Biles, J., Deravin, L., McMillan, A. M., Anderson, J., Sara, G., & Biles, B. (2023). Aboriginal and Torres Strait Islander nurses and midwives culturally safe mentoring programmes in Australia: A scoping review. *Contemporary Nurse: A Journal for the Australian Nursing Profession*, 59(2), 173–183. https://doi.org/10.1080/10376178.2023.2175700

Bradford, H., Hines, H. F., Labko, Y., Peasley, A., Valentin-Welch, M., & Breedlove, G. (2022). Midwives mentoring midwives: A review of the evidence and best practice recommendations. *Journal of Midwifery & Women's Health*, 67(1), 21–30. https://doi.org/10.1111/jmwh.13285

Bradshaw, C., Pettigrew, J., & Fitzpatrick, M. (2019). Safety first: Factors affecting preceptor midwives experiences of competency assessment failure among midwifery students. *Midwifery*, 74, 29–35. https://doi.org/10.1016/j.midw.2019.03.012

Chenery-Morris, S., & Divers, J. (2024). Midwifery higher education: Who are we and Who do we teach? *British Journal of Midwifery*, 32(1), 32–37. https://doi.org/10.12968/bjom.2024.32.1.32

Clement, S. (2014). The use of virtual mentoring in nursing education. *Online Journal of Nursing Informatics, 18*(2). Retrieved from https://www.proquest.com/openvi ew/0fb3e3258d37af68607656fa6b800139/1?pq-origsite=gscholar&cbl=2034896

Downer, T., & Slade, C. (2019). Starting early: Using ePortfolios to prepare first-year midwifery students for professional practice. In *Ensuring Quality in Professional Education Volume I*, edited by K. Trimmer, T. Newman, and F. Padro. Cham: Palgrave Macmillan.

Dragon, N. (2019). 10 tips to effective mentorship. *Australian Nursing and Midwifery Journal*. https://anmj.org.au/10-tips-to-effective-mentorship/

Edwards, G., Gordon, U., & Atherton, J. (2005). Network approach boosts midwives' public health role. *British Journal of Midwifery, 13*(1), 48–53. https://doi. org/10.12968/bjom.2005.13.1.17325

Gray, M., & Downer, T. (2021). Midwives' perspectives of the challenges in mentoring students: A qualitative survey. *Collegian (Royal College of Nursing, Australia), 28*(1), 135–142. https://doi.org/10.1016/j.colegn.2020.05.004

Gray, M., Downer, T., & Capper, T. (2019). Australian midwifery student's perceptions of the benefits and challenges associated with completing a portfolio of evidence for initial registration: Paper based and ePortfolios. *Nurse Education in Practice, 39*, 37–44. https://doi.org/10.1016/j.nepr.2019.07.003

Gray, M., Downer, T., & Capper, T. (2020). Midwifery student's perceptions of completing a portfolio of evidence for initial registration: A qualitative exploratory study. *Nurse Education in Practice.* 43. https://doi.org/10.1016/j.nepr.2020.102696

Greatbatch, D. (2016). A false economy, cuts to continuing professional development funding for nursing, midwifery, and the allied health professions in England (accessed 11 November 2024). https://www.magonlinelibrary.com/doi/full/10.12968/bjom. 2024.32.1.32

Hill, S. E. M., Ward, W. L., Seay, A., & Buzenski, J. (2022). The nature and evolution of the mentoring relationship in academic health centers. *Journal of Clinical Psychology in Medical Settings, 29*(3), 557–569. https://doi.org/10.1007/s10880-022-09893-6

Houghton, T. (2016). Assessment and accountability: Part 2 – Managing failing students. *Nursing Standard, 30*(41), 41–49. https://doi.org/10.7748/ns.30.41.41.s44

Hughes, A. J., & Fraser, D. M. (2011). "There are guiding hands and there are controlling hands": Student midwives experience of mentorship in the UK. *Midwifery, 27*(4), 477–483. https://doi.org/10.1016/j.midw.2010.03.006

International Confederation of Midwives (ICM). (2020). *Mentoring Guidelines for Midwives.* https://internationalmidwives.org/resources/mentoring-guidelines-for-midwives/

Jefford, E., Nolan, S., Munn, J., & Ebert, L. (2021). What matters, what is valued and what is important in mentorship through the Appreciative Inquiry process of co-created knowledge. *Nurse Education Today, 99*, 104791–104791. https://doi. org/10.1016/j.nedt.2021.104791

Kramer, D. (2024). Mentor training. In: *A Guide for Developing a Culture of Caring Through Nursing Peer Mentorship Programs.* Springer. https://doi-org.ezproxy. usc.edu.au/10.1007/978-3-031-66139-6_5

Kranz, A., & Abele, H. (2024). The impact of artificial intelligence (AI) on midwifery education: A scoping review. *Healthcare (Basel), 12*(11), 1082. https://doi. org/10.3390/healthcare12111082

Mathope, K., du Preez, A., & Scheepers, N. (2023). Mentorship needs in an intrapartum setting – Mentor-centred approach: A qualitative descriptive study. *Nurse Education in Practice, 71*, 103727–103727. https://doi.org/10.1016/j.nepr.2023.103727

Nolan, S., Baird, K., & McInnes, R. J. (2022). What strategies facilitate & support the successful transition of newly qualified midwives into practice: An integrative literature review. *Nurse Education Today, 118*, 105497–105497. https://doi. org/10.1016/j.nedt.2022.105497

NSW Ministry of Health. (2023). *Mentoring in Midwifery Facilitators Guide.* https://www.health.nsw.gov.au/nursing/culture/Publications/mentoring-facilitators-guide.pdf

NSW Ministry of Health. (2024). *Mentoring in Midwifery Resource Book.* https://www.health.nsw.gov.au/nursing/culture/Publications/mentoring-resource-book.pdf

Nursing and Midwifery Council (NMC). (2023). *Standards for Student Supervision and Assessment.* https://www.nmc.org.uk/globalassets/sitedocuments/standards/2024/standards-for-student-supervision-and-assessment.pdf

O'Connor, S. (2022). Teaching artificial intelligence to nursing and midwifery students. *Nurse Education in Practice, 64,* 103451–103451. https://doi.org/10.1016/j.nepr.2022.103451

O'Connor, S., Yan, Y., Thilo, F. J. S., Felzmann, H., Dowding, D., & Lee, J. J. (2023). Artificial intelligence in nursing and midwifery: A systematic review. *Journal of Clinical Nursing, 32*(13–14), 2951–2968. https://doi.org/10.1111/jocn.16478

Panda, S., Dash, M., John, J., Rath, K., Debata, A., Swain, D., Mohanty, K., & Eustace-Cook, J. (2021). Challenges faced by student nurses and midwives in clinical learning environment – A systematic review and meta-synthesis. *Nurse Education Today, 101,* 104875–104875. https://doi.org/10.1016/j.nedt.2021.104875

Power, A., & Jewell, L. (2018). Students in practice: The role of the student support midwife. *British Journal of Midwifery, 26*(7), 475–477. https://doi.org/10.12968/bjom.2018.26.7.475

Sheehan, A., Dahlen, H. G., Elmir, R., Burns, E., Coulton, S., Sorensen, K., Duff, M., Arundell, F., Keedle, H., & Schmied, V. (2023). The implementation and evaluation of a mentoring program for Bachelor of Midwifery students in the clinical practice environment. *Nurse Education in Practice, 70,* 103687–103687. https://doi.org/10.1016/j.nepr.2023.103687

Sheehan, A., Elmir, R., Hammond, A., Schmied, V., Coulton, S., Sorensen, K., Arundell, F., Keedle, H., Dahlen, H., & Burns, E. (2022). The midwife-student mentor relationship: Creating the virtuous circle. *Women and Birth: Journal of the Australian College of Midwives, 35*(5), e512–e520. https://doi.org/10.1016/j.wombi.2021.10.007

South Eastern Sydney Local Health District (SESLHD). (2020). *Mentoring Toolkit.* https://www.seslhd.health.nsw.gov.au/sites/default/files/groups/Nursing_and_Midwifery/Nightingale%20Challenge/Mentorship/SESLHD%20Mentoring%20Toolkit%20Feb%202020.pdf

Stefaniak, M., & Dmoch-Gajzlerska, E. (2020). Mentoring in the clinical training of midwifery students – A focus study of the experiences and opinions of midwifery students at the Medical University of Warsaw participating in a mentoring program. *BMC Medical Education, 20*(1), 394–394. https://doi.org/10.1186/s12909-020-02324-w

Stefaniak, M., & Dmoch-Gajzlerska, E. (2021). Evaluation of a mentor training program for midwives in two hospitals in Warsaw, Poland – A qualitative descriptive study. *BMC Medical Education, 21*(1), 1–345. https://doi.org/10.1186/s12909-021-02769-7

Sweet, L., Henderson, A., Fleet, J., Graham, K., Fox, D., Bowman, R., Ebert, L., Bull, A., Bass, J., Downer, T., & Bazargan, M. (2019). Development and validation of the Australian Midwifery Standards Assessment Tool (AMSAT) to the Australian midwife standards for practice 2018. *Woman and Birth, 32*(2), 135–144. https://doi.org/10.1016/j.wombi.2019.08.004

Thumm, E. B., & Flynn, L. (2018). The five attributes of a supportive midwifery practice climate: A review of the literature. *Journal of Midwifery and Women's Health, 64*(1), 90–103. https://doi.org/10.1111/jmwh.12707

Tuomikoski, A.-M., Ruotsalainen, H., Mikkonen, K., Miettunen, J., Juvonen, S., Sivonen, P., & Kaaariainen, M. (2020). How mentoring education affects nurse mentors' competence in mentoring students during clinical practice – A quasi-experimental study. *Scandinavian Journal of Caring Sciences*, *34*(1), 230–238. https://doi.org/10.1111/scs.12728.

West, F., Homer, C., & Dawson, A. (2016). Building midwifery educator capacity in teaching in low and lower-middle income countries. A review of the literature. *Midwifery*, *33*, 12–23. https://doi.org/10.1016/j.midw.2015.06.011

Wissemann, K., Bloxsome, D., De Leo, A., & Bayes, S. (2022). What are the benefits and challenges of mentoring in midwifery? An integrative review. *Women's Health*, *18*, 17455057221110141. https://doi.org/10.1177/17455057221110141

World Health Organization. (2021). *Ethics and Governance of Artificial Intelligence for Health*. https://www.who.int/publications/i/item/9789240029200

27

MIDWIFERY MENTORSHIP

The Impact on Participating Midwives

Georgie Haver and Lisa Charmer

Introduction

Background

The midwifery profession in Australia faces significant challenges due to widespread staff shortages and high attrition rates (Catling & Rossiter, 2020). Studies have revealed a concerning number of midwives intending to leave the profession, which could have serious implications for the care provided to women and newborns during the perinatal period (Harvie et al., 2019; Pugh et al., 2013). Addressing these issues requires identifying and implementing strategies that support and sustain the midwifery workforce, both now and in the future (Hildingsson et al., 2016). Research indicates that inadequate staffing levels, limited managerial support, and poor workplace culture contribute to feelings of disempowerment and disengagement among midwives, leading to decreased job satisfaction and increased turnover (Catling & Rossiter, 2020). Key elements that positively impact midwives' work experiences include adequate resources, effective leadership, and a supportive work environment that fosters collegial relationships (Sullivan et al., 2011). Strategies such as leadership development and enhanced support systems have been proposed as essential for improving workforce retention (Callander et al., 2021).

Mentoring has been widely acknowledged as a potential strategy to retain midwives within the profession (Bradford et al., 2022; Kakyo et al., 2022; Wissemann et al., 2022). Mentoring is especially valuable in health professions, where mentors serve as a buffer for recent graduates navigating complex clinical environments (Pairman, 2016). Studies have shown that mentees

DOI: 10.4324/9781003533733-28

who work within a supportive mentorship structure experience increased confidence, knowledge growth, and overall reassurance (Pairman, 2016). In an integrative review, Wisemann et al. (2022) found that mentoring within midwifery fosters professional growth, leadership skills, and a supportive workforce environment, enhancing collegiality and professional satisfaction. In New Zealand, the mandatory "Midwifery First Year of Practice Program" has demonstrated that new midwives involved in structured mentorship report increased confidence, job satisfaction, and, importantly, higher retention rates (Bradford et al., 2022). Furthermore, mentoring has been shown to benefit mentors themselves by enhancing their communication skills, self-confidence, career growth, and job satisfaction, thus positively impacting the profession (Kakyo et al., 2022; Wissemann et al., 2022).

A key element of successful mentorship is the relationship between mentor and mentee, which thrives on mutual trust, safety, and professional belonging as discussed in chapter 6. Mentors who offer support beyond the clinical context, helping mentees navigate a midwifery unit's cultural and social aspects, significantly contribute to positive mentoring experiences (Jefford et al., 2021). Reciprocal, relationship-centred practices in mentoring have been shown to enhance workplace learning and foster growth (Dewar et al., 2020).

Mentoring in Midwifery Programme (MiM)

In 2022, the NSW Health Nursing and Midwifery Office introduced the MiM programme to attract, develop, and retain skilled midwives in NSW, focusing on supporting students and early-career midwives (Lennon, 2022). The MiM model is grounded in three relationship-centred frameworks, including Appreciative Inquiry (AI), discussed in more detail in section III *Mentoring, Leadership and Education in Practice: Australia*, Chapter 25. Studies suggest that AI-based mentorship may strengthen connections among colleagues, foster leadership, and support reflective practices that improve clinical settings (Stulz et al., 2021). MiM also applies the Caring Conversations framework by Dewar and MacBride (2017), which focuses on promoting listening, communication, and acknowledgement of achievements to enrich learning and development. Additionally, the programme utilises the Senses framework, also elaborated in Chapter 25. The Senses Framework proposes that environments where individuals feel secure, connected, and purposeful lead to stronger, more positive professional relationships and team dynamics (Dewar et al., 2020).

The Study

While extensive research supports the benefits of mentorship in midwifery, studies specifically exploring mentorship models based on AI are limited.

A gap exists in understanding whether AI-based mentorship can sustain long-term benefits and positively transform midwifery teams over time. Recognising the importance of effective support strategies for midwife retention and the advantages of relationship-centred mentorship, this study aimed to describe the programmes impacts on the midwives by assessing both the benefits and challenges perceived by participants and identifying key factors to successful mentoring in midwifery. Although the research intended to address the gap in understanding AI's sustained impact in midwifery over time, changes in the participant cohort, specifically, the completion of pre- and post-surveys by different groups, limited the feasibility of a longitudinal approach.

Methods

A qualitative methodology was chosen for this study, utilising a pre–post cross-sectional comparison design. The study aimed to explore the experiences of participants in the MiM programme through the analysis of open-ended survey responses.

Participants and Recruitment

Participants were recruited using convenience sampling, inviting all individuals involved in the MiM programme to participate in the appropriate data collection for their group, either as mentors or mentees. Participation in the study was voluntary. The mentors included midwives working in maternity units within a regional Australian local health district who had completed MiM training. The mentees included midwives or student midwives who expressed interest in mentorship, matched based on the capacity of trained mentors to accommodate them.

Data Collection

Surveys were distributed pre-mentoring on the initial workshop's completion and then repeated at four to six months post-mentoring. Rolling data collection was implemented as workshops occurred throughout the year. Data were collected through a series of surveys that incorporated both scaled and open-ended questions. Although the surveys were initially designed to collect both quantitative and qualitative data, the study's limited sample size meant that quantitative data would not yield meaningful or reliable results. Therefore, the focus was placed exclusively on qualitative data, specifically the responses to the open-ended survey questions. These questions allowed participants to share their thoughts and experiences freely, aligning with the study's aim to gain a deeper understanding of the mentorship experience from both mentors' and mentees' perspectives.

Data Analysis

Qualitative data analysis was conducted using Braun and Clarke's (2021) six-phase reflexive thematic analysis framework. This inductive approach facilitated the identification and interpretation of themes within the open-ended survey responses. Braun and Clarke's methodology emphasises researcher reflexivity and flexibility, ensuring that the analysis remains grounded in the participants' experiences. The six phases included:

1 **Familiarisation:** Immersion in the data by reading and re-reading responses.
2 **Generating Initial Codes:** Systematic coding of significant features across the dataset.
3 **Searching for Themes:** Collating codes into potential themes based on patterns and meanings.
4 **Reviewing Themes:** Refining themes to ensure they accurately reflect the dataset.
5 **Defining and Naming Themes:** Clearly articulating the essence of each theme.
6 **Producing the Report:** Synthesising themes to construct a coherent narrative that addressed the research questions.

Free-text survey responses were chosen as the primary data source due to their ability to capture participants' thoughts and experiences in an open and unstructured manner (Rouder et al., 2021). This approach provided rich qualitative data to explore the nuanced experiences of both mentors and mentees in the MiM programme.

Themes Identified

Several themes were identified in the pre-mentoring dataset, highlighting both the expected benefits and potential barriers of the MiM Programme as perceived by participants. Six themes were identified as anticipated benefits of the program, reflecting areas where MiM could positively impact midwifery practice. These themes are illustrated in Figure 27.1 and included:

'Creating Space for Self-Reflection,' 'Confidence Building for Personal and Professional Growth,' 'Skill Building and Knowledge Sharing,' 'Gaining and Giving Support,' 'Fostering Connection: Collegiality for a Positive Work Environment,' and 'Revitalising Purpose: Meaningful Impact in Midwifery.'

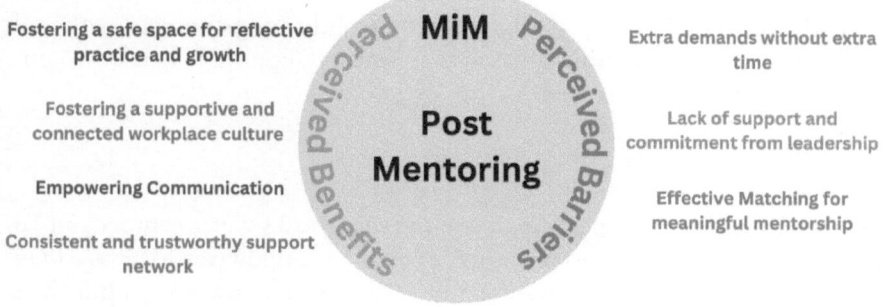

FIGURE 27.1 MiM Pre-Mentoring

Additionally, three themes were highlighted as envisaged challenges to the programme's effectiveness and reflect areas where MiM could negatively impact midwives. These are namely:

'The Time Challenge: Navigating Workload Pressures,' 'Commitment and Support: Drivers for Success,' and 'Personality Clashes and Communication Challenges.'

In the post-mentoring data, four themes were identified as current perceived benefits and impact midwives positively. As illustrated in Figure 27.2, these included:

'Fostering a Safe Space for Reflective Practice and Growth,' 'Fostering a Supportive and Connected Workplace Culture,' 'Empowering Communication,' and 'Consistent and Trustworthy Support Network.'

Conversely, in the post-mentoring data, three themes outlined perceived barriers within the programme and impact midwives negatively:

'Extra Demands Without Extra Time,' 'Lack of Support and Commitment from Leadership,' and 'Effective Matching for Meaningful Mentorship.'

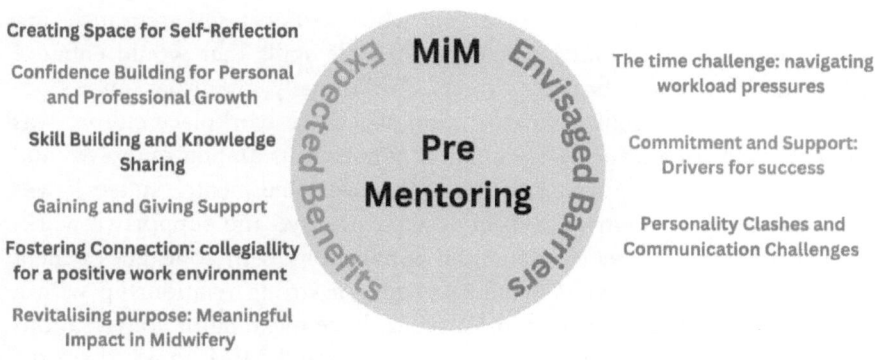

FIGURE 27.2 MiM Post-Mentoring

These themes collectively provide insight into how MiM is viewed within the midwifery community, spotlighting its strengths in fostering growth and connection and highlighting areas where further support is needed to enhance programme effectiveness.

Results

Of the 47 midwives that participated in the surveys, 31 were mentors and 16 were mentees. Out of the 31 mentors, 15 had been midwives for more than 15 years. Mentees were predominantly early-career midwives within their first year of practice.

A cohort of 35 midwives completed the pre-mentoring surveys (22 mentors, 13 mentees), while 18 participated in the post-mentoring surveys (11 mentors, 7 mentees). Of the 47 midwives surveyed, only 4 mentees and 2 mentors completed both the pre- and post-surveys, limiting the feasibility of a longitudinal comparison. Consequently, a pre–post cross-sectional comparison was employed. The pre-survey data were analysed to assess participants' expected benefits and envisaged barriers to the programme, while the post-survey data focused on evaluating the perceived benefits and barriers to the programme.

Findings Pre-Mentoring

Participants in the MiM programme identified several anticipated positive outcomes as well as potential barriers that could impact its success. Key benefits included the creation of a secure environment for self-reflection, which allowed both mentees and mentors to process their experiences and emotions openly, fostering personal and professional growth. Mentees anticipated having "a safe space to reflect with a more experienced midwife" and discuss their challenges without judgment while mentors valued the opportunity to reinforce their roles "be a role model and learn more about others and myself" and further develop their skills. Confidence-building was also highlighted, with participants expecting MiM to boost self-assurance, improve communication, and provide transferable skills that would enhance both their practice and broader careers. Additionally, the programme's potential to foster collegiality, support, and a positive workplace culture was seen as crucial for nurturing meaningful connections among midwives and revitalising a sense of purpose in the profession. One mentee stated it was "an opportunity to contribute to building a positive and supportive working environment" whereby meaningful connections with colleagues benefit the team. Mentees felt MiM would provide "a strong relationship with a colleague" or "a friend in the workplace to have meaningful conversations with". This was echoed by the mentors who stated MiM could "help the culture of my workplace grow into a more supportive, inclusive environ-ment", "improve my relationships with colleagues", and "foster meaningful and caring connection extending beyond clinical teamwork".

However, participants also anticipated several challenges that could hin-der the programme's effectiveness. "Not being given space to meet with men-tees during work hours" and the lack of "time being allocated to mentoring sessions due to high workload" would hinder the success of the programme. Time constraints and balancing the demands of mentoring with their exist-ing workload were common concerns, as mentors worried about insufficient time allocation for mentoring sessions within their work hours. The need for genuine management support was emphasised, with participants fearing the programme would suffer if not actively backed by leadership. Mentors also acknowledged potential risks of personality clashes and communication issues that could disrupt the mentor-mentee relationship. These challenges underscore the importance of sufficient support and resources to sustain the programme.

Findings Post-Mentoring

The post-mentoring participants highlighted both positive outcomes and per-ceived challenges with the MiM programme. It is important to note that the cohort of midwives was different to the midwives that participated in the pre-mentoring survey.

Participants valued MiM's ability to create a safe space for reflection, growth, and connection, which facilitated personal and professional devel-opment. As noted by one mentee, the MiM programme offered the "space to reflect on growth and contributions as a new midwife".

By "allow[ing] time to reflect on practice and life", as one mentor noted, midwives can consider both their clinical skills and their personal well-being, facilitating professional development and deeper self-awareness. Importantly, mentors expressed that having a non-judging environment or to "open up and explore in particular about negative experiences in a safe setting is valu-able" and enabled midwives to process challenges.

The programme fostered a supportive workplace culture, strengthened communication skills, and provided a trustworthy support network. These benefits promoted midwives' connection within their teams. As one mentee stated, "someone I can turn to for help about everything" ensured they felt supported both personally and professionally. Another midwife stated that having "a named person makes it easier to access support", indicating it cre-ates a clear and accessible pathway for guidance.

Participants, however, also identified challenges, particularly the lack of time for mentoring within already demanding schedules and insufficient sup-port from leadership. Many expressed frustrations at having to participate in the programme on personal time without compensation, feeling undervalued as a result. As one mentor noted, "requesting health care professionals who are already burned out within the system to contribute more time, energy, and effort... without any form of extra support, time, or financial compensation" is an unsustainable expectation. While the programme was appreciated for its supportive potential, the barriers related to time constraints, and lack of managerial support presented obstacles.

Discussion

The findings of this study reveal that the participants gained personal and professional benefits from the MiM programme; however, they perceived barriers that would impact the long-term engagement and sustainability of the programme. Benefits highlighted by the participants of MiM align with broader research on the advantages of mentoring in midwifery. An integrative review by Wisemann et al. (2022) highlighted that mentoring fosters professional growth, leadership development, and collegiality while helping to establish a supportive workforce environment, benefits that were indicated by participants of MiM. Furthermore, mentoring in midwifery is known to impact midwives by improving communication skills and boosting self-confidence among midwives (Bradford et al., 2022), which concurs with the findings from this study. This is beneficial to the midwifery profession as creating a supportive workforce environment not only attracts student midwives to the profession but also strengthens retention of the current workforce, nurturing the next generation of leaders and innovators in care (Jefford et al., 2021).

Moreover, the results of this study align with existing literature that suggests the model of AI fosters space for reflective practice, enhances workplace culture, empowers communication, and provides reliable support networks for early-career and student midwives (Callander et al., 2021; Catling & Rossiter, 2020; Merriel et al., 2022; Stulz et al., 2021; Trajkovski et al., 2013; Watkins et al., 2016). Notably, these benefits of MiM resonate with research indicating that strong collegial relationships within the workforce can impact midwives by acting as a protective mechanism against job stress and enhancing job satisfaction (Cull et al., 2020). If the benefits of MiM have the potential to counteract key stressors such as burnout, high stress levels, and negative workplace culture, programmes such as MiM may also play a crucial role in improving retention and reducing attrition within the midwifery workforce (Callander et al., 2021; Catling & Rossiter, 2020).

While the expected benefits of MiM, such as professional growth and fostering collegiality, aligned with many of the post-mentoring outcomes, mentors initially expressed a desire to feel more valued in their roles beyond financial rewards. Unfortunately, this aspiration was not reflected in the post-mentoring feedback, where mentors highlighted feelings of being under-valued, largely due to the absence of financial compensation. The impact on midwives of realising the lack of support from management – and the implicit shift in responsibility to them to enhance workplace morale and culture deep-ened their awareness of feeling undervalued within the profession. Further-more, unsupported mentors risk becoming disengaged, leading to negative mentoring experiences for both mentors and mentees (Lasater et al., 2021). This perceived lack of managerial support emphasises the broader issue of insufficient recognition for midwives' contributions (Bloxsome et al., 2019; Catling & Rossiter, 2020) and highlights a gap in the leadership's commit-ment to fostering a supportive work environment. As a result, midwives are left not only to manage their clinical responsibilities but also to shoulder the additional emotional and professional labour of building a positive culture, without adequate resources or support. This shift places undue pressure on midwives, who recognise the essential role that the MiM programme could play in cultivating a sustainable workforce if given adequate support. The lack of investment from leadership in MiM sends a disheartening message, further reinforcing the perception that midwives – and their efforts to mentor and support one another – are undervalued. This dynamic risks diminishing morale and impedes the MiM programme's potential to effectively contribute to workforce sustainability.

It is important to recognise that the cyclical and iterative nature of a men-toring programme based on the AI model demands deep, ongoing engage-ment to be truly effective (Carter et al., 2007). This raises concerns about MiM's capacity to meet these requirements, especially in light of the per-ceived lack of sustained support and incentives reported by participants in this study. Participants identified a perceived lack of facilitation and follow-up support as significant barriers to the long-term sustainability of MiM. This concern is particularly relevant when considering the demands of im-plementing an AI model. Effective facilitation of AI requires not only time and commitment but also skilled facilitators (Watkins et al., 2016). Watkins et al. (2016) warn that if expert facilitation is indeed critical to the success of AI strategies, it could present considerable challenges in healthcare settings, where the shortage and expense of hiring such experts may hinder the pro-gramme's feasibility in midwifery. This further complicates MiM's potential for sustained effectiveness, especially when coupled with the issues of mentor engagement and financial support.

If strategies such as MiM are unsupported and mentorship is not valued by leadership, the benefits highlighted in this study may not be realised to their full potential. A model that healthcare policymakers could look to for guidance is New Zealand's "Midwifery First Year of Practice Program", a government-funded initiative offering mentorship to early-career midwives. Mentors in this program are compensated for up to 56 hours of their time annually and provided with mentor education, a toolkit, and professional development resources for their mentees (Bradford et al., 2022). The success of this programme, evidenced by increased confidence and high retention rates among mentees, suggests that similar support could benefit the MiM programme.

Given that both MiM and AI require ongoing, resource-intensive efforts and substantial funding, their ability to bring about meaningful, long-term improvements in midwifery may be limited, particularly in resource-constrained public health systems. While MiM offers valuable opportunities to impact midwives' experiences and foster a positive work environment, practical and financial constraints may hinder its broader implementation. The lack of support from leadership has impacted midwives by reinforcing feelings of being undervalued, undermining their motivation and engagement with the programme. To fully realise the benefits of the MiM programme and ensure its sustainability, healthcare leaders must recognise the importance of investing in MiM as a strategic approach to workforce development. Providing essential resources, such as financial incentives and dedicated time for mentoring, is crucial for maintaining mentor engagement, countering the perception of being undervalued and ensuring the programme's long-term success. This support will enhance midwives' professional practice and contribute to building a resilient and sustainable midwifery workforce.

Conclusion

The MiM programme provided personal and professional growth for participants, reinforcing broader research on mentoring's positive impact on midwives, such as fostering development, leadership, and support. AI, a foundational element of MiM, enabled a strengths-based approach that encouraged reflective practice and supportive relationships. However, barriers to MiM's sustainability including lack of remuneration, time allocation, and ongoing facilitation impacted participants sense of being valued and highlight the need for additional support to maximise engagement and long-term impact. Adequate resources and protected time for mentorship would enhance MiM's ability to strengthen midwifery resilience.

Limitations in the study design, including cross-sectional data from different cohorts, a lack of validated tools, and a small sample size, affect the generalisability of results and underscore the need for longitudinal research and validated measures in future studies. Addressing these constraints and increasing midwife engagement in research could further reveal MiM's potential to foster a positive workplace culture and improve workforce retention.

REFLECTIVE ACTIVITY 1

Reflect on challenges that might arise in implementing and maintaining a Mentoring in Midwifery program within your team or organisation.

For each identified barrier, propose one actionable solution you could implement to mitigate its impact and support the programme's success.

References

Bloxsome, D., Ireson, D., Doleman, G., & Bayes, S. (2019). Factors associated with midwives' job satisfaction and intention to stay in the profession: An integrative review. *Journal of Clinical Nursing, 28*(3–4), 386–399. https://doi.org/10.1111/jocn.14651

Bradford, H., Hines, H. F., Labko, Y., Peasley, A., Valentin-Welch, M., & Breedlove, G. (2022). midwives mentoring midwives: A review of the evidence and Best practice recommendations. *Journal of Midwifery & Women's Health, 67*(1), 21–30. https://doi.org/10.1111/jmwh.13285

Braun, V., & Clarke, V. (2021) *Thematic Analysis: A Practical Guide.* Sage Publishing. https://au.sagepub.com/en-gb/oce/thematic-analysis/book248481

Callander, E., Sidebotham, M., Lindsay, D., & Gamble, J. (2021). The future of the Australian midwifery workforce – Impacts of ageing and workforce exit on the number of registered midwives. *Women and Birth: Journal of the Australian College of Midwives, 34*(1), 56–60. https://doi.org/10.1016/j.wombi.2020.02.023

Carter, C. A., Ruhe, M. C., Weyer, S., Litaker, D., Fry, R. E., & Stange, K. C. (2007). An appreciative inquiry approach to practice improvement and transformative change in health care settings. *Quality Management in Health Care, 16*(3), 194–204. DOI: 10.1097/01.QMH.0000281055.15177.79.

Catling, C., & Rossiter, C. (2020). Midwifery workplace culture in Australia: A national survey of midwives. *Women Birth, 33*(5), 464–472. https://doi.org/10.1016/j.wombi.2019.09.008

Cull, J., Hunter, B., Henley, J., Fenwick, J., & Sidebotham, M. (2020). "Overwhelmed and out of my depth": Responses from early career midwives in the United Kingdom to the work, health and emotional lives of midwives study. *Women and Birth: Journal of the Australian College of Midwives, 33*(6), e549–e557. https://doi.org/10.1016/j.wombi.2020.01.003

Dewar, B., & MacBride, T. (2017). Developing caring conversations in care homes: An appreciative inquiry. *Health & Social Care in the Community, 25*(4), 1375–1386. https://doi.org/10.1111/hsc.12436

Dewar, B., Stulz, V., Buliak, A., Connolly, L., McLaughlin, D. K., Newport, K., Rebolledo, S., Stephenson, L., MacBride, T., Lennon, K., & Drayton, N. (2020). Exploring and developing student midwives' experiences (ESME) – An appreciative inquiry study. *Midwifery, 91*, 102844–102844. https://doi.org/10.1016/j.midw.2020.102844

Harvie, K., Sidebotham, M., & Fenwick, J. (2019). Australian midwives' intentions to leave the profession and the reasons why. *Women and Birth: Journal of the Australian College of Midwives, 32*(6), e584–e593. https://doi.org/10.1016/j.wombi.2019.01.001

Hildingsson, I., Gamble, J., Sidebotham, M., Creedy, D. K., Guilliland, K., Dixon, L., Pallant, J., & Fenwick, J. (2016). Midwifery empowerment: National surveys of midwives from Australia, New Zealand and Sweden. *Midwifery, 40*, 62–69. https://doi.org/10.1016/j.midw.2016.06.008

Jefford, E., Nolan, S., Munn, J., & Ebert, L. (2021). What matters, what is valued and what is important in mentorship through the appreciative inquiry process of co-created knowledge. *Nurse Education Today, 99*, N.PAG. https://doi-org.ezproxy.scu.edu.au/10.1016/j.nedt.2021.104791

Kakyo, T. A., Xiao, L. D., & Chamberlain, D. (2022). Benefits and challenges for hospital nurses engaged in formal mentoring programs: A systematic integrated review. *International Nursing Review, 69*(2), 229–238. https://doi.org/10.1111/inr.12730

Lasater, K., Smith, C., Pijanowski, J., & Brady, K. P. (2021). Redefining mentorship in an era of crisis: Responding to COVID-19 through compassionate relationships. [Redefining mentorship. *International Journal of Mentoring and Coaching in Education, 10*(2), 158–172. https://doi.org/10.1108/IJMCE-11-2020-0078

Lennon, M. K. (2022). Us, together- co-creating a mentoring in midwifery program in NSW. *Women and Birth: Journal of the Australian College of Midwives, 35*, 29. https://doi.org/10.1016/j.wombi.2022.07.079

Merriel, A., Wilson, A., Decker, E., Hussein, J., Larkin, M., Barnard, K., O'Dair, M., Costello, A., Malata, A., & Coomarasamy, A. (2022). Systematic review and narrative synthesis of the impact of Appreciative Inquiry in healthcare. *BMJ Open Quality, 11*(2), e001911. https://doi.org/10.1136/bmjoq-2022-001911

Pairman, S. (2016). The midwifery first year of practice programme: Supporting New Zealand midwifery graduates in their transition to practice. *Journal (New Zealand College of Midwives), 52*(52), 12–19. https://doi.org/10.12784/nzcomjnl52.2016.2.12-19

Pugh, J. D., Twigg, D. E., Martin, T. L., & Rai, T. (2013). Western Australia Facing critical losses in its midwifery workforce: A survey of midwives' intentions. *Midwifery, 29*(5), 497–505. https://doi.org/10.1016/j.midw.2012.04.006

Rouder, J., Saucier, O., Kinder, R., & Jans, M. (2021). What to do with all those open-ended responses? Data visualization techniques for survey researchers. *Survey Practice*. https://doi.org/10.29115/SP-2021-0008

Stulz, V., Francis, L., Pathrose, S., Sheehan, A., & Drayton, N. (2021). Appreciative inquiry as an intervention to improve nursing and midwifery students transitioning into becoming new graduates: An integrative review. *Nurse Education Today, 98*, 104727–104727. https://doi.org/10.1016/j.nedt.2020.104727

Sullivan, K., Lock, L., & Homer, C. S. E. (2011). Factors that contribute to midwives staying in midwifery: A study in one area health service in New South Wales, Australia. *Midwifery, 27*(3), 331–335. https://doi.org/10.1016/j.midw.2011.01.007

Trajkovski, S., Schmied, V., Vickers, M., & Jackson, D. (2013). Using appreciative inquiry to transform health care. *Contemporary Nurse: A Journal for the Australian Nursing Profession, 45*(1), 95–100. https://doi.org/10.5172/conu.2013.45.1.95

Watkins, S., Dewar, B., & Kennedy, C. (2016). Appreciative Inquiry as an intervention to change nursing practice in in-patient settings: An integrative review. *International Journal of Nursing Studies, 60*, 179–190. https://doi.org/10.1016/j.ijnurstu.2016.04.017

Wissemann, K., Bloxsome, D., De Leo, A., & Bayes, S. (2022). What are the benefits and challenges of mentoring in midwifery? An integrative review. *Women's Health, 18*, 174550572211101–17455057221110141. https://doi.org/10.1177/17455057221110141

28

MIDWIFERY MENTORING AND SUPERVISION

Annette Briley

Support in the Early Period Post-Initial Registration

Preceptorship

In the United Kingdom (UK), preceptorship has long been implemented to facilitate students and newly graduated midwives to become accountable independent, knowledgeable, skilled practitioners in clinical settings (Nursing and Midwifery Council (NMC), 2020). Preceptorship provides structured support for new midwives to successfully transition to competent and confident healthcare professionals. A period of preceptorship lays strong foundations for lifelong reflection and capacity for continuing professional development needs throughout a career as a midwife (Nursing and Midwifery Council (NMC), 2020). For more details on mentorship in the UK, please see Chapter 12: Midwifery Mentorship in the UK.

Organisational cultures that support preceptorship foster collaborative, collegial, impartial, fair, and kind environments, where good interprofessional and multi-agency relationships exist and thrive. There is organisational understanding, and processes and systems in place to build the confidence of newly qualified staff (Nursing and Midwifery Council (NMC), 2020). Adherence to the Principle of Preceptorship is evidenced in all programmes, which are identified as key activities within the organisation. Preceptees are empowered by this tailored programme, as they receive appropriate resources to enhance their confidence, including support for their individual learning needs, with a named preceptor and opportunities to reflect and seek feedback as required. Advantages for the preceptor include personal professional

DOI: 10.4324/9781003533733-29

development, the opportunity to be a role model, ongoing support, and the opportunity to share effective practice and learn from others.

As part of the National Health Service (NHS) Long Term Plan, those commencing their careers as registered nurses or midwives in the NHS in England are supported and guided by the National Preceptorship Framework for Nursing (NHS England, 2022) and a National Preceptorship Framework for Midwifery (NHS England, 2023). This commences within one year of registration and lasts for a minimum of 12 months but can extend to two years. In the UK, there are two models of midwifery preceptorship:

Model 1: There is a lead preceptor named for all midwife preceptees, and this is usually a senior midwife who is responsible for overseeing the programme. This person is supported by buddies, who are midwives with at least 12 months of experience, and an education team and/or midwifery skills educators. Buddies work clinically alongside the preceptees facilitating formal meetings quarterly to track progress.

Model 2: Clinically based midwives support preceptees as part of their everyday role, undertaking quarterly meetings to track progress.

One core component of the preceptorship period is supernumerary status for all newly registered preceptees for a minimum of 4 weeks (150 hours) over the 12-month period. Typically, these are the first two weeks of rotation to each new clinical area.

Those undertaking the preceptor role should have at least 8 hours, and preferably 12 hours, protected time per year, to undertake progress meetings and peer support needs.

The costs of these programmes are incurred by the NHS Trusts that employ new graduate midwives. Investment in such programmes is considered a major strategy to increase retention rates for newly registered midwives (NHS England, 2023). Similar initiatives exist in other parts of the UK.

Transition to Professional Practice Programme (TPPP)/Graduate Midwife Programme

In Australia, as in some other countries, newly qualified midwives can apply for a TPPP and other Graduate Programmes (SA Health, 2024; The Royal Women's Hospital, Victoria Australia, 2024). These are structured programmes which support new graduates in the first year of practice. Each provides opportunities to further develop skills and apply knowledge in all areas of care. Additionally, there are opportunities for self-directed learning and relevant professional development days. For midwifery, topics may include violence against women, reproductive loss, foetal surveillance, and perinatal mental health to name just a few. In these programmes, new graduates receive performance review assessments and have support from experienced midwifery educators and clinicians. Time and support are allocated and provided by the Local Health Networks that employ new graduate midwives.

Not all countries have either a framework or identified programme to support new graduate midwives, but in many places, informal mentoring occurs from experienced midwives keen to ensure their junior colleagues are confident and competent in clinical practice and understand the organisational structures and procedures inherent within all healthcare systems and health facilities.

Ongoing Support in Clinical Practice

Where they exist, once the initial period of a formal programme is completed, many organisations initiate a system whereby junior colleagues are supported and mentored by more senior clinicians or clinical experts. Some of these initiatives are formal and others are informal. Definitions are varied but in general:

- **Mentor**
- An experienced and trusted advisor (noun)
- **Mentorship**
- Someone who teaches or gives help and advice to a less experienced, and often younger, person.

In an organisational setting, a mentor influences the personal and professional growth of a mentee.

The importance of mentorship has long been described with the experience and structure influenced by engagement in the mentoring relationships by mentors and mentees, affecting the 'amount of psychosocial support, career guidance, role modelling and communication that occurs' (Fagenson-Eland and Marks, 1997). Effective mentoring has been identified as having a positive influence on personal development, career choice, and guidance (Burgess et al., 2018).

Mentoring involves both coaching and educational roles. It requires generosity of time, willingness to share knowledge and skills, empathy, and a desire to see others succeed (Burgess et al., 2018). Many organisations provide training opportunities for mentors, and within health systems, undertaking this role has been identified as optimising professional development and professionalism whilst shaping knowledge, skills, and attitudes of future healthcare professionals (Ramani et al., 2023). But not all mentorship relationships are successful. Some are adversely impacted by ethical issues such as conflicts of interest, power imbalance, and unrealistic expectations (Burgess et al., 2018). Difficulties within the mentorship relationship should be highlighted and referred to in a timely manner through the systems within the organisation to enable.

The establishment of ground rules at the start of a mentoring relationship is advised. These include setting out the expectations of both parties, ensuring all discussions are career-focused, valuing each parties' time by prioritising meetings and rearranging as soon as possible if they need to be cancelled, mutual respect for cultural, religious, gender, age, and other diversity and being adequately prepared for meetings, with identified questions or opportunities to discuss (Australian Nurses and Midwives Clinical Trials Network, 2024).

Ongoing Support when Changing Area of Practice or Job Roles

Health professionals can work in diverse settings and sectors including primary and tertiary healthcare providers, community, not-for-profit organisations, in the public private and voluntary sectors. As midwives, we tend to rotate around the clinical areas, so we can work to the full scope of our practice, so although one might become very proficient in one area, orientation, and induction into another aspect of clinical care might be warranted. In addition, midwives and nurses can work in educational institutions in undergraduate and postgraduate situations. Following induction and orientation sessions to new workplaces and roles, mentorship can be offered and is important as it includes development of knowledge and skills, in addition to an understanding of the professional culture within organisations. In other words, in all these situations, some degree of mentorship should be provided, at least initially. In many situations, the mentor/mentee relationship ends after a specified time or due to changing circumstances or demands of the job and new employees.

Developing Mentor Relationships for the Longer Term

As you develop in your career, there are always people with more specialised clinical or institutional knowledge and therefore know better than you. But sometimes enduring relationships are the secret to ongoing success, for both the mentor and mentee. Being a trusted advisor, who knows a person's professional history and potential trajectory is a privilege and watching them gain professional knowledge and expertise and develop into confident competent midwives is very special. For the mentee, having someone who knows you and understands the impact of your professional history on your current practice is invaluable in supporting reflexivity and identifying areas for professional development. Therefore, it can be mutually beneficial to promote and extend this relationship beyond the initial period.

Academic Mentoring

Academia can be a challenging environment, especially for those from clinical backgrounds. It can appear competitive and cut-throat, with a very different set of priorities. The importance in supporting the required period of adjustment with mentorship has been advocated (Gray et al., 2024). People enter academia for different reasons, it could be to focus on teaching and education delivery or on research or to undertake a higher degree, and the period of adaptation to this new environment, when an individual is usually very experienced and confident in the clinical context, can be challenging.

Whilst those undertaking a higher degree will have a supervisory team, academic supervision is not quite the same as mentorship. Supervision tends to be task-orientated, whereas mentorship focuses on broader scholarly and career development issues (Ong and Swift, 2018).

Research Mentoring

Mentoring in a research environment enables those with specialist experience to pass on their knowledge, but also to support and guide other midwives to thrive in this different environment as well as learn from each other (Pye et al, 2023). For the mentee, it provides the opportunity to hear unbiased advice from someone in the field but not directly involved with, or conflicted by, the demands of the clinical trial.

When working on a research project, inevitably the investigators have their own agenda, mostly notably to ensure the project (trial) is completed to time and target and the results are robust and appropriately disseminated. Most research positions last for the duration of a project, and therefore can be short term with any renewal of contract, or transfer to another project, contingent on further successful funding acquisition. For midwives, this can be very different to their previous employment status.

Research networks are beginning to develop mentorship programmes for clinicians undertaking research roles. In England, the NIHR Midwife Champion Group was developed through the local Clinical Research Networks (CRNs) to develop a peer group of midwives working in national clinical trials in reproductive health and childbirth. This group enables mentoring clinical midwives working in clinical trials.

In Australia, the Australian Nurses and Midwives Clinical Trial network (ANMCTN) has established a Mentoring programme for mid-career researchers who want to become research leaders in applied areas of clinical studies (Australian Nurses and Midwives Clinical Trials Network, 2024). This comprises six sessions, each lasting one hour, and their overview of mentoring (www.anmctn. com.au) provides very clear outcomes regarding expectations for mentors and mentees. But, for many entering these roles, outside the parameters of a higher degree by research (HDR) seeking a mentoring relationship can be difficult. Despite this, it is important to develop these wherever possible.

Although still not a common career trajectory, there are increasing opportunities to work in research, either concurrently with clinical load, or for a temporary or fixed-term contract, without committing to undertaking a higher degree. Similarly, there are now midwives and nurses who have worked in research, either currently or for a particular project, who have experience of the different skills and application of knowledge required in a research position (Tinkler and Robinson, 2018). Most midwives who have or are holding these posts are very willing to share their experiences and help guide others. Not least to support those on a fixed-term contract to settle into a research post efficiently and maximise their opportunities during this time.

Informal Mentorship

The concept of mentoring in midwifery and nursing gained prominence in the late 20th century (McCloughen et al., 2006); however, historical records show it is intrinsically rooted in the professions. Evidence shows Florence Nightingale actively mentored specific individuals, maintaining consistent contact with them throughout their careers, mainly through letters, but with occasional face-to-face meetings (Lorentzon and Brown, 2003).

Informal mentoring involves the spontaneous initiation of a mentor/mentee relationships with the specific aim of providing support and guidance, with little or no intervention by an organisation (NIHR, 2023). Whilst it has been associated with negative experiences, particularly in low-resource settings (Kakyo et al., 2024), where informal mentoring is successful, it has been identified as positively impacting career confidence and progression and patient care. With mentees reporting greater satisfaction both with their mentor but also with their professional role (NIHR, 2023).

When considering finding a mentor, it is important to be cognisant of your needs and expectations:

- Do you have a particular reason for wanting to engage with a mentor?
- What specific knowledge are you seeking information and guidance for?
- What do you want in your mentor?

  - Professional/career development.
  - Skills development.
  - Institutional/sector knowledge or insight.
  - Confidence and self-esteem.
  - Change management.

- Why should a mentor engage with you?

  - What makes you a 'good' mentee?

When identifying a potential mentor, you should look at those around you:

- Professional circle

  - Previous manager.
  - Previous lecturer/educator.
  - Co-workers in another department or hospital.

- Professional bodies

  - Mentoring registers, for example, the ANMCTN.

- Personal communication

  - People known to those in your immediate network ('friends of friends').

- Internet sources

  - LinkedIn.

Selection of a mentor should be a thoughtful, reflexive process. Most importantly, you should identify someone who believes in you and shares your values and goals. Consider mentors who can grow with you, this relationship could be a mutually beneficial, career-long partnership.

Once you have identified a potential mentor, you may want to find out more about them. Depending on your selection you could have an initial conversation or send them an email to gauge their suitability and willingness to take on this role.

Paying it Forward

Mentoring in any environment is a privilege and can be beneficial for both the mentor and mentee. Honesty is always the best policy and mutual respect and trust are important in this relationship. Figuratively, 'holding the hand' of a colleague through change and beyond enables the mentee to thrive and provides the mentor a unique opportunity to contribute to the career of another. For the mentor, working with mentees provides additional job satisfaction and enables them to hear different viewpoints and develop a relationship that fosters debate and discussion around professional issues.

By mentoring, midwives are 'paying it forward' for future generations of midwives and women. When today's novices, in any area, are effectively mentored they become experts in their chosen area, completing the care nexus, optimising care provided to women and babies, which is underpinned by robust research and high-quality education for midwifery students and midwives of the future. Furthermore, they are more likely to remain in the midwifery profession and undertake higher degrees or clinical specialist education.

References

Australian Nurses and Midwives Clinical Trials Network. Mentoring program ANMCTN 2024. www.anmctn.com.au

Burgess A, van Diggele C, Mellis C. Mentorship in the health professions: a review. Clinical Teacher 2018; 15(3): 197–202.

Fagenson-Eland EA, Marks MA, Amendola K. Perceptions of mentoring relationships. Journal of vocational Behaviour 1997; 51(1): 29–42.

Gray M, De Leo A, Baker M, Jefford E. The lived experiences of midwives' transitioning form a clinical role into teaching in higher education in one jurisdiction in Australia: a pilot study. Nurse Education in Practice 2024; 79: 104071.

Kakyo TA, Xiao LD, Chamberlain D. Exploring the dark side of informal mentoring: experiences od nurses and midwives working in hospital settings in Uganda. Nursing Inquiry 2024; 31: e12641.

Lorentzon M, Brown K. Florence Nightingale as 'mentor of matrons'. Correspondence with Rachel Williams at St Mary's Hospital. Journal of Nursing Management 2003; 11(4): 266–74.

McCloughen A, O'Brien L, Jackson D. Positioning mentorship within Australian nursing contexts: a literature review. Contemporary Nurse 2006; 23(1): 120–34.

NHS England. National Preceptorship framework for nursing NHS People Plan, Nursing midwifery and care, Workforce. NHS England 2022.

NHS England. National preceptorship framework for midwifery. NHS England 2023. www.england.nhs.uk/long-read/national-preceptorship-framework-for-midwifery/

National Institute for Health and Care Research. Accessing informal mentoring 2023. Version January 2023. www.nihr.ac.uk/accessing-informal-mentoring#

Nursing and Midwifery Council (NMC) Principles of preceptorship. NMC 2020 London. https://www.nmc.org.uk/globalassets/sitedocuments/nmc-publications/nmc-principles-for-preceptorship-a5.pdf

Ong H, Swift C. Mentoring and supervision in academia: establishing distinctions to manage expectations. Haematology Communications 2018; 2 (12): 1419–20.

Pye C, Tinkler L, Metwally M. Clinical research nurse and midwife as an integral member of the Trial management group (TMG): much more than a resource to manage and recruit patients. BMJ Leader 2023; 7: 152–5.

Ramani S, Kusurker RA, Lyon-Maris J, et al. Mentorship in health professions education_ an AMEE guide for mentors and mentees. AMEE Guide N0. 167. Medical Teacher 2023; 46(8): 999–1011.

SA Health Transition to Professional Practice Program (TPPP) 2024. https://www.sahealth.sa.gov.au/wps/wcm/connect/public+content/transition+to+professional+practice+program

The Royal Women's Hospital, Victoria Australia. Graduate Midwife Program 2024. https://www.thewomens.org.au/health-professionals/clinical-education-training/nursing-midwifery-edtraining/graduate-midwife-program

Tinkler L, Robinson L. Clinical research nursing and factors influencing success: a qualitative study describing the interplay between individual and organisational leadership influences and their impact on the delivery of clinical research in healthcare. Journal of Research in Nursing 2020; 25: 361–77.

29

MIDWIFERY MENTORSHIP

Future Directions

Lyn Ebert and Elaine Jefford

Introduction

This chapter draws together findings from the world of mentoring within the midwifery context. An overview of how midwifery clinicians, academics, clinical educators, researchers, leaders, and clinicians, from around the world, view the current mentoring in midwifery situation and how the different countries and midwifery professional groups currently support midwives in their professional and practice development is provided. In concluding this book, we present possible initiatives or strategies to be implemented to support the development of mentoring in midwifery programmes that are sustainable; thus, improving the future midwifery workforce, quality care provision and, therefore, maternal, and infant care outcomes.

Mentoring in the Midwifery Context, a Global Perspective

Midwives face emotional and professional challenges when their maternity service fails to provide the appropriate resources or support required to continuously support them to be woman-centred practitioners, facilitate student midwife learning, mentor new staff, and aid their own professional growth. While current midwives (mentors) and future midwives (mentees) require support from healthcare facilities and management, they also require advocacy from their professional bodies. Continuous professional development is required by many regulatory bodies globally. In Australia, the Australian Health Practitioner Regulation Agency (AHPRA), as a requirement for annual registration as a midwife, requires all registered midwives to confirm that they meet the standards for registration. These standards include the recency

DOI: 10.4324/9781003533733-30

of practice, continuing professional development (CPD) and professional indemnity insurance registration standards (Australian Health Practitioner Regulation Agency (AHPRA), 2023). In addition to these generic standards of practice, there are discipline-specific professional standards. The practice standards for the registered midwife in Australia require the midwife to:

- (Standard 3.4) **contribute to a culture that supports learning, teaching,** knowledge transfer, and critical reflection
- (Standard 6.4) **provide** and accept effective and **timely direction, allocation, delegation, teaching, and supervision** (Registered Midwife Practice Standards, Nurses and Midwives Board of Australia [NMBA], 2018)

Such a requirement is not unique to Australia, rather many countries' regulatory organisations around the world require midwives to support their fellow midwives and/or student midwives in developing the knowledge and skills of midwifery, as well as undertake their own professional development. Yet, as demonstrated in Chapter 26 – *The role of supporting mentorship in Midwifery*, and Chapter 27 – *Midwifery Mentorship: The Impact on Participating Midwives*, midwives do not feel they have time to teach others or continue to learn. It could therefore be suggested; professional development of self and others is not valued within the discipline or workplace culture where time is not provided to undertake professional learning, thus resulting in devaluing midwives and midwifery. Furthermore, the global push for e-learning by local health districts, e-portfolios, and clinical supervision, to be provided in the midwife's own time, is seen as an additional burden by midwives. Maternity service management and the country's specific professional body need to support local midwives in the clinical environment to continue their professional development in a manner that facilitates, and values continued learning. Equally, midwives need to be supported to guide and guard student midwives in their learning, demonstrating a valuing of midwifery time to supporting each other in professional development. Professional development is held sacred in other professions such as medicine, social work, and education. For example, Australian school teachers working for the New South Wales Department of Education have mandated pupil-free days for staff development. Midwives need to be valued sufficiently by the New South Wales Ministry of Health and other States and Territories and our professional body to secure scheduled woman-free days or blocks of time to enable professional development, clinical supervision, and other support mechanisms. This should be applied to midwifery irrespective of geographical location.

Currently, it appears it is the individual midwife, who is responsible for enabling a student or mentee to feel safe and valued to learn within the maternity care context. This is an additional burden placed on the midwife; to facilitate conditions to communicate trust and respect, despite the workload, model of care, or midwifery context or geographical location around the world. Only when a midwife has the capacity and time to create a safe environment in which the mentee is more able to connect emotionally, can both parties engage in shared learning. For the midwife–mentor to be available for the mentee, to create the conditions in which the mentee can feel valued and safe to learn and grow professionally, the midwife must have the resources and conditions in which they can feel valued in their midwifery choices and safe in their midwifery voices (Ebert, 2012). Midwifery management that makes available the resources and conditions that support midwives to be available for both the childbearing woman and mentee learning to be a midwife demonstrates a valuing of women, midwifery, and learning.

REFLECTIVE ACTIVITY 1: LOOK UP YOUR PROFESSIONAL BODY'S REGULATION AND LEGISLATION DOCUMENTS

If you have not already done so, take the time now to explore your local, regional, and national professional documents that underpin your practice as a midwife. For example:

- Standards for Practice/Registration Standards
- Code of Ethics
- Code of Conduct
- Professional Development Requirements

Note any requirements for recency of practice, evidence of professional development, the obligation to engage in teaching and learning of self and/or others, the responsibility to seek or provide clinical supervision, and accountability for providing midwifery leadership.

The Future of Mentoring in the Midwifery Context

The impact of maternity service management failing to value midwives' professional development is apathy towards teaching and learning, which effects the role they play in educating the next generation of midwives. When future midwives (students or mentees) understand that midwifery ways of being are not valued in the clinical environment, they do not feel safe to create space and time to teach while also providing care in maternity service units/departments with high workloads. Mentees need to understand they are valued and considered with respect by their future midwifery colleagues and the organisation in which they work and learn. There is potential for improved mentee learning and application of midwifery theoretical knowledge in the clinical environment with better guidance from mentor–midwives. Maternity services therefore need to better support mentor–midwives to be available for student midwife and mentee learning. Improving a health professional's and in particular mentees and student's sense of being accepted and valued within the clinical environment will improve their clinical competence and critical thinking skills and therefore improve patient safety (Wissemann et al., 2022). Understanding that new staff, students, and mentees are likely to take on the behaviours and values of mentor–midwives with whom they work (Norman, 2015), it is important that all midwives feel valued and are inspired to create time and space for all those in the workplace that require learning support, including self and mentees.

Strategies to Support Sustainable Mentoring Programmes in Midwifery

Recommendations or future workforce directions presented here are suggestions based on the findings from the chapters in this textbook and current research. They are offered as support strategies in the implementation of sustainable mentoring programmes in the midwifery environment, with the aim of improving the future midwifery workforce. Mentoring programmes valued and supported by management, mentors, and mentees have the potential to increase workforce retention, reduce workplace stress and improve staff morale (Wissemann et al., 2022). Enhancing the workplace environment is a priority as improved job satisfaction and increased retention positively correlates with improved health outcomes for women and babies and overall reduced healthcare costs (Roder-DeWan et al., 2020).

The International Confederation of Midwives (ICM) is the global voice of midwifery representing over 136 midwives' associations in 117 countries. In 2020, the ICM with the support of UNFPA, provided a mentoring guide for midwives which offers a theoretical overview of mentoring including principles, definitions, a mentoring cycle, and benefits. Yet, it fails to address how to negotiate time to mentor within a maternity service organisation or how to instil a work culture of learning that is valued. Yet, as countries around the globe look for guidance from the ICM documents for regulation, and professional practice, therefore as these fundamental aspects of mentorship are missing, it is perhaps not surprising professional development of self and others is viewed as not being valued within the discipline or workplace culture around the globe, including Australia. A recommendation, therefore, is for the ICM to take the lead in placing the practice of mentorship on everyone's agenda so time can be provided and valued within the workplace culture.

Midwifery Education

Globally, midwifery curricula are designed to meet the region's or country's professional standards as well as guidelines from the ICM. As stated in Chapter 23 – Midwifery Mentorship in Australian Curricula, "the ICM clearly articulate the role of the clinical midwife in supporting student development." Local professional standards, however, may provide little to no guidance for the role of the clinical midwife in supporting student development, specifically through mentorship roles. Currently, as revealed in the chapters in section two of this book (mentorship, leadership, and education in midwifery: A Global Perspective), there appears to be a discrepancy in the education requirements, number of years of experience as a midwife before accepting the role of mentor, or preparation to effectively support students on practice placement.

The ICM essential competencies for midwifery practice document provides a minimum set of knowledge, skills, and professional behaviour required to be attained prior to being entitled to use the title of midwife (ICM, 2024). Although mentorship and supporting the education of others (student midwives) are mentioned in this document, there are no action plans, strategies, or recommendations as to how these skills, professional behaviours, and knowledge are to be acquired, retained or practised, or evaluated. Many countries use these competencies as a building block to develop their own educational standards for programmes leading to registration as a midwife. In Australia, midwifery curricula are assessed and accredited against the Midwife Accreditation Standards by the Nursing and Midwifery Accreditation Council (ANMAC) and have their curricula approved by the Nursing and Midwifery Board of Australia (NMBA). Universities use these standards to design their educational programme. Nowhere within the standards is mentorship mentioned. This lack of inclusion of such a vital element of midwifery when educating the next generation of midwives is reflected in Australian midwifery programmes with most university's not having dedicated mentorship courses (units/subjects/modules).

The first recommendation to improve the support available to midwives is to build the culture of mentoring into our professional psyche from entry into the world of midwifery. In other words, to incorporate content relating to mentorship in pre-registration midwifery curricula and to integrate teaching and learning activities that develop the knowledge, skills and professional behaviour required to be effectively mentored as a student and understand the roles and responsibilities of a mentor. Together, this will provide future midwives with the knowledge and skills to be effective mentors. While it is important to increase student midwives or mentees' knowledge and skills related to effective mentoring elements and attributes, registered midwives need to understand or value what students are taught in their curriculum and how that knowledge might be applied in practice.

The second recommendation to build a culture of mentorship is for midwifery education providers and health services to form closer partnerships. It is important that the registered midwives who mentor their future colleagues, understand what is involved in student midwife education. Working collaboratively with the education provider enhances continued professional development of the midwife and relationships with the students. This empowers the midwife to better guide and guard students/mentees in their learning in order to align midwifery theory and clinical practice. Registered midwife mentors with curricula knowledge are better able to support the learning needs of their mentees and tailor learning to where the mentee is in their journey.

Not only is it important to educate future midwives or mentees about CPD and support strategies that can shape a mentoring culture, the midwives taking up the role of mentor need support and education to ensure they are able to be effective in the role and do not burn out from what some see as additional tasks on their already heavy clinical workload (see Chapter 27 – *Midwifery Mentorship: The Impact on Participating Midwives*). When reading Chapter 12 – *Midwifery Mentorship in the United Kingdom,* it is clear the United Kingdom (UK) may be considered a role model in how to facilitate students and newly graduated nurses and midwives (mentees) in becoming accountable independent, knowledgeable, skilled practitioners in clinical settings (Nursing and Midwifery Council (NMC), 2020). The UK Nursing and Midwifery Council (NMC) has implemented the standards "Support Learning and Assessment in Practice" (SLAIP), Preparation for mentors, practice teachers and teachers. The SLAIP standards "set out clear expectations of the requirements for mentor preparation programmes which included academic level (HE Intermediate); Length of time (minimum of 10 days of which 5 days were protected learning time); learning both in academic and practice settings; relevant work-based learning (mentoring a student under supervision of a qualified mentor with the opportunity to reflect on the experience); and normally completed within 3 months" (for more information, see Chapter 12).

The third recommendation to ensure sustainable models of midwifery mentorship is the implementation of standards for mentoring programmes or education in all midwifery contexts around the globe. Mentoring programmes should have criteria as to who can elect to become a mentor, what skills and knowledge must be learnt within a university-level mentoring programme, and how these skills and knowledge are assessed in practice and evaluated by the stakeholders (mentees).

REFLECTIVE ACTIVITY 2: INTEGRATING MENTORING INTO THE MIDWIFERY CURRICULUM/TEACHING/FACILITATION

As you read about the recommendations for developing a culture of mentoring in midwifery through education, reflect on how you might integrate teaching and learning activities into your:

- Curriculum,
- Classroom teaching, or
- Clinical facilitation

Make some notes that describe how you can build a culture of mentoring for student midwives, new graduate midwives and midwives who ask for, or need, support in their professional development or clinical practice. Consider:

- Where, in the curriculum, will mentoring be taught and assessed? (if you are in midwifery academia)
- How will you discuss mentoring in the classroom as a professional development strategy for midwives?
- How will you promote and role model mentoring as a professional development strategy when teaching in the clinical environment?

Midwifery Management

In the previous section of this final chapter, we discussed how education providers, who provide midwifery programmes, and midwifery educators, in the clinical context, might develop a culture of mentoring within the world of midwifery. However, to implement and sustain mentoring in midwifery settings, midwives need to see the position as valued by management. For midwife/mentors to fully engage in effective mentoring relationships, to provide authentic, honest conversations and commit to openness and shared trust, with sufficient time for compassion and reflection (ICM, 2020) time and resources are required. Mentoring needs to be seen, by management, as an essential requirement for the provision of quality care and safety, professional development, and a cost-effective strategy to improve and increase workforce capacity.

In Chapter 28 – *Midwifery Mentoring and Supervision*, the author describes how time is allocated to ensure mentees can actively participate in their professional development. A "core component of the preceptorship period is supernumerary status for all newly registered preceptees for a minimum of four weeks (150 hours) over the 12 months period. Typically, this is the first two weeks rotation to each new clinical area." Not only do mentees understand that the role is valued with time allocated, but the mentors are also allocated time to undertake their role. "Those undertaking the preceptor role should have at least eight hours, and preferably twelve hours, protected time per year, to undertake progress meetings and peer support needs. The costs of these programs are incurred by the NHS Trusts that employ new graduate midwives. Investment in such programs is considered a major strategy to increase retention rates for newly registered midwives (NHS England, 2023). Similar initiatives exist in other parts of the UK" (for more information see Chapter 28).

The call for these initiatives are pronounced in Chapter 24 – Midwifery Mentorship in Practice: An Organisational Perspective, where the authors deliberate how midwifery leaders and leadership is essential in valuing, embedding, and sustaining a culture of mentorship. They argue that "midwifery leaders are pivotal in fostering successful mentorship programs by enabling environments that value and prioritise professional development. This includes establishing clear organisational strategies that support time for mentorship activities, developing formal recognition systems for mentors, and integrating mentorship into career development pathways" (for more information, see Chapter 24).

The return on investment in running mentorship programmes can be measured through various metrics, including improved staff retention rates (Fleming, 2023), increased leadership capability, and enhanced organisational performance indicators (Bamford, 2011; Feyissa et al., 2019; Liff & Rovio-Johansson, 2025). However, as stated by Lennon and Tierney, in Chapter 24, "the most significant returns often come through developing a more engaged, confident, and capable midwifery workforce that can drive innovation and improvement in maternity services."

Recommendation four, when endeavouring to implement a sustainable mentoring culture into your maternity service, is to demonstrate an understanding of the value of mentoring. To provide staff time and organisational resources to commit to the role and responsibilities essential when engaging in a mentee–mentor partnership. To acknowledge the leadership role inherent in mentoring staff and provide professional recognition and/or career pathways for those mentoring. This willimprove the organisation's key performance indicators.

REFLECTIVE ACTIVITY 3: IMPLEMENTING A SUSTAINABLE MENTORING PROGRAMME IN YOUR UNIT/WARD

As you read about the recommendations for developing a culture of mentoring in a maternity unit, reflect on how you might implement and support a sustainable mentoring programme in the ward.

Make some notes that describe how you can build a culture of mentoring for student midwives, new graduate midwives and midwives who ask for, or need, support in their professional development or clinical practice. Consider:

- Who the key stakeholders are when designing, or introducing a programme?
- How will staff be involved or engaged in the programme?
- What strategies will you implement to ensure the programme is sustainable?
- How will you evaluate the success of the programme (short and long term)?
- How will you promote and role model mentoring as a professional development strategy in the clinical environment?
- What resources do you have to invest in professional development?
- How will you acknowledge those undertaking the responsibility to mentor your future workforce?

Midwifery Professional Practice

Chapters in this textbook have highlighted that midwives around the globe understand the value of mentoring the next generation of midwives, and the requirement to continue to professionally develop self and others. However, recent research and discussions conveyed in this textbook have also revealed midwives, by and large, feel stressed and overworked (Catling & Rossiter, 2020; Fenwick et al., 2018; Geraghty et al., 2019; Wissemann et al., 2022). The midwifery profession, therefore, is challenged by workplace stress and burnout with midwives often viewing the mentorship role as an additional task to undertake on top of their clinical roles and responsibilities. As stated in Chapter 4 – *Midwifery Mentorship: The Context,* midwives understand their work is not valued when their maternity service fails to provide appropriate resources, support, or time to continuously deliver individualised support for women, student midwife learning, mentoring of other staff, and their own professional development. This leads to further professional dissonance and lower levels of job satisfaction. This view was echoed in Chapter 27 – *Midwifery Mentorship: The Impact on Participating Midwives.* To build resilience in the workforce and improve job satisfaction and workforce retention, Chapter 25 – *Midwifery Mentorship – Mentee perspective*, endorsed the implementation of sustainable mentoring programmes to prevent early attrition from the workforce, build confidence and resilience, and increase skill acquisition and a quality workforce.

Recommendation five to ensure midwives have capacity to facilitate learning, teaching, and mentoring in the clinical context requires a shift in workplace culture. A culture where mentoring, teaching, and continued professional development is considered as important as capability in clinical skills. Mandated CPD hours aligned with mentoring or teaching should be required to ensure all midwives have the capacity to support learning, teaching, and knowledge transfer and create opportunities for midwifery students and midwives under supervision to learn. For recommendation 5 to be fulfilled, recommendations 1–4 must concurrently be implemented.

Building midwives' capacity to facilitate learning, teaching, and mentoring needs to be underpinned by professional regulatory bodies. In Australia, the midwife's scope of practice is underpinned by registration requirements to:

3.4 **contribute to a culture that supports learning, teaching, knowledge transfer, and critical reflection,** and
6.4 **provide and accept effective and timely direction, allocation, delegation, teaching, and supervision** (Registered Midwife Practice Standards, *NMBA*, 2018)

It is the responsibility of all midwives to create opportunities for midwifery students and midwives under supervision to learn, as well as benefit from oversight and feedback. In their teaching and supervisor roles, midwives must:

5.1.a. **seek to develop the skills, attitudes, and practices of an effective teacher and/or supervisor.**

Furthermore, assessing colleagues and students is an important part of making sure the highest standard of practice is achieved across the profession. In assessing the competence and performance of colleagues or students, midwives must:

5.2.a. **be honest, objective, fair, without bias and constructive, and not put women at risk of harm by inaccurate and inadequate assessment,** and
5.2.b. **provide accurate and justifiable information promptly...** (Midwives Code of Conduct, *NMBA,* 2018).

Finally, the ICM requires midwives to advance midwifery knowledge and practice through the contribution to the formal education of midwifery students and ongoing education of midwives (ICM, 4 2024).

However, for midwives to create safe environments in which they can cultivate the learning of self and others. Management needs to provide enabling environments, where midwives can work to their full scope of practice, act as role models, and teach midwifery ways of being "with woman" to mentees, students, and less experienced maternity care staff.

REFLECTIVE ACTIVITY 4: IMPLEMENTING A CULTURE OF MENTORING IN YOUR MIDWIFERY PRACTICE

As you read about the requirements for sustaining effective mentor–mentee relationships, reflect on how you might promote and role model mentoring as a professional development and support strategy for colleagues, students, and new staff. Make some notes that describe how you will build your mentoring practice and evaluate your mentorship role. Consider:

- What skills and knowledge you need to be an effective mentor?
- How will you evaluate your practice?
- What barriers might you face in sustaining your mentoring relationships, and
- What strategies will you implement to overcome the identified barriers?
- Who can you approach to assist in developing a mentoring culture where you work?

Conclusion

Midwifery has a long history of being subjugated to medicine and nursing and in some countries this hard-fought success has resulted in midwifery being recognised profession in its own right. Other countries, however, are far behind in this struggle, for example, as noted in Chapter 16: Midwifery Mentorship in Mexico. We must support the continuing fight for all countries to acknowledge midwifery as its own profession.

Yet, drawing upon the chapters within this textbook, research, knowledge, and skills, the editors of, and authors of several chapters this textbook, including this final chapter, have made recommendations on what regulatory and professional bodies, maternity service providers, midwives (mentors), and mentees need to do to make education and leadership fundamental aspects of mentorship. Together as the global family of midwifery, we must now include mentorship in this fight. As without valuing the empowering role of effective mentorship in guiding the next generation of midwives, then the midwifery profession will continue to struggle with all aspects of the workforce challenges noted above and its impact on effective high-quality safe care for women and babies around the world and the right to use the title "Midwife" and be part of a well-respected, knowledgeable, and skilled profession.

Final Word

Firstly, Elaine and Lyn would like to thank every author who contributed to this textbook. It has been a great experience for us to view midwifery ways of working from different countries, regions, and perspectives. It has also been insightful and thought provoking to see how midwives are supporting those in their professional development or just embarking on their midwifery career.

We hope you, the reader, have gained as much from the book as we have, and can use some of the information in this book to initiate or improve ways to support your midwifery colleagues. We have enjoyed the process in birthing this textbook and hope to leave you with one thought ….

Be the mentor you wished you had at the start of your midwifery career.

References

Australian Health Practitioner Regulation Agency (AHPRA). (2023). Available from: https://www.ahpra.gov.au/Registration/Registration-Standards.aspx Accessed March 7, 2025.

Bamford, C. (2011). Mentoring in the twenty-first century. *Leadership in Health Services* (2007), 24(2), 150–163. https://doi.org/10.1108/17511871111125710

Catling, C., & Rossiter, C. (2020). Midwifery workplace culture in Australia: A national survey of midwives. *Women Birth, 33*(5), 464–472. https://doi.org/10.1016/j.wombi.2019.09.008

Ebert, L. (2012). *Woman-centred care and the socially disadvantaged woman: an Interpretative Phenomenological Analysis* [Doctoral dissertation, University of Newcastle]. https://openresearch.newcastle.edu.au/search?q=Ebert

Fenwick, J., Lubomski, A., Creedy, D. K., & Sidebotham, M. (2018). Personal, professional and workplace factors that contribute to burnout in Australian midwives. *Journal of Advanced Nursing, 74*(4), 852–863. https://doi.org/10.1111/jan.13491

Feyissa, G. T., Balabanova, D., & Woldie, M. (2019). How effective are mentoring programs for improving health worker competence and institutional performance in Africa? A systematic review of quantitative evidence. *Journal of Multidisciplinary Healthcare, 12*, 989–1005. https://doi.org/10.2147/JMDH.S228951

Fleming, K. (2023). Reducing staff turnover through the implementation of a peer mentoring program. *Nursing Management, 54*(1), 32–39. https://doi.org/10.1097/01.NUMA.0000905016.75550.3f

Geraghty, S., Speelman, C., & Bayes, S. (2019). Fighting a losing battle: Midwives experiences of workplace stress. *Women and Birth: Journal of the Australian College of Midwives, 32*(3), e297–e306. https://doi.org/10.1016/j.wombi.2018.07.012

ICM. (2020). *Mentoring Guidelines for Midwives*. Available from: https://internationalmidwives.org/resources/mentoring-guidelines-for-midwives Accessed March 14, 2025.

ICM. (2024). *Essential Competencies for Midwifery Practice*. International Confederation of Midwives. Licence: CC BY-NC-SA 4.0. Available from: https://internationalmidwives.org/resources/essential-competencies-for-midwifery-practice/ Accessed March 13, 2025.

Liff, R., & Rovio-Johansson, A. (2025). Mentoring as a management practice to retain newly certified professionals in healthcare organisations. *Journal of Health Organization and Management*, *39*(9), 54–70. https://doi.org/10.1108/JHOM-12-2023-0370

Norman, K. (2015). How mentors can influence the values, behaviours, and attitudes of nursing staff through positive professional socialisation. *Nursing Management*, *22*, 33–38. DOI: 10.7748/nm.22.8.33.s28.

Nurses and Midwives Board of Australia [NMBA]. (2018). *Registered Midwife Practice Standards 2018*. Available from: https://www.nursingmidwiferyboard.gov.au/Registration-Standards.aspx Accessed March 7, 2025.

Nursing and Midwifery Council (NMC). (2020). *Principles of Preceptorship*. NMC. https://www.nmc.org.uk/globalassets/sitedocuments/nmc-publications/nmc-principles-for-preceptorship-a5.pdf

Roder-DeWan, S., Nimako, K., Twum-Danso, N. A. Y., Amatya, A., Langer, A., & Kruk, M. (2020). Health system redesign for maternal and newborn survival: Rethinking care models to close the global equity gap. *BMJ Global Health*, *5*, e002539. https://doi.org/10.1136/bmjgh-2020-002539

Wissemann, K., Bloxsome, D., De Leo, A., & Bayes, S. (2022). What are the benefits and challenges of mentoring in midwifery? An integrative review. *Women's Health (London, England)*, *18*, 17455057221110141. https://doi.org/10.1177/17455057221110141

INDEX